W9-DEU-290

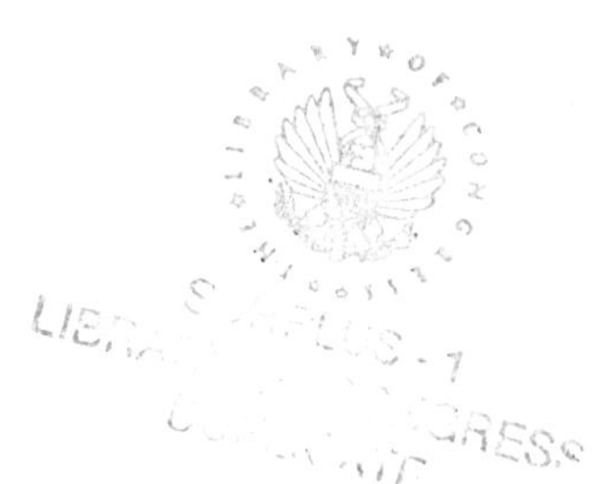

Roberto Patarca-Montero, MD, PhD

Chronic Fatigue Syndrome, Genes, and Infection
The Eta-1/Op Paradigm

Pre-publication
REVIEWS,
COMMENTARIES,
EVALUATIONS . . .

"*Chronic Fatigue Syndrome, Genes, and Infection* is the first book that I am aware of that discusses in great detail the infectious and at times genetic basis of ME/CFS. This is a book that you should have in your library, and recommend to physicians. Chapter 3, 'Induction or Direct Use of Eta-1/Op Protein As a Potential for Therapy for CFS,' is worth the price of the whole book. This book is also useful for patients who are involved in legal problems resulting from their disabilities."

Byron M. Hyde, MD
Chairman, Nightingale Foundation,
Ottawa, Canada

"By providing knowledge of early T-cell activation-1/osteopontin (Eta-1/Op), this book lets us look into the immune system. If individuals who are genetically susceptible to chronic infections are infected by particular microbial agents, they may get immune disturbances and develop CFS. The author gives us an exhaustive scientific coverage of Eta-1/Op and presents an interesting view of its possible role in chronic syndromes such as CFS as well as malignancy. The knowledge presented in the book bears witness to a unique understanding of CFS, which may also be used for formulating treatment."

Carl-Gerhard Gottfries, MD
Professor Emeritus,
Department of Clinical Neuroscience,
University of Göteborg,
Sweden

NOTES FOR PROFESSIONAL LIBRARIANS AND LIBRARY USERS

This is an original book title published by The Haworth Medical Press®, an imprint of The Haworth Press, Inc. Unless otherwise noted in specific chapters with attribution, materials in this book have not been previously published elsewhere in any format or language.

CONSERVATION AND PRESERVATION NOTES

All books published by The Haworth Press, Inc. and its imprints are printed on certified pH neutral, acid free book grade paper. This paper meets the minimum requirements of American National Standard for Information Sciences-Permanence of Paper for Printed Material, ANSI Z39.48-1984.

Chronic Fatigue Syndrome, Genes, and Infection
The Eta-1/Op Paradigm

THE HAWORTH MEDICAL PRESS®
Haworth Research Series
on Malaise, Fatigue, and Debilitation

Roberto Patarca-Montero, MD, PhD
Senior Editor

Concise Encyclopedia of Chronic Fatigue Syndrome by Roberto Patarca-Montero

CFIDS, Fibromyalgia, and the Virus-Allergy Link: Hidden Viruses, Allergies, and Uncommon Fatigue/Pain Disorders by R. Bruce Duncan

Adolescence and Myalgic Encephalomyelitis/Chronic Fatigue Syndrome: Journeys with the Dragon by Naida Edgar Brotherston

Phytotherapy of Chronic Fatigue Syndrome: Evidence-Based and Potentially Useful Botanicals in the Treatment of CFS by Roberto Patarca-Montero

Autogenic Training: A Mind-Body Approach to the Treatment of Fibromyalgia and Chronic Pain Syndrome by Micah R. Sadigh

Enteroviral and Toxin Mediated Myalgic Encephalomyelitis/Chronic Fatigue Syndrome and Other Organ Pathologies by John Richardson

Treatment of Chronic Fatigue Syndrome in the Antiviral Revolution Era by Roberto Patarca-Montero

Chronic Fatigue Syndrome, Christianity, and Culture: Between God and an Illness by James M. Rotholz

The Concise Encyclopedia of Fibromyalgia and Myofascial Pain by Roberto Patarca-Montero

Chronic Fatigue Syndrome and the Body's Immune Defense System by Roberto Patarca-Montero

Chronic Fatigue Syndrome, Genes, and Infection: The Eta-1/Op Paradigm by Roberto Patarca-Montero

The Psychopathology of Functional Somatic Syndromes: Neurobiology and Illness Behavior in Chronic Fatigue Syndrome, Fibromyalgia, Gulf War Illness, Irritable Bowel Syndrome, and Premenstrual Syndrome by Peter Manu

Handbook of Chronic Fatiguing Illnesses by Roberto Patarca-Montero

Chronic Fatigue Syndrome, Genes, and Infection
The Eta-1/Op Paradigm

Roberto Patarca-Montero, MD, PhD

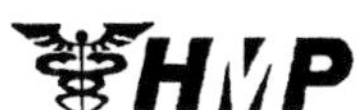

The Haworth Medical Press®
An Imprint of The Haworth Press, Inc.
New York • London • Oxford

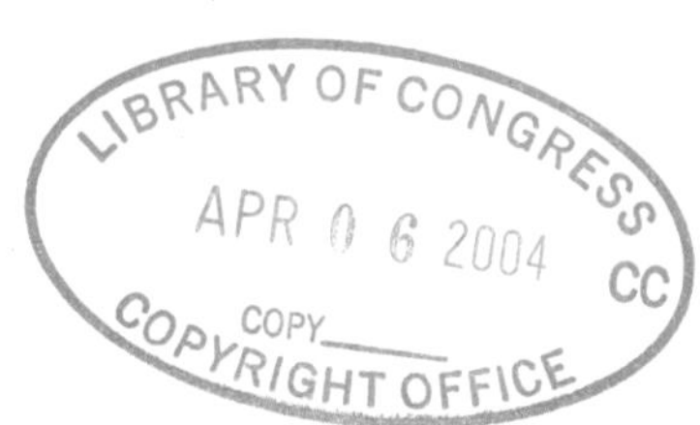

Published by

The Haworth Medical Press®, an imprint of The Haworth Press, Inc., 10 Alice Street, Binghamton, NY 13904-1580.

PUBLISHER'S NOTE
This book has been published solely for educational purposes and is not intended to substitute for the medical advice of a treating physician. Medicine is an ever-changing science. As new research and clinical experience broaden our knowledge, changes in treatment may be required. While many potential treatment options are made herein, some or all of the options may not be applicable to a particular individual. Therefore, the author, editor and publisher do not accept responsibility in the event of negative consequences incurred as a result of the information presented in this book. We do not claim that this information is necessarily accurate by the rigid scientific and regulatory standards applied for medical treatment. **No Warranty, Express or Implied, is furnished with respect to the material contained in this book. The reader is urged to consult with his/her personal physician with respect to the treatment of any medical condition.**

The author has exhaustively researched all available sources to ensure the accuracy and completeness of the information contained in this book. The publisher and author assume no responsibility for errors, inaccuracies, omissions, or any inconsistency herein.

Cover design by Marylouise E. Doyle.

Library of Congress Cataloging-in-Publication Data

Patarca-Montero, Roberto.
Chronic fatigue syndrome, genes, and infection : the Eta-1/Op paradigm / Roberto Patarca-Montero.
p. ; cm.
Includes bibliographical references and index.
ISBN 0-7890-1793-8 (hardcover : alk. paper)—ISBN 0-7890-1794-6 (softcover : alk. paper)
1. Chronic fatigue syndrome—Genetic aspects. [DNLM: 1. Fatigue Syndrome, Chronic—genetics. 2. Sialoglycoproteins—genetics. 3. Fatigue Syndrome, Chronic—immunology. WB 146 C294ca 2003] I. Title.
RB150 .F37 P378 2003
616'.0478—dc21

2002012398

CONTENTS

ABOUT THE AUTHOR

Roberto Patarca-Montero, MD, PhD, HCLD, is Assistant Professor of Medicine, Microbiology, and Immunology and also serves as Research Director of the E. M. Papper Laboratory of Clinical Immunology at the University of Miami School of Medicine. Previously, he was Assistant Professor of Pathology at the Dana-Farber Cancer Institute and Harvard Medical School in Boston. Dr. Patarca serves as Editor of *Critical Reviews in Oncogenesis* and the *Journal of Chronic Fatigue Syndrome.* He is also the author or co-author of more than 100 articles in journals or books, as well as the *Concise Encyclopedia of Chronic Fatigue Syndrome* and *Chronic Fatigue Syndrome: Advances in Epidemiologic, Clinical, and Basic Science Research.* He is currently conducting research on immunotherapy of AIDS and chronic fatigue syndrome. Dr. Patarca is a member of the Board of Directors of the American Association for Chronic Fatigue Syndrome and the Acquired Non-HIV Immune Diseases Foundation.

Chapter 1

Microbial Infections, Chronic Fatigue Syndrome, and Microbial Infection Resistant Host Genes

Many debilitating chronic illnesses are characterized by the presence of fatigue (Morrison, 1980), and chronic fatigue is the most commonly reported medical complaint of all patients seeking medical care (Kroenke et al., 1988). Fatigue syndromes, such as chronic fatigue syndrome (CFS), have complex chronic signs and symptoms, including fatigue, muscle pain, headaches, memory loss, nausea, gastrointestinal problems, joint pain, vision problems, breathing problems, depression, low-grade fevers, skin disorders, tissue swelling, and chemical sensitivities, among others (Patarca, 1999). Although there is a lack of definitive laboratory or clinical tests that could identify the cause(s) of these illnesses, there is growing awareness that chronic fatigue illnesses can be associated with an infectious agent that is responsible (causative) for the illness; a cofactor for the illness; or appears as an opportunistic infection(s) responsible for aggravating patient morbidity (Nicolson et al., 1999). There are several reasons for this notion (Nicolson, 1998), including the nonrandom or clustered appearance of the illness, often in immediate family members, and the course of the illness and its response to therapies in many patients based on treatment of infectious agents (Patarca, 1999).

Over the course of two decades, a large number of studies have been conducted to unravel the pathogenesis of chronic fatigue syndrome (Patarca, 1999). Although several studies investigating the precipitating factor for CFS reveal a high percentage of patients who associate the onset of their disorder to an apparently infectious illness (Bock and Whelan, 1993; Komaroff and Buchwald, 1991; Lloyd et al.,

1990; MacDonald et al., 1996; Salit, 1997; Schluederberg et al., 1992), there is no consensus among researchers or clinicians as to a possible microbial etiology (Ablashi et al., 1988; Buchwald and Komaroff, 1991; Buchwald et al., 1987, 1992; De Freitas et al., 1991; Gold et al., 1990; Gow et al., 1994; Heneine, 1994; Josephs et al., 1991; Khan et al., 1993; Kitani et al., 1996; Klonoff, 1992; Landay et al., 1991; Levine et al., 1992; Luka et al., 1990; Martin, 1997; Nakaya et al., 1996, 1997, 1999; Swanink et al., 1998). Moreover, although chronic microbial infections often present with very similar symptoms to those seen in CFS patients, their diagnosis can be problematic because the physician may not associate the clinical manifestations with these hidden infections, and because laboratory tests needed to diagnose them lack sensitivity (Bottero, 2000; Jadin, 2000).

Even if they prove not be causative, microbial agents such as *Rickettsia, Coxiella, Mycoplasma, Chlamydia, Brucella,* and possibly others, such as the novel Human Blood Bacterium (Linder and MacPhee, U.S. Patent 6,255,467 B1, July 3, 2001), cause patient morbidity or exacerbation of the major signs and symptoms observed in patients with chronic illness, including chronic fatigue syndrome. For instance, lipid-soluble-membrane-damaging toxin production by skin coagulase-negative staphylococci (CoNS) has been associated with myofascial pain syndrome and, in CFS patients, the number of δ-toxin producing strains of CoNS correlates positively with general CFS symptom scores (Butt et al., 1998; McGregor et al., 1996). As another example, both human immunodeficiency virus (HIV)-infected and CFS patients have increased carriage of L-form bacteria such as *Mycoplasma* spp. (Choppa et al., 1998; Horowitz et al., 1998; Vojdani et al., 1998), and Nicolson et al. (1998) suggested that the number of detectable *Mycoplasma* spp. increases with duration of illness, two criteria that comply with a typical comorbid pathogen for both CFS and HIV infection.

The inability to identify a microbial agent in a chronic illness does not necessarily mean that a microbe infection did not take place. Levy (1994) proposed a "hit and run" effect, whereby a microbe may infect the host, trigger immune abnormalities leading to CFS, and then be eliminated, leaving the immune system in an activated state. The latter postulate is based on the fact, exemplified in several paragraphs later in this chapter, that several microbes have been associated with the development of autoimmune processes, and on studies of systemic autoimmune disease that have led to the view that initiation and progression of the disease process reflects chronic and sustained lymphocyte activation by unidentified polyclonal activating agents (Blaese et al., 1980; Budman et al., 1977; Hang et al., 1985; Klinman and Steinberg, 1987; Ueda et al., 1989). This abnormal lymphocyte response is thought to lead to production of autoantibodies that mediate immunologic tissue destruction (Klinman et al., 1988).

Mycoplasmal infections are associated with various autoimmune disorders, such as multiple sclerosis, amyotrophic lateral sclerosis, lupus, autoimmune thyroid disease, and possibly others (Nicolson et al., 2000). The autoimmune manifestations could result from intracellular pathogens such as mycoplasmas escaping from cellular components and incorporating into their structure pieces of host cell membranes that contain important host antigens. Mycoplasmal surface components may also directly stimulate autoimmune responses, possibly secondary to molecular mimicry of host antigens (Dallo et al., 1996). Chronic airway disorders, such as asthma, airway inflammation, and bronchial hyperreactivity (known to be present in CFS patients), are also known to be associated with mycoplasmal infections (Cassell, 1998; De Meirleir, 1999; Gil et al., 1993; Kraft et al., 1998). *Mycoplasma fermentans* has also been found to promote apoptosis (Gong et al., 1999; Paddenberg et al., 1998), and Nicolson et al. (1998) report that four antibiotics are useful for the treatment of mycoplasma-positive CFS patients, and suggest that these be used in multiple six-week courses: doxyclycline (200 to 3,000 mg/day), azithromycin (500 mg/day), minocyclin (200 to 300 mg/day), and ciprofloxacin (1,000 to 15,000 mg/day).

Chlamydiae are intracellular bacteria frequently associated with fatigue in infected patients (Chia and Chia, 1999). *Chlamydia pneumoniae* is transmitted by the respiratory route (Grayston, 1995) and is a widely recognized pathogen in atherosclerosis (Airenne et al., 1999; Grayston, 1995; Penttila et al., 1999; Roedel et al., 2000; Rottenberg et al., 2000), sinusitis (Rottenberg et al., 2000), bronchitis (Airenne et al., 1999; Rottenberg et al., 2000), pneumonia (Rottenberg et al., 2000), and adult-onset asthma (Airenne et al., 1999; Roedel et al., 2000) as well as myocarditis, pericarditis, and endocarditis (Grayston, 1995; Penttila et al., 1999). *Chlamydia pneumon-*

iae has been suggested to contribute to morbidity in subsets of chronic fatigue syndrome (Salit, 1997) and fibromyalgia (Machtey, 1997) patients, and Chia and Chia (1999) demonstrated the presence of chronic *Chlamydia pneumoniae* infection in a subset of CFS patients who responded well to treatment with the antibiotic azythromycin. However, positive serology for chlamydia is not a good indicator for antibiotic therapy because there is a high prevalence of antichlamydial seropositivity in asymptomatic patients (Grayston, 1995).

Rickettsiae are small gram-negative bacteria. *Rickettsiae* are transmitted by the bite of ticks, lice, fleas, or, in certain special circumstances, by exposure to infected dust, cows, sheep, goats, and by drinking raw milk. The principal *Rickettsiae* in Europe are *Rickettsia conotii, R. prowazekii, R. mooserii,* and *Coxiella burnetti*. *Rickettsiae* have a long period of survival in the reticular endothelial system and the walls of blood vessels, and are liable to be activated by an acute or hidden infection after delays of differing duration, thereby initiating chronic pathology. *Rickettsiae* and chlamydiae are involved in chronic psychopathology with concomitant vascular problems or neurological illnesses (Bottero, 2000; Loo and Menier, 1962, 1993; Masbernard, 1963). Treatment with tetracyclines and other antibiotics of rickettsial infections that had been diagnosed by immunofluorescence testing in patients with persistent fatigue resulted in 84 to 96 percent recovery (Jadin, 2000).

Jadin (2000) highlighted several congruent features between CFS and chronic rickettsial infection: similar symptomatology; epidemic CFS was first reported in Incline, Nevada, the same location of origin of Rocky Mountain spotted fever in 1916 [Jadin, 1953]; similarities between CFS and the disease that affected Florence Nightingale, who worked surrounded by lice, fleas, and ticks during the Crimean War (Hennessy, 1994), in which soldiers presented with epidemic typhus, the common disease of wars, regularly reported since the time of Hannibal; similar immunological findings in sheep with tickborne diseases, CFS patients, and patients with Q-fever endocarditis or the so-called post-Q-fever fatigue syndrome (Marmion and Shannon, 1996). Post-Q-fever fatigue syndrome is characterized by inappropriate fatigue, myalgia and arthralgia, night sweats, and changes in mood and sleep patterns following about 20 percent of laboratory-proven cases of acute primary Q-fever, a condition caused by the rickettsial organism *Coxiella burnetii* (Ayres et al., 1998; Bennett et al., 1998; Penttila et al., 1998), which can be transmitted through ticks, droplets, or raw milk from infected animals. *Coxiella burnetti* also can be transmitted by the wind, and a substantial proportion of patients have reported no direct contact with animals (Bernit et al., 2002). Although improvement of similar symptoms of this zoonotic condition occurs rapidly, resolution of fatigue takes longer and is associated with improvement in cell-mediated immunity as measured by delayed-type hypersensitivity skin responses (Penttila et al., 1998).

Genetic endowment may explain why some individuals may develop chronic disease after microbial infection and others do not. Early protection against bacterial infection is generally thought to depend on a nonspecific host response that includes production of acute phase proteins such as complement and C-reactive protein, as well as nonspecific reaction of macrophages and granulocytes (Rosenstreich et al., 1982). Subsequent protection comes from the development of a specific immune response that usually depends on T cells (Rosenstreich et al., 1982). This division of labor does not easily account for the host response to bacteria such as *Rickettsia tsutsugamushi,* a gram-negative intracellular bacterium that is the etiologic agent of human scrub typhus (Groves et al., 1980). This model of bacterial infection has been studied extensively because resistance to the lethal effects of acute infection is under unigenic dominant control by the *Ric* locus (Groves et al., 1980). Susceptible mouse strains allow local and systemic bacterial growth during the first week of infection and die within 10 to 12 days. By contrast, resistant mouse strains show minimal levels of bacterial infection over the first week and survive infection (Jerrells and Osterman, 1982; Nacy and Groves, 1981). Although the *Ric* locus affects early resistance to *Rickettsia tsutsugamushi* infection, mice bearing the resistant genotype are converted to the sensitive one if T-cell development is genetically impaired by the *nu* mutations (Jerrells and Eismann, 1983; Murata and Kawamura, 1977).

There is considerable evidence for genetic control of resistance to infections by bacteria, viruses, and protozoa (Rosenstreich et al., 1982). One class of genes confers resistance by nonimmunological mechanisms. Notable examples are the Duffy and *Mx* genes, which affect resistance to the malarial parasite *Plasmodium vivax* and influenza virus, respectively (Hadley et al., 1986; Staeheli et al., 1986). A second class of genes that may confer resistance by immunological mechanisms has been inferred from the responses of inbred mice to a variety of infectious agents (Rosenstreich et al., 1982). Examples of the second class of genes are loci in the major histocompatibility complex (Rosenstreich et al., 1982) and the early T-cell activation-1/osteopontin (Eta-1/Op) gene, which encodes a cytokine and is the focus of the present book. Although lymphocytes can be specifically activated by cells that express peptide/major histocompatibility complex (MHC) associated with infection by bacteria or viruses, they are not usually equipped to rapidly eliminate infected target cells. An effective immune response depends on the elaboration of soluble mediators (cytokines) that can attract macrophages and other effector cells to the site of infection and enhance their capacity to destroy ingested microbes (Churchill et al., 1975; Kleinerman et al., 1983). Production of the Eta-1/Op cytokine is part of an early T-cell-dependent response after *Rickettsia tsutsugamushi* infection of resistant mouse strains but not of susceptible hosts.

As with other cytokines, insight into Eta-1/Op has come from several independent lines of research:

1. studies of a phosphoprotein expressed by a variety of virally and spontaneously transformed cell lines, termed transformation-related phosphoprotein 2ar (Smith and Denhardt, 1987) and subsequently designated secreted phosphoprotein-1 (Spp-1) (Senger et al., 1989), indicated that this protein may be a marker of neoplastic transformation (Craig et al., 1988; Senger et al., 1983, 1989). High levels of this phosphoprotein also are found in the serum of patients with certain carcinomas and in patients with sepsis (Senger et al., 1988);
2. independent studies of bone matrix proteins led to the purification of a hydroxyapatite-binding phosphoprotein with a variable apparent molecular weight, designated 44 kDa-phosphoprotein, pp69, bone sialoprotein I, and, most recently, osteopontin (Butler, 1989; Glimcher, 1989; Oldberg et al., 1986; Reinholt et al., 1990); and
3. efforts to define genes involved in immunological resistance to microbial infection led to the description of a murine gene desig-

nated Eta-1 (Patarca et al., 1989), which is expressed by T cells early after activation by antigen.

Eta-1 is also expressed in vivo as part of an early response to bacterial infection and mapped with 100 percent confidence to the *Ric* locus controlling protective immunity to certain intracellular bacteria, such as *Rickettsia tsutsugamushi* (RT) (Patarca et al., 1989). The 2ar/Ssp-1 mouse gene subsequently also was mapped to the same locus (Fet et al., 1989). Reports of the sequence of osteopontin cDNAs from different species then showed that mouse osteopontin (2ar) is virtually identical to Eta-1 (Craig et al., 1989; Patarca et al., 1989). The gene and its product will be referred to as Eta-1/Op (for early T-cell activation protein-1/osteopontin) throughout this book.

It could be possible that individuals who are infected with particular microbial agents and carry gene variants of resistance genes which make them susceptible to chronic infection and its untoward effects may account for the development of chronic diseases, such as chronic fatigue syndrome. The characterization and study of genes whose protein products confer natural resistance to particular infections is therefore of paramount importance to understanding the etiopathogenesis of chronic diseases. These gene products also could be used as therapeutic modalities, as a simile to the use of interferon-a in the treatment of hepatitis C virus infection. Subsequent chapters address the properties of Eta-1/Op in etiopathogenesis and treatment of CFS and other maladies.

Chapter 2

Definition of the Role of the Eta-1/Op Gene in Genetic Resistance to Bacterial and Viral Infections

MAPPING OF THE ETA-1/OP GENE TO A BACTERIAL RESISTANCE LOCUS AND CHARACTERIZATION OF FUNCTIONAL ALLELES

There is considerable evidence for genetic control of resistance to infections by bacteria, viruses, and protozoa (Rosenstreich et al., 1982). However, with the exception of loci within the major histocompatibility complex (Rosenstreich et al., 1982), the relevant genes and their products had escaped molecular definition. Eta-1/Op was mapped to mouse chromosome 5 using hamster somatic cell hybrids (Patarca et al., 1989). Analysis of EcoRV/XbaI restriction fragment length polymorphisms (RFLPs) from recombinant inbred strains revealed that Eta-1/Op was a single copy gene having at least two structural alleles. It mapped 0 to 1 cm from a locus on chromosome 5, which controls inborn resistance to lethal infection by certain intracellular bacterial parasites including *Rickettsial tsutsugamushi* (RT) (Patarca et al., 1989). Inbred mouse strains that expressed the Eta-1/Op^{a} allele were resistant to infection, whereas inbred mouse strains expressing the Eta-1/Op^{b} allele were susceptible (Patarca et al., 1989).

Since these initial studies, the RFLP survey has been extended to other inbred mouse strains and determined that the RT-resistant strains BDP/J, 1/LnJ, AU/SsJ, C57L/J, CE/J, and A/HeJ also bear the Eta-1/Op^{a} allele (Table 2.1). In agreement with the mapping of the Eta-1/Op to the *Ric* locus, no variation of the Eta-1/Op RFLP was found in the presence of mutations of surrounding loci (Table 2.1), including the *Pgm-1* (phosphoglucomutase-1), *rd* (retinal degeneration), *Ph* (patch marker), and *W* (dominant spotting) loci (Groves et al., 1980). A third allele of Eta-1/Op, the *c* allele, was then characterized using the restriction enzyme StuI in susceptible DBA strains (Table 2.1) (Miyazaki et al., 1990; Patarca et al., 1993). Taken together, these results indicate that Eta-1/Op and *Ric* show 100 percent concordance in their allelic distribution and chromosome localiza-

TABLE 2.1. Allelic Distribution of Eta-1/Op in Inbred Mouse Strains

Rickettsia resistant	**Rickettsia sensitive**	
Allele *a*	**Allele *b***	**Allele *c***
1/LnJ	CBA/J	DBA/J
A/HeJ	C3H/HeJ	DBA/1La
AKR/J	SJL/J	DBA/2HaJ
AU/SsJ	STS/A	DBA/2DeJ
BALB/clut		DBA/2J
BALB/cJ		
BDP/J		
CBA/CaJ		
CBA/CaHTeJ		
C57BL/6J-Ph		
C57BL/6J		
C57BL/10J		
C57L/J		
CE/J		
MWT/Le		
P/J		
PL/J		
SWR/J		

tion, and that DBA strains bear a third allele, Eta-1/Op^c, which is distinct from Eta-1/Op^b expressed by other RT-susceptible strains. Although the mutations in the two susceptible alleles, *b* and *c,* appear to be in different locations, both have the common effect of abrogating early inducibility of the Eta-1/Op gene in response to RT infection. These results are consistent with those of Fet et al. (1989), who used an RFLP that distinguished two 2ar alleles in C57BL/6J and DBA/2J mice to assign the 2ar (Eta-1/Op) gene to the *Ric* locus on chromosome 5.

The human Eta-1/Op gene was mapped to human chromosome 4 using human-rodent cell hybrids (Young et al., 1990). A single copy gene with an approximate length of 5.4 to 8.2 kb was localized to band 4q13 near the centromere by in situ hybridization of metaphase chromosomes using Eta-1/Op cDNA as the probe (Young et al., 1990). This location is consistent with the notion that human chromosome 4 is similar to mouse chromosome 5 over an extended region (from 4p16.3 to 4q21). The human dentin matrix acidic phosphoprotein gene (DMP1) maps to the dentinogenesis imperfecta type II critical region at chromosome 4q21 close to but not overlapping the Eta-1/Op locus (Aplin et al., 1995; Crosby et al., 1995). The porcine genes encoding interleukin 2, alcohol dehydrogenase (class I) γ polypeptide, and Eta-1/Op map to chromosome 8 by linkage analysis, and Ellegren et al. (1993) described an extensive syntenic homology with human chromosome 4.

ANALYSIS OF RESISTANCE PHENOTYPES CONFERRED BY ALLELES OF THE ETA-1/OP GENE

The degree of resistance conferred by the Eta-1/Op polymorphism is substantial. Inbred mouse strains that carry the resistant allele suppress local growth of RT following intraperitoneal inoculation of 10^5 to 10^6 organisms, whereas susceptible strains fail to suppress peritoneal growth and die from widespread infection within 10 to 14 days after infection by as few as 10^3 organisms (Groves and Osterman, 1978; Patarca et al., 1989). Determination of levels of Eta-1/Op gene expression in both resistant and susceptible mouse strains infected with RT, namely in two mouse strains CBA/CaJ (Eta-1/Op^a) and CBS/J (Eta-

1/Op^b) that are genetically similar but differ at the Eta-1/Op locus, revealed that Eta-1/Op expression increased within 24 hours of RT infection of CBA/CaJ (Eta-1/Op^a) mice and remained elevated over the next six days (Patarca et al., 1989). Peritoneal cells obtained from these mice five days after infection contained 0 to 1 RT bacterium per cell. In contrast, cells from infected CBA/J (Eta-1/Op^b) mice did not express significant levels of Eta-1/Op for the first three days after infection, and peritoneal cells from these mice five days after infection contained more than 200 RT bacteria per cell. Failure of CBA/J mice to express the Eta-1/Op^b allele early after RT infection did not reflect a generalized transcriptional defect of this allele because inoculation of CBA/J mice with the T-cell mitogen concanavalin A resulted in strong induction of Eta-1/Op RNA within 24 hours (Patarca et al., 1989).

The *Ric* locus was successfully mapped because it exerted unigenic control of resistance to rickettsial infection. In contrast, resistance to other intracellular bacterial pathogens is under multigenic control and has been more difficult to define (Rosenstreich et al., 1982). Determination of the role of the Eta-1/Op gene in genetic resistance to other bacterial infections using the CBA substrains revealed that challenge of CBA/Ca (Eta-1/Op^a) but not CBA/J (Eta-1/Op^b) mice with *Listeria monocytogenes* (LM) results in a strong Eta-1/Op response (Patarca et al., 1993). In preliminary experiments, this is associated with increased resistance to the lethal effects of LM infection in CBA/Ca hosts compared with CBA/J hosts.

The Eta-1/Op protein has an RGD cellular adhesion motif that contributes to binding activity of the ligand to macrophages and may affect the migration and activation state of these cells in vivo (Rodan, 1995; Singh, Patarca, et al., 1990). The interaction between Eta-1/Op and macrophages is inhibited by an Eta-1/Op RGD-containing peptide and also may be influenced by sialic acid-binding receptors of macrophages, termed sialoadhesin (Crocker et al., 1991), and sialic acid residues on the ligand. In view of the lipopolysaccharide (LPS) inducibility of Eta-1/Op in macrophages (Miyazaki et al., 1990), it also is possible that Eta-1/Op can mediate resistance to gram-negative bacteria via a macrophage pathway. Sublethal and lethal doses of LPS endotoxin differentially induce splenic and hepatic expression of Eta-1/Op as compared with interferon-γ in CBA/CaJ, CBA/J, and MRL/n mice, and the level of induction varies according to the Eta-

1/Op allele present (Patarca et al., 1993). It is also noteworthy that Eta-1/Op production probably does not contribute to LPS toxicity because a nontoxic derivative of LPS also induced high levels of Eta-1/Op and there was no difference in Eta-1/Op induction between LPS-resistant and LPS-sensitive C3H substrains (Patarca and Cantor, unpublished observations). Instead, toxicity correlated with hepatic expression of tumor necrosis factor (TNF), which was consistent with previous reports (Fong et al., 1990). These observations also may explain the presence of high levels of circulating Eta-1/Op in patients with sepsis (Senger et al., 1988) and may be relevant to apparent beneficial effects of endotoxin in the development of host resistance to bacterial (both gram-negative and gram-positive), fungal, parasitic, and viral infections.

Prior to these studies, early resistance to bacterial infection had been attributed to nonspecific host responses mediated by macrophages and acute phase proteins (Rosenstreich et al., 1982). Indeed, the early and rapid expression of Eta-1/Op after RT infection preceded expression of other T-cell cytokines, such as interferon-γ, by four to five days. Mice bearing the *nu/nu* mutation, which lack normal T cells, were used to determine if the Eta-1/Op response is T-cell dependent. *Nu/nu* mice did not express significant levels of Eta-1/Op 48 hours after RT infection unless they had received T cells from syngeneic donors immediately before infection (Patarca et al., 1989). These studies, along with the findings that large numbers of T cells can recognize certain bacterial proteins termed superantigens (Janeway et al., 1989), indicate that infections by bacteria such as RT may mobilize rapid and vigorous T-cell responses in vivo. Conversely, deactivation of macrophage functions plays an important role in the establishment of chronic human infectious and inflammatory diseases (Staege et al., 2001). Analysis of gene expression of human mononuclear phagocytes deactivated with interleukin (IL)-4, IL-10, and dexamethasone (DEX), in the absence and presence of infection with *Listeria monocytogenes (Listeria),* revealed

1. pronounced IL-4-induced up-regulation of ABCG2, an ATP-binding cassette transporter highly expressed in the placenta, which mediates multidrug resistance of cancer cells but is otherwise of unknown function;

2. both DEX- and IL-4-mediated down-regulation of Eta-1/Op, an important factor of host resistance against intracellular infections;
3. inhibition of the CC-chemokine I-309 mRNA expression by all three deactivators in the presence of *Listeria* infection; and
4. up-regulation by *Listeria* infection of the interferon-stimulated gene ISG20 of unknown function, whose product localizes with nuclear dots. (Staege et al., 2001)

POTENTIAL ROLE OF ETA-1/OP IN RESISTANCE TO FLAVIVIRUSES

Flaviviruses are a subgroup of RNA viruses that include yellow fever, West Nile encephalitis, Japanese B encephalitis, St. Louis encephalitis, and hepatitis C and G viruses. Studies of genetic resistance to this group of viruses resulted in the early identification of a resistant mouse strain, the Princeton Swiss mouse (PRI). Goodman and Koprowski (1962) introduced the resistance gene from PRI mice to the C3H/He strain, resulting in the new strain C3H/RV, which is congenic to the C3H/He strain except for a locus conferring flavivirus resistance as a single autosomal dominant trait (Goodman and Koprowski, 1962). This pair of strains was subsequently found to differ at the locus conferring resistance to infection by RT (Jerrells and Osterman, 1981). These findings suggest that resistance to flaviviruses also may be controlled by Eta-1/Op. At present, the basis for resistance to this group of viruses is not well understood. Early studies suggested that the growth of flavivirus in macrophages from genetically resistant strains was associated with increased production of defective virus particles, which interfered with virus replication (Jerrells and Osterman, 1981). One intriguing possibility involves an interaction between Eta-1/Op and intracellular viral proteins leading to decreased viral growth.

POTENTIAL ROLE OF ETA-1/OP IN RESISTANCE TO HIV INFECTION

Double negative $CD4^-$ $CD8^-$ T cells express Eta-1/Op, a fact that first became apparent from in vitro studies of a $CD4^+$ T-cell clone

(Patarca, Wei, et al., 1990). A variant of this clone, termed Ar5v, arose during in vitro growth, retained expression of CD1, and expressed neither CD4 nor CD8. In addition, the variant, but not the parent clone, expressed CD45R according to immunofluorescence analysis and thus had acquired the typical surface phenotype of mature double negative (DN) T cells. Unstimulated Ar5v cells did not express detectable levels of IL-2, IL-3, IL-4, IFN-γ, or Eta-1/Op. However, the DN Ar5v cell line constitutively expressed very high levels of Eta-1/Op mRNA and showed a less pronounced but significant expression of IFN-γ mRNA (Patarca, Wei, et al., 1990).

$CD4^-$ $CD8^-$ (DN T cells), bearing the α/β T-cell receptor and specific for CD1 (a family of nonmajor histocompatilibility complex-encoded, nonpolymorphic, β2-microglobulin-associated glycoproteins) and expressing high levels of Eta-1/Op, recognize bacterial nonpeptidic antigens such as mycolic acid (a family of α-branched, β-hydroxy, long-chain fatty acids), lipoarabinomannam (LAM), and TUBag4 (a 5' triphosphorylated thymidine-containing compound) and are therefore important in bacterial immunity (Beckman et al., 1994; Bendelac et al., 1995; Constant et al., 1995; Sieling et al., 1995). Eta-1/Op could also interact directly with bacteria through the cellular adhesion Arg-Gly-Asp motif that is also present in the extracellular matrix protein fibronectin. Bacteria such as *Escherichia coli, Staphylococcus, Streptococcus, Treponema,* and mycobacteria bind to the Arg-Gly-Asp-containing extracellular matrix proteins. In this respect, preliminary studies have pointed to a direct antibacterial role of an Eta-1/Op-derived decamer peptide that includes the Arg-Gly-Asp motif (Patarca and Cantor, unpublished observations).

T-cell receptor $\alpha\beta^+$ $CD4^-$ $CD8^-$ T cells differentiate extrathymically in an lck-independent manner and participate in early response against *Listeria monocytogenes* infection through interferon-γ and Eta-1/Op production (Kadena et al., 1997; Song et al., 1995). The α/β T-cell receptor-bearing $CD4^-$ $CD8^-$ T cells that produce Eta-1/Op are a population of mature T cells that has been shown to generate from $CD8^+$ T cells in the presence of interleukin-4 in mice (Erard et al., 1993). Patarca et al. (1996) reported increased proportions of DN T cells in association with declining proportions of $CD4^+$ T cells in pediatric acquired immunodeficiency syndrome (AIDS) slow progressors, but not in rapid progressors. The latter finding appears to mimic the increase in the proportion of DN lymphocytes in lymph nodes of mice depleted of circulating CD4+ lymphocytes by injection of anti-CD4 monoclonal antibody (Goronzy et al., 1986). An increase in the proportion of DN T cells may therefore provide a compensatory advantage to declining CD4+ T-cell proportions in pediatric slow progressors because these cells have strong cytotoxic activity (Arase et al., 1993) and secrete cytokines such as Eta-1/Op.

POTENTIAL ROLE OF ETA-1/OP IN NATURAL RESISTANCE TO HERPESVIRUSES

After intraperitoneal infection with murine cytomegalovirus (MCMV), numbers of CD3+ CD4− CD8− (DN) T-cell receptor (TCR) αβ+ T cells increase in peritoneal cavity (peak levels around day 5), liver and spleen in both resistant C57BL/6 and susceptible BALB/c mice (Hossain et al., 2000). The peritoneal DN TCR αβ+ T cells express highly skewed TCRVβ8 on day 5 after infection compared with the uninfected mice, but those in spleen and liver show moderate and low skewed TCRVβ8, respectively. The percentages of NK1.1+ DN TCRαβ+ T cells gradually decrease as does modulation of some of their activation markers consistent with an activated cell phenotype. The peritoneal DN TCRαβ+ T cells on day 5 after infection express the genes of Eta-1/Op, interferon (IFN)-γ, tumor necrosis factor-α, and MCP-1 (monocyte chemoattractant protein 1) but lack expression of interleukin-4 (IL-4). After in vitro stimulation with phorbol 12-myristate 13-acetate and calcium ionophore in the presence of Brefeldin A, higher frequencies of intracellular IFN-γ+ DN TCRαβ+ T cells are detected in all three organs of infected mice compared with those of uninfected mice. Stimulation of peritoneal DN TCRαβ+ T cells with plate-bound anti-TCRβ monoclonal antibodies show proliferation and also production of IFN-γ but not IL-4. These results suggest that DN TCRαβ+ T cells are activated and may have an antiviral effect through the production of IFN-γ, Eta-1/Op, and other macrophage-activating factors during an early phase of MCMV infection (Hossain et al., 2000).

POTENTIAL ROLE OF ETA-1/OP IN NATURAL RESISTANCE TO MYCOBACTERIAL INFECTIONS

Eta-1/Op expression correlates with clinical outcome in patients with mycobacterial infection (Nau et al., 2000). Eta-1/Op is expressed in chronic inflammatory diseases including tuberculosis, and its deficiency in mice predisposes them to more severe mycobacterial infections. There is an inverse correlation between Eta-1/Op levels and disease progression after inoculation of *Mycobacterium bovis* bacillus Calmette-Guerin (BCG) vaccine in humans: Patients with regional adenitis and good clinical outcomes had abundant Eta-1/Op in infected lymph nodes. This pattern of Eta-1/Op accumulation was also observed in patients infected by *M. avium-intracellulare*. In contrast, patients with disseminated infection and histologically ill-defined granulomas had no significant Eta-1/Op accumulation in infected lymph nodes; these patients had either deficiencies in the interferon-γ receptor 1 or idiopathic immune defects. The level of Eta-1/Op protein expression was inversely correlated with disseminated infection and with death of the patient. Therefore, Eta-1/Op expression correlates with an effective immune and inflammatory response when humans are challenged by a mycobacterial infection, and Eta-1/Op contributes to human resistance against mycobacteria (Nau et al., 2000).

Part of the relevance of Eta-1/Op in mycobacterial disease stems from the fact that cells in granulomas of various origins express Eta-1/Op, and Eta-1/Op functionally contributes to the formation of granulomatous lesions (Chiba et al., 2000). In this respect, cardiomyopathic hamsters express Eta-1/Op, and form granulomatous lesions in heart tissue in both albumin-immunized and untreated animals. In addition, immunization induces expression of Eta-1/Op in lung and lymph nodes of cardiomyopathic (but not normal) hamsters, and also induces granuloma formation in these organs. Intratracheal administration of an adenoviral vector containing the murine Eta-1/Op gene into the lungs of normal hamsters induced pulmonary granuloma formation (Chiba et al., 2000).

Eta-1/Op levels are elevated in granulomas caused by *Mycobacterium tuberculosis* (Nau et al., 1999). *Mycobacterium tuberculosis* infection of primary human alveolar macrophages causes a substantial increase in Eta-1/Op gene expression (Nau et al., 1997). Eta-1/Op protein was identified by immunohistochemistry in macrophages, lymphocytes, and the extracellular matrix of pathologic tissue sections of patients with tuberculosis (Nau et al., 1997). When infected with *Mycobacterium bovis* BCG, mice lacking a functional Eta-1/Op gene have more severe infections characterized by heavier bacterial loads and a delayed clearance of the bacteria. The Eta-1/Op-null mice have greater granuloma burdens consistent with the elevated bacterial load. The ability of Eta-1/Op to facilitate the clearance of mycobacteria is most pronounced early after infection and appears to be independent of known mediators of resistance to infection by mycobacteria: antigen-specific T-cell immunity, interferon-γ production, and nitric oxide production. BCG grows more rapidly in macrophages derived from Eta-1/Op-null mice than in those from wild-type mice, demonstrating that the null phenotype is secondary to an intrinsic macrophage defect. These results indicate that Eta-1/Op augments the host response against mycobacterial infection and that it acts independently from other antimycobacterial resistance mechanisms (Nau et al., 1999).

Chapter 3

Induction or Direct Use of Eta-1/Op Protein As Potential Therapy for CFS

Although chronic fatigue syndrome (CFS) is an ailment of as yet unknown etiology, it is characterized in at least a subgroup of patients, mostly among those with an acute onset, i.e., following a flu-like illness, by evidence of activation of the immune army, an observation which lends support to the hypothesis that CFS is caused by an infection that either lingers chronically or leaves an autoimmune sequel. In this respect, it is known that microbes can cause damage to their human hosts either directly or indirectly. While attacking a microbe, some microbial components may resemble human components, and the body may end up generating antibody bullets that can also recognize bodily components, a process termed molecular mimicry that can lead to autoimmune disease manifestations. The latter process is also favored by genetic predisposition in the form of particular variants of the human leukocyte antigen (HLA) molecules, the proteins that antigen-presenting cells use to present foreign and self particles to the T cells.

It is curious that although the immune army is activated in a subset of CFS patients, the soldiers of the immune army, particularly the T cells and natural killer cells, function poorly. T cells from CFS patients have a decreased capacity to divide and generate new T cells, and the natural killer cells have significantly decreased "killing" or cytotoxic activity. In CFS, not only is the function of the T cells impaired but the repertoire of T-helper cells is also biased, as in autoimmune diseases, toward a Th2-type (humoral immunity dominant) response. Activated T-helper cell generals from CFS patients produce less interferon-γ, a Th1-type (cellular immunity dominant) cytokine, and more interleukin-5, a Th2-type cytokine. These features combine to create a pervasive immunological battlefield-like environment in CFS patients that is Th2-type predominant with compromised cellular immunity and the ability of the body to deal with microbes along with the presence of autoantibodies. The triggers and maintenance factors of the Th2-type predominance are unknown but could include infections, toxins, prior immunizations, hormonal status changes, or a combination thereof.

As mentioned in Chapter 2, Eta-1/Op is a key cytokine in cell-mediated and granulomatous inflammation (Cantor, 1995; O'Regan and Berman, 2000; O'Regan, Hayden, et al., 2000; O'Regan, Nau, et al., 2000; Uede et al., 1997; Weber and Cantor, 1996). A comprehensive gene expression profile analysis of human activated Th1- and Th2-polarized cells from cord blood revealed that human activated Th1-polarized, but not Th2-polarized, cells highly express Eta-1/Op (Nagai et al., 2001) along with proteins, such as IFN-γ, lymphotactin, MIP-1α, MIP-1β, perforin, β-catenin, and CD55 (Nagai et al., 2001; Swanson et al., 1989). The comprehensive identification of genes selectively expressed in human-activated Th1 or Th2 cells should contribute to our understanding of the molecular basis of Th1/Th2-dominated human diseases and may provide genetic information to diagnose these diseases (Kasprowicz et al., 2000; Kohm et al., 2000; Nagai et al., 2001).

Mice deficient in Eta-1/Op gene expression have severely impaired type-1 immunity to viral infection (herpes simplex virus-type 1 [KOS strain]) and bacterial infection *(Listeria monocytogenes)* and do not develop sarcoid-type granulomas (Rittling and Denhardt, 1999). Interleukin-12 (IL-12) and interferon-γ production is diminished, and IL-10 production is increased. A phosphorylation-dependent interaction between the amino-terminal portion of Eta-1/Op and its integrin receptor stimulated IL-12 expression, whereas a phosphorylation-independent interaction with CD44 inhibited IL-10 expression. Eta-1/Op is a key cytokine that sets the stage for efficient type-1 immune responses through differential regulation of macrophage IL-12 and IL-10 cytokine expression (Ashkar et al., 2000). Expression of Eta-1/Op mRNA is up-regulated during activation of GMG cells, which are differentiated natural killer (NK) lineage cells that share phenotypic, functional, and morphologic characteristics with adherent interleukin-2 (IL-2)-activated NK cells (Pollack et al., 1994).

Studies have demonstrated that early IL-12 and IFN-γ expression is required to induce a protective response to many intracellular pathogens (O'Regan, Hayden, et al., 2000; O'Regan, Nau, et al., 2000). Eta-1/Op stimulation augments the ability of anti-CD3 monoclonal antibody to induce CD40 ligand (CD40L) and IFN-γ expression on human T cells, resulting in CD40L- and IFN-γ-dependent IL-12 production in vitro. These findings suggest a functional role for Eta-1/Op in early Th1 responses, namely regulation of T-cell-dependent IL-12 production. Furthermore, Eta-1/Op up-regulation of CD40L provides mechanistic support for the association of Eta-1/Op with polyclonal B-cell proliferation and humoral autoimmune disease (Cantor, 2000; O'Regan, Hayden, et al., 2000; O'Regan, Nau, et al., 2000). The latter feature calls for caution in the level of cytokine induction in immunotherapeutic interventions because untoward effects may develop at higher doses, a warning that is addressed at the end of this chapter through expanding on the role of Eta-1/Op expression dysregulation in autoimmune disease.

Based on the observations described, several therapeutic interventions being tested are aimed at favoring a shift of the T-helper cell responses of CFS patients from a Th2- to a Th1-type predominant pattern. These approaches are based on the use of *Staphylococcus* vaccine, influenza and/or rubella virus vaccines, *Mycobacterium vaccae* vaccine, poly I-C, and autologous reinfusion of lymph node cells that had been expanded and activated outside the body with Th-1-type inducing cytokines, such as interleukin-2. Some of these therapeutic interventions are based on the old medical wisdom of curing one infection by giving another to the patient, and most appear in published patents. These immunotherapies have shown promising results with clinical improvement as assessed by functional status and cognitive measures. Some other interventions are based on the use of herbal products, such as *Panax ginseng*, which have been associated with improved Th1-type responses. Further studies will allow the elucidation of the factors that mediate Th-2 response predominance in CFS, as well as the association of particular cytokines with different CFS symptoms. The two bacteria-based interventions are expanded in the following sections. A third one suggested by the findings described in this book would entail direct administration of Eta-1/Op. The latter therapies would be particularly useful when no evidence of chronic infection is apparent, i.e., when antibiotic treatment would not be useful, and when there is evidence of immunological dysregulation, possibly as a result of an initial infection.

MYCOBACTERIUM VACCAE

As described in international published patent number WO-09826790 by Rook, Stanford, and Zumla, preparations of killed *Mycobacterium vaccae* are able to effect a nonspecific systemic Th1-type response bias, in particular by down-regulation of Th2-type activity without concomitant up-regulation of Th1-type activity. As mentioned in Chapter 2, mycobacteria induce Eta-1/Op expression and resistance to mycobacterial infection by some individuals is associated with higher levels of this cytokine.

In experimental animals, a nonspecific systemic bias away from Th2-type activity on administration of *M. vaccae* can be seen as a reduction in the titer of an IL-4 (Th2)-dependent antibody response to ovalbumin (an allergen unrelated to *M. vaccae* itself), in mice preimmunized so as to establish a Th2-type response. A single injection of *M. vaccae* is able to cause this effect, and further injections can enhance it. The effect is nonspecific because it does not require the presence of any component of ovalbumin in the injected preparation. Briefly, Balb/c mice six to eight weeks old were immunized with 50 μg ovalbumin emulsified in oil (incomplete Freund's adjuvant) on days 0 and 24. This is known to evoke a strong Th2-type pattern of response, accompanied by IgE production, and priming for release of two Th2-type cytokines, IL-4 and IL-5. Animals then received saline or 10^7 autoclaved *M. vaccae* on days 53 and 81 by subcutaneous injection. Injections of *M. vaccae* reduced the rise in IgE levels caused by immunization with ovalbumin. The reduction caused by treatment with *M. vaccae* was significant at all time points tested. Similarly, spleen cells from the immunized animals failed to release IL-5 in vitro in response to ovalbumin if the donor animals had been treated with *M. vaccae,* while spleen cells from immunized animals treated with saline released large quantities of IL-5 in response to ovalbumin. The latter data show that *M. vaccae* will reduce a Th2-type pattern of response, even when given after immunization with a potent allergen, and without epitopes of the Th2-inducing molecule. There is therefore a nonspecific systemic down-regulation of the Th2-type pattern of response, not dependent upon a direct adjuvant effect on the allergen itself.

In cancer patients, the effect of *M. vaccae* injection has been demonstrated by the appearance in the peripheral blood of lymphocytes that spontaneously secrete IL-2 (a characteristic Th1 cytokine) and the decrease in T cells that secrete IL-4 (a characteristic Th2 cytokine) after stimulation with phorbol myristate acetate and calcium ionophore. The percentage of lymphocytes showing this activated Th1-type phenotype increases progressively after each successive injection of *M. vaccae,* reaching a plateau in many individuals after three to five injections of 10^9 organisms (days 0, 15, 30, and then monthly).

The *M. vaccae* used for these therapies is grown on a solid medium including modified Sauton's medium solidified with 1.3 percent agar. The medium is inoculated with the microorganisms and incubated aerobically for ten days at 32°C to enable growth of the microorganism to take place. The microorganisms are then harvested, weighed, and suspended in diluent to give 100 mg of microorganisms/mL of diluent. The suspension is then further diluted with buffered saline to give a suspension containing 10 mg wet weight (about 10^{10} cells) of microorganisms/mL of diluent and dispensed into 5 mL multidose vials. The vials containing the live microorganisms are then autoclaved (115-125°C) for ten minutes at 69 kPa to kill the microorganisms. The therapeutic agent thus produced is stored at 4°C before use. Then 0.1 mL of the suspension, containing 1 mg wet weight (about 10^9 cells) of *M. vaccae,* is shaken vigorously immediately before being administered by intradermal injection over the left deltoid muscle.

In the same patent publication, Rook, Stamford, and Zumla describe their experience with CFS patients treated with *M. vaccae*. For instance, a CFS patient reported improvement after two injections of a *M. vaccae* preparation. A second one reported that, since she had begun receiving a *M. vaccae* preparation at two-month intervals, her CFS symptoms and food allergy had improved considerably and she believes she will be very well as long as she continues with her regular injections.

STAPHYLOCOCCAL VACCINE

In international published patent number WO-09829133 by Goteborg University Science Invest AB, Carl-Gergard Gottfries and Bjoern Regland describe the use of staphylococcal vaccine to favor a Th-1-type predominance. The treatment is preferably conducted as a series of administrations with increasing doses during a specific period. Preferably, the vaccine is administered in eight to ten increasing doses for four to twelve weeks, preferably for eight to ten weeks. The reason for the increasing doses is that during the first week or weeks, the patient will probably suffer from side effects, and it is therefore advantageous to start with a low dose. The side effects will diminish after some time. The first series of administrations is followed by repeated administrations given approximately once a week for five to 15 weeks, preferably for ten weeks. To prevent recurrence, the repeated administrations are then followed by a maintenance treatment with administrations approximately once a month, which preferably are continued for several years, such as one to ten years, but preferably approximately five years. The doses in the repeated administrations of the maintenance treatment are preferably constant and relatively high. Vitamin B_{12} and/or folacin are preferably administered simultaneously or in parallel with the staphylococcal preparation.

If the known staphylococcal vaccine Staphypan Berna from the Serum and Vaccine Institute, Bern, Switzerland, is used, a typical treatment schedule may be as follows: eight to ten administrations are made during a period of four to 12 weeks, preferably eight to ten weeks, wherein the dose of the staphylococcal preparation is gradually increased from 0.1 to 1 mL of the pure vaccine. The increase depends on the response from the patient. It may be, for example, 0.1, 0.2, 0.3, 0.4, 0.5, 0.6, 0.7, 0.8, 0.9, and 1.0 mL, respectively. If the patient shows a strong local reaction, it is possible to repeat a dose before increasing it. The dose of staphylococcal preparation in the repeated administration and in maintenance treatment is 1 mL.

As described in the published patent, after a pilot study comprising eight patients was made, a double-blind placebo-controlled study was performed, using a group of 24 women patients fulfilling both the criteria for fibromyalgia and for chronic fatigue syndrome. Seven of the 13 patients who received the staphylococcal preparation were assessed as being minimally improved, three as being much improved, and the remaining three were unchanged. In the placebo group, three patients were minimally improved, while the remaining eight were unchanged. The improvement in the group with active treatment was statistically significant ($p < 0.05$) compared to the improvement in the placebo group. Following the controlled study, 24 patients chose to continue with the treatment and 20 of these have been treated for one and two years. Nineteen of these 20 patients were on the sick list or received sickness pension prior to the start of treatment, and one patient was employed part-time. At a one-year follow-up after the completed study, nine of the 20 patients were in full- or part-time paid employment, while one patient was taking part in a work experience program and one was in the middle of a two-year training program to become a nurse. The treatment strategy used in this study is a series of administrations of staphylococcal preparations given approximately once a week during a period of some months, for example, three months, and thereafter long-term treatment with monthly administrations. This Swedish group is conducting further studies.

It is noteworthy that *Staphylococcus aureus* expresses a major histocompatibility complex (MHC) class II analog (Jonsson et al., 1995). The deduced protein consists predominantly of six repeated domains of 110 residues. Each of the repeated domains contains a subdomain of 31 residues that share striking sequence homology with a segment in the peptide binding groove of the ß chain of the MHC class II proteins from different mammalian species. The purified staphylococcal recombinant protein binds several mammalian proteins, including recombinant Eta-1/Op (Jonsson et al., 1995; Ryden et al., 1989).

CAVEATS IN THE USE OF ETA-1/OP AS A THERAPEUTIC AGENT: ETA-1/OP AND AUTOIMMUNE DISEASE

Cell-mediated (type-1) immunity is necessary for immune protection against most intracellular pathogens but, when excessive, can mediate organ-specific autoimmune destruction (Ashkar et al., 2000). Expansion of double negative (DN) $CD4^{-}$ $CD8^{-}$ cells described in

Chapter 2 is also characteristic of autoimmune disease in MRL/lpr mice, which harbor a mutation in the fas ligand (CD95) (Cantor, 2000). The MRL/lpr inbred mouse strain spontaneously develops a systemic autoimmune disease with histopathological features of human systemic lupus erythematosus (SLE) and rheumatoid arthritis (Theofilopoulos and Dixon, 1985; Wuthrich, 1998; Wuthrich et al., 1998). Although the development of autoimmune disease is heralded by the appearance of large numbers of DN cells in peripheral lymphoid tissues, there had been little information on the potential contribution of these cells to the sustained activation of immunological effector cells that may mediate the autoimmune process. This prompted the determination of whether the expanded population of DN cells in peripheral lymphoid tissues of MRL/lpr mice showed evidence of dysregulated Eta-1/Op expression. A 25-fold increase in Eta-1/Op expression was noted when compared with levels of a cellular housekeeping gene, glyceraldehydephosphate dehydrogenase (GAPDH), over the period from 2.5 to 4.5 months after birth (Patarca, Wei, et al., 1990). Moreover, the absolute increase in Eta-1/Op expression in lymph node (LN) tissue during this time was substantially higher because of the development of severe lymphadenopathy: total levels of Eta-1/Op mRNA in the peripheral LN of MRL/lpr but not of MRL/n mice increased by approximately four orders of magnitude. The following observations suggest that elevated Eta-1/Op expression represents a highly specific genetic marker of the developmental defect associated with this murine autoimmune disease, namely a defective fas ligand that leads to expansion of DN cells, which in turn produce excessive amounts of Eta-1/Op:

1. No elevated levels of IL-2, IL-3, or IL-4 were detected in MRL/lpr (Mori et al., 1994; Patarca, Wei, et al., 1990). A modest elevation in the levels of IFN-γ occurred in some but not all animals tested relatively late in the course of the disease (Patarca, Wei, et al., 1990).
2. Increased levels of Eta-1/Op mRNA were first apparent at three months of age and reached maximal levels by five months. Lymphadenopathy and signs of autoimmune disease in MRL/lpr mice began at approximately three months of age and reached

maximum levels by five to six months of age (Patarca, Wei, et al., 1990).

3. Eta-1/Op expression also was elevated in association with abnormal expression of DN T cells in C3H/lpr and C57B6/lpr strains, but increased expression in these two lpr-congenic strains was intermediate between normal inbred strains and the MRL/lpr strain (Patarca, Wei, et al., 1990), consistent with the milder form of autoimmune disease they display.
4. NZB, NZB/W, and BxSB, which develop an autoimmune disease that reflects an intrinsic B-cell abnormality according to cell transfer studies (Theofilopoulos et al., 1981), do not display increased Eta-1/Op expression compared to age- and sex-matched nonautoimmune strains, despite evidence of massive B-cell and macrophage expansion and activation toward the end of the disease process (Patarca and Cantor, unpublished observations).
5. Mori et al. (1994) demonstrated that DN T cells, the major cell population in MRL/lpr mice, failed to express IL-3, IL-4, IL-5, and IL-6 genes that influence B-cell growth and activation. In contrast, DN T cells expressed the Eta-1/Op gene, which is shown to augment polyclonal activation of B cells and immunoglobulin production (Mori, 1994; Mori et al., 1994).

Enhanced expression of the chemotactic protein Eta-1/Op by renal tubular cells is a prominent feature of murine lupus nephritis and might be promoted by the proinflammatory cytokine environment in MRL-lpr (Mori et al., 1994; Wuthrich, 1998; Wuthrich et al., 1998). The chronic up-regulation of Eta-1/Op could participate in the recruitment of monocytes in the kidney of MRL/lpr mice, thereby contributing to the pathogenesis of autoimmune renal disease. In this respect, immunofluorescence staining revealed prominent expression of Eta-1/Op by proximal tubules in MRL/lpr mice but not in MRL/++ control mice. Northern blot analysis demonstrated that steady-state transcript levels for Eta-1/Op mRNA were also significantly increased in MRL/lpr kidneys compared with control kidneys. Furthermore, in situ hybridization showed massive Eta-1/Op mRNA transcripts in proximal tubules in MRL/lpr mice but not in controls. The diffuse macrophage infiltration in the kidney of MRL/lpr correlated with the enhanced Eta-1/Op expression. Eta-1/Op secretion in vitro by cultured renal tubular epithelial cells was up-regulated by TNF-α and 1,25(OH)2-vitamin D3, whereas no regulation was observed in a control macrophage cell line (Wuthrich, 1998; Wuthrich et al., 1998).

Studies of systemic autoimmune disease have led to a consensus that the initiation and progression of the disease process reflects chronic and sustained polyclonal B-cell activation. In some cases (NZB, BxSB), B-cell hyperactivity may reflect differentiation defects intrinsic to this class of lymphocyte. In the case of MRL/lpr disease, chronic activation of B cells is likely to be caused by T cells because thymectomy or treatment of animals with anti-CD4 antibody prevents development of this disorder (Santoro et al., 1988; Steinberg et al., 1980; Theofilopoulos et al., 1981). Other studies have suggested that the abnormal DN T cells in these animals constitutively produce a soluble factor termed MRL B-cell differentiation factors (L-BCDF), which causes B-cell activation and immunoglobulin (Ig) production in vitro (Prud'homme et al., 1983).

The Eta-1/Op gene product may represent the soluble factor L-BCDF (Lampe et al., 1991). Supernatant fluids of COS cells after transfection with pCD-Eta-1/Op, but not pCD alone, stimulate B cells to produce both IgM and IgG. To directly determine the effects of Eta-1/Op on Ig production in B cells in the absence of other COS cell proteins, this protein was purified to homogeneity from supernatant fluids of the T-cell line Ar5v, which produces extremely large amounts of the Eta-1/Op protein (Singh, Patarca, et al., 1990). Addition of purified Eta-1/Op to B-cell cultures resulted in an increase in IgM and IgG that was directly proportional to the concentrations of Eta-1/Op present in cultures (Lampe et al., 1991). Analysis of IgG isotypes induced by Eta-1/Op shows a tenfold enhancement of the IgG2a+b response, whereas the IgG3 response was not affected (Lampe et al., 1991). This induction profile is characteristic of T-cell-dependent induction and is similar to the profile of IgG isotypes spontaneously produced by splenic B cells directly explanted from MRL/lpr mice (Slack et al., 1984).

The concentration of serum Eta-1/Op protein is elevated not only in autoimmune-prone MRL/lpr mice but also in patients with systemic lupus erythematosus (Iizuka, 1998; Iizuka et al., 1998; Mori et al., 1994). Eta-1/Op induces the polyclonal activation of B cells, resulting in the augmented production of immunoglobulin, indicating that Eta-1/Op plays some role in the development of autoimmune disease. In two kinds of Eta-1/Op-overexpressing transgenic mice, one carrying the immunoglobulin (Ig) enhancer/SV40 promoter and the other carrying the cytomegalovirus enhancer/chicken β-actin (CAG) promoter, the B1 cell population in the peritoneal cavity was markedly increased, and titer of IgM and IgG3 antibodies in the serum was considerably higher than that in wild-type mice. Most important, the titer of the IgM class of anti-double-stranded DNA antibody was significantly elevated in transgenic mice. These results strongly suggest that Eta-1/Op has an important role in the propagation and differentiation of B1 cells and production of autoantibodies (Iizuka, 1998; Iizuka et al., 1998). Moreover, Eta-1/Op itself has been shown to be an autoantigen of somatostatin cells in human islets, as evinced from identification by screening random peptide libraries with sera of patients with insulin-dependent diabetes mellitus (Fierabracci et al., 1999).

The observations in MRL/lpr mice and in patients with systemic lupus erythematosus bring attention to the fact that excess expression of cytokines may also cause pathology, a phenomenon that is important to bear in mind when designing cytokine-based therapies. For instance, Eta-1/Op could contribute to formation of the verrucoma induced by the bacteria *Bartonella bacilliformis* (Caceres-Rios et al., 1995) because Eta-1/Op, which is produced by DN T cells stimulated by bacterial nonpetidic antigens, promotes vascular cell and macrophage adhesion and spreading (Liaw et al., 1994), and is a substrate for the angiogenic factor XIII (Prince et al., 1991). *Bartonella bacilliformis* is the bacterial agent responsible for human bartonellosis (Caceres-Rios et al., 1995), and it is closely related to the etiologic factor for bacillary angiomatosis, a rickettsial illness, in AIDS (Cockerell et al., 1991). *Bartonella bacilliformis* probably also induces the expression of other soluble immune mediators such as tumor necrosis factor (TNF)-α, basic fibroblast growth factor, interleukin-8 or factor XIII, all of which have angiogenic properties (Fajardo et al., 1992; Koch et al., 1992; Leibovich et al., 1987; Mignatti et al., 1989; Nemeth and Penneys, 1989; Schaumberg-Lever et al., 1994; van Deventer et al., 1993). The angiogenic action of TNF-α may arise from direct stimulation of endothelial or stromal cells, which would in turn result in the release of secondary mediators. In particular, prostaglandins (Fajardo et al., 1992) and platelet-activating factor (1-O-alkyl-2-acetyl-sn-glycero-3-phosphocholine) (Camussi et al., 1995; Montrucchio et al., 1994) have been proposed to mediate TNF-α-induced angiogenesis. Moreover, TNF-α transiently induces c-*ets 1* gene expression in endothelial cells, and the c-*ets 1* protein induces Eta-1/Op expression (Hultgardh-Nilsson et al., 1996). The c-*ets 1* protein is believed to regulate transcription of the genes coding for matrix-degrading proteases, which are necessary for angiogenesis (Wernert et al., 1992). More recently, TNF-α has been shown to induce B61, an endothelial cell gene product that is angiogenic and can also function as an endothelial cell chemotaxin that interacts with the endothelial cell Eck receptor protein tyrosine kinase (Pandey et al., 1995). Interestingly, B61 expression is also induced by interleukin-1β and lipopolysaccharide (Holzman et al., 1990; Shao et al., 1995). Therefore, *Bartonella bacilliformis* could induce expression of B61, which in turn could be involved both in angiogenesis and endothelial cell proliferation. An additional candidate cell product that could be induced by *Bartonella bacilliformis* is the angiogenic oncogene int-2, which belongs to the fibroblast growth factor family and the expression of which is dysregulated in Kaposi's sarcoma lesions (Huang et al., 1993).

Chapter 4

Structure and Regulation of the Eta-1/Op Gene and Protein

STRUCTURE OF THE ETA-1/OP GENE

The mouse Eta-1/Op gene spans approximately 4.8 kb and contains six exons and five introns. There is a high level of similarity (72 percent) between the exon regions of the mouse and human Eta-1/Op genes, but, as expected, less interspecies similarity (51 percent) between the flanking introns (Crosby et al., 1996; Ono et al., 1995). The human Eta-1/Op gene consists of seven exons that are similar to those of the mouse gene, although the human Eta-1/Op gene is longer than the mouse homologue (Yamamoto, Hijiya, et al., 1995). This difference is attributable to an insertion of about 1750 bp immediately before exon 4, in intron 3, in the human Eta-1/Op gene (Hijiya et al., 1994). A region of approximately 285 bp immediately upstream of the human Eta-1/Op transcription initiation site is highly conserved and contains a number of potential *cis* regulatory consensus sequences (Hijiya et al., 1994; Yamamoto, Hijiya, et al., 1995). Length polymorphism in an intron of the porcine Eta-1/Op gene is caused by the presence or absence of a SINE (PRE-1) element (Knoll et al., 1999; Wrana et al., 1989).

EXPRESSION OF THE ETA-1/OP GENE

Although Eta-1/Op is expressed by activated T cells and can bind to macrophages, several nonimmunological cell types also express it (see also Chapter 5). The gene may be transcribed in activated T cells (Patarca et al., 1989), activated macrophages (Cummings et al., 2001;

Miyazaki et al., 1990; Newman, Brunn, Mistry, 1995; Newman, Brunn, Porter, et al., 1995; Yamada et al., 2001), bone cells (preosteoblasts, osteoblasts, and osteocytes in the areas of cartilage-to-bone transition) (Kitazawa et al., 1999; Mark, Butler, et al., 1988; Mark, Prince, et al., 1988; Moore et al., 1991), granulated metrial gland cells of the decidua and placenta (Nomura et al., 1988), embryonic epithelial tissues including the endolymphatic sac and semicircular canals of the inner ear, postnatal kidney proximal convoluted tubules, uterine epithelium (Mark, Butler, et al., 1988; Mark, Prince, et al., 1988; Swanson et al., 1989; Yoon et al., 1987), and neuroepithelial cells (Mark et al., 1988). Immunohistochemical studies have revealed that Eta-1/Op is deposited as a prominent layer at the luminal surfaces of specific populations of epithelial cells of the gastrointestinal tract, gallbladder, pancreas, urinary and reproductive tracts, lung, breast, salivary glands, and sweat glands (Brown et al., 1992). Northern blot analyses identified the gallbladder as a major site of Eta-1/Op gene transcription comparable in magnitude with that of the kidney, and immunoblotting identified the Eta-1/Op protein in bile. In situ hybridization localized Eta-1/Op gene transcripts predominantly to the epithelium of a variety of organs as well as to the ganglion cells of bowel wall (Brown et al., 1992).

Eta-1/Op effects on gene expression include the suppression of the induction of nitric oxide synthase by inflammatory mediators (Guo et al., 2001). Eta-1/Op can also reduce cell peroxide levels, promote the survival of cells exposed to hypoxia, and inhibit the killing of tumor cells by activated macrophages (Denhardt et al., 1995). In terms of T-cell differentiation, Eta-1/Op may be expressed constitutively by $CD4^-CD8^-$ double negative (DN) mature T cells (Patarca, Wei, et al., 1990) and immature pre-T-cell lines (NCKA and KKE), which have undergone rearrangement of the T-cell receptor genes but do not express TCR transcripts (Patarca et al., 1993). Eta-1/Op can be detected in cells within the marrow of developing limb bones and calvaria at 14.5 days of gestation (Nomura et al., 1988, 1989). The Eta-1/Op protein has also been purified from human milk (Senger et al., 1989). Cytokine expression by nonimmunological cells, including bone and kidney tissue, is not limited to Eta-1/Op. For instance, bone tissue produces IL-6 (Freyen et al., 1989) and kidney tissue expresses both IL-6 and IL-7 (Namen et al., 1988; Van Snick, 1990). Moreover, a renal ligand that regulates the circulating levels of a number of cytokines, including IL-1 and tumor necrosis factor, has been defined (Hession et al., 1987).

REGULATION OF ETA-1/OP GENE EXPRESSION: THE PROMOTER REGION

The following is a summary of published data and an analysis of the potential transcriptional regulatory elements in the 5' flanking region of the mouse Eta-1/Op gene (Behrend et al., 1993; Craig and Denhardt, 1991; Miyazaki et al., 1990).

TATA Box

Several TATA-like sequences are located approximately 20 to 40 nucleotides upstream from each of the transcription initiation sites mapped by S1 nuclease protection analysis (Miyazaki et al., 1990) from the published cDNA sequence (Patarca et al., 1989). Craig and Denhardt (1991) found another exon located 5' to the "exon 1" reported by Miyazaki et al. (1990). The DNA upstream from this 5' exon functions as a promoter in epidermal fibroblast and osteoblast-like cells (Craig and Denhardt, 1991). The initiation site for Eta-1/Op in activated T cells is the one farthest upstream. This organization of initiation sites is reminiscent of the IL-6 gene, which also contains at least two cap sites (May et al., 1989).

The TATA sequence, TTTAAA, is present at positions –26 to –31 of the porcine Eta-1/Op gene (Zhang et al., 1992). However, the highest transcription rate was observed in a construct extending 180 bp upstream that included a CCGCCC Sp1 binding sequence (–63 to –68), and an AP1 site (–74 to –80) (Zhang et al., 1992). Promoter activity was also exhibited by a region containing a TTTAAA sequence in the first intron of the porcine Eta-1/Op gene that corresponded to the putative promoter site reported for mouse Eta-1/Op in macrophages (Miyazaki et al., 1990).

Phorbol Ester-Responsive Elements

Optimal expression of Eta-1/Op in the T-cell tumor cell line EL-4 requires both phorbol ester and calcium ionophore (CaI), although phorbol ester alone is sufficient to induce significant levels of Eta-1/Op gene expression (Patarca, Wei, et al., 1990). A single application of the phorbol ester 12-O-tetradecanoylphorbol-13-acetate (TPA) also can transiently induce Eta-1/Op gene expression in mouse epidermal cells in vitro, and in mouse epidermis in vivo (Senger et al., 1983). Accumulation of mRNA may not necessarily be secondary to transcriptional activation of the gene. For example, TPA can modulate an mRNA degradation pathway that regulates levels of granulocyte monocyte-colony stimulating factor (GM-CSF) and other cytokine transcripts (Shaw and Kamens, 1986; Thorens et al., 1987). However, the consensus *cis*-acting sequence required for the latter posttranscriptional effect is not present in the 3' translated region of Eta-1/Op mRNA (Shaw and Kamens, 1986).

The possibility that the inductive effects of TPA may reflect transcriptional regulation is consistent with the presence of a consensus TPA-responsive element (TRE) (TGACTCA) in an inverted orientation downstream from the transcription initiation site of the cDNA derived from activated T cells (Table 4.1). Although the downstream location is unusual, it does not preclude a physiological role for this

TABLE 4.1. Regulatory Domains of the 5' Region of the Eta-1/Op Gene

Domain	Location relative to the major transcription initiation site (+1)	Reference
TATA box	20-40 bases upstream of each of the multiple transcription initiation sites	Miyazaki et al., 1990
TRA-responsive element	50-56 bases	Patarca et al., 1993
Oct-1 binding site	–211 to –204	Miyazaki et al., 1990
HiNF-D binding site	–420 to –416	Stein et al., 1989
NF-AT binding site	–541 to –534	Patarca et al., 1993
Interferon regulatory factor I	–207 to –202	Miyazaki et al., 1990
	–570 to –565	
	–589 to –584	

element. For example, downstream phorbol myristate acetate (PMA)-responsive elements can regulate expression of the tissue plasminogen activator (tPA) gene (Medcalf et al., 1990). A complex composed of the transcription factors AP-1/Jun and c-fos may bind to TRE with high affinity, leading to efficient transactivation of associated genes (Ullman et al., 1990). Since c-fos is induced within 30 minutes of T-cell activation, this pathway may contribute to induction of Eta-1/Op via its *cis*-acting TRE sequences.

CCAAT Box

A consensus CCAAT box in the inverted orientation (AATTGG) is located approximately 60 nucleotides upstream from a transcription initiation site (Miyazaki et al., 1990). CCAAT boxes have been shown to act as enhancer elements and can act as binding sites for the transcription factor CAAT enhancer binding protein (C/EBP). The family of immunologically related transcription factors known as C/EBPs or ATF (Hai et al., 1988; Lin and Green, 1988) also is involved in the activation of cAMP and adenovirus E1A-inducible genes (Montminy et al., 1986).

Expression in HT1080 fibrosarcoma cells of v-src, a transforming viral oncogene product encoded by Rous sarcoma virus (RSV), significantly stimulates mouse Eta-1/Op promoter activity through the inverted CCAAT box located at –53 to –49 from the transcription start site (Tezuka et al., 1996). Mutations of the CCAAT box disrupt protein-DNA interaction and diminish both v-src stimulation and basal promoter activity. A CCAAT box-containing fragment corresponding to –155 to –122 of RSV long terminal repeat competes with the –72 to –38 fragment of mouse Eta-1/Op promoter for specific protein binding in the gel shift assay. A polyclonal antibody against CAAT-binding factor (CBF), a CCAAT box-binding factor, supershifts in gel shift assays the protein-DNA complex formed by the nuclear extract of HT1080 with either the RSV CCAAT box fragment or with the Eta-1/Op –72 to –38 fragment. Moreover, both Eta-1/Op mRNA levels and enhancer activity of CCAAT box-containing the –72 to –38 fragment were significantly elevated in v-src-transformed NIH 3T3 cells relative to parental cells. These findings suggest that the elevated Eta-1/Op expression in transformed cells could be secondary, at least in part, to v-src stimulation of the Eta-1/Op promoter and that this effect is mediated by a CBF-like factor (Tezuka et al., 1996).

The v-src oncogene induces expression of a number of genes that are involved in tumor growth and metastasis, including Eta-1/Op and others (Kim and Sodek, 1999). In the bone sialoprotein (BSP), an early marker of differentiated osteoblasts that has been implicated in the nucleation of hydroxyapatite crystal formation during de novo bone formation and that is also expressed ectopically by carcinomas that exhibit microcalcification and which metastasize to bone with high frequency, the v-src activity is targeted to an inverted CCAAT box located immediately upstream from an inverted TATA box in the BSP promoter. Nuclear factor-Y (NF-Y) is the principal nuclear factor that binds to the CCAAT box (Kim and Sodek, 1999).

Nuclear factor-IL-6 (NF-IL6) belongs to the CCAAT/enhancer binding protein family of transcription factors (Matsumoto et al., 1998). NF-IL6 binds to the regulatory regions of many genes induced in activated macrophages in vitro, and inducible expression of NF-IL6 is able to increase endogenous gene expression of Eta-1/Op, macrophage inflammatory protein (MIP)-1a, and CD14 in M1 cells, a monocytic leukemia cell line (Matsumoto et al., 1998).

Oct-1 Binding Site and Related Sites

Studies of cytokine expression patterns associated with T-cell activation indicate that Eta-1/Op is more efficiently expressed than other cytokines after T-cell receptor (TCR) ligation and may represent a genetic marker for low affinity interactions between T cells and major histocompatibility complex (MHC) products (Patarca, Wei, et al., 1990). Miyazaki et al. (1990) have detected an Oct-1 binding site (ATGCAAAT) within the Eta-1/Op promoter region. These sites are thought to play a role in gene expression in response to signals generated by antigen-receptor ligation or stimulation with TPA. The Oct-1 binding protein has been shown to regulate tissue-specific transcription of immunoglobulin heavy and light chain genes. Transcriptional activation through the Oct-1 site usually depends on the contribution of additional proteins that interact with a second closely spaced heptamer motif not present in the Eta-1/Op promoter region.

Deletion and mutagenesis analyses of the human Eta-1/Op promoter region identified a proximal promoter element (–24 to –94 relative to the transcription initiation site) that is essential for maintaining high levels of Eta-1/Op expression in the U-251MG and U-87MG human malignant astrocytoma cell lines (Wang, Yamamoto, et al., 2000). This element, designated RE-1, consists of two *cis*-acting elements, RE-1a (–55 to –86) and RE-1b (–22 to –45), which act synergistically to regulate the activity of the Eta-1/Op promoter. Gel shift assays using nuclear extracts of U-251MG cells demonstrated that RE-1a contains binding sites for transcription factors Sp1, the glucocorticoid receptor, and the E-box-binding factors, whereas RE-1b contains a binding site for the octamer motif-binding protein (Oct-1/Oct-2). Inclusion of antibodies directed toward Myc and Oct-1 in the gel shift assays indicate that Myc and Oct-1 participate in forming DNA-protein complexes on the RE-1a and RE-1b elements, respectively (Wang, Yamamato, et al., 2000).

Nuclear Factor of Activated T-Cell (NF-AT) Binding Sites

The 5'-flanking region contains the sequence AACCAGGA (at position –541) (see Table 4.1), which matches a purine-rich motif (Pu box) associated with the SV40 promoter enhancer in lymphoid cells (Petterson and Schaffner, 1987). Although this sequence is located relatively far from the transcription initiation sites of Eta-1/Op, Pu boxes located at –255 to –300 from the IL-2 and HIV-1 transcription initiation sites exert significant regulatory effects on these genes. NF-AT is expressed shortly after T-cell activation (Shaw et al., 1988). Interaction of this factor with the Pu box of the 5'-flanking region of the Eta-1/Op gene may therefore contribute to its expression in activated T cells. The immunosuppressant drugs cyclosporin A (CsA) and FK506 are potent blockers of NF-AT translocation, resulting in inhibition of transcription of several T-cell genes, including IL-2. The previous considerations suggest that CsA and FK506 also may inhibit T-cell expression of Eta-1/Op.

Smad- and Hox-Binding Elements

Members of the transforming growth factor (TGF) superfamily are known to transduce signals via the activation of Smad proteins. Ligand binding to transmembrane cell surface receptors triggers the phosphorylation of pathway-specific Smads. Smad2 and Smad3 are downstream transforming growth factor (TGF)-β signaling molecules. Upon phosphorylation by its type I receptor, Smad2 or Smad3 forms a complex with Smad4, and translocates to the nucleus where the complex activates target gene transcription (Hullinger et al., 2001; Shi et al., 2001). Smads 1 and 4 mediate bone morphogenetic protein (BMP) activation of the Eta-1/Op promoter by inhibiting the interaction of Hoxc-8 protein with a Hox-binding element (HBE). Functional analyses demonstrated that both the HBE- and Smad-binding region (containing the sequence AGACTGTCTGGAC) were involved in BMP-2-induced activation of the Eta-1/Op promoter, whereas, the HBE appeared to be the primary region involved in activation by TGF-β. Deletion of the first nine bases in the Smad-binding region substantially reduced BMP-2-mediated activation of the promoter. These results strongly suggest that both the Hox- and the Smad-binding regions play a role in BMP-2-induced activation of the Eta-1/Op promoter (Hullinger et al., 2001; Shi et al., 1999; Yang et al., 2000). Indeed, Shi et al. (2001) reported that Smad3 binds directly to the Eta-1/Op promoter and that Smad4 interacts with the Hox protein and displaces it from its cognate DNA binding site in response to TGF-β stimulation. In gel shift assays, the glutathione S-transferase-Smad3 fusion protein bound to a 50-base pair DNA element (–179 to –229) from the Eta-1/Op promoter. Also, both Hoxc-8 and Hoxa-9 bound to a Hox binding site adjacent to Smad3 binding sequence. Interestingly, Smad4, the common partner for both bone morphogenic protein and TGF-β signaling pathways, inhibited the binding of Hox protein to DNA. FLAG-tagged Smad4 coimmunoprecipitated with HA-tagged Hoxa-9 from cotransfected COS-1 cells, demonstrating an interaction between Smad4 and Hoxa-9. Transfection studies showed that Hoxa-9 is a strong transcriptional repressor: it suppresses the transcription of the luciferase reporter gene driven by a 124-base pair Eta-1/Op promoter fragment containing both Smad3 and Hox binding sites (Shi et al., 2001).

Smad6 and Smad7, a subgroup of Smad proteins, antagonize the signals elicited by TGF-β (Bai et al., 2000). These two Smads, induced by TGF-β or BMP stimulation, form stable associations with their activated type I receptors, blocking phosphorylation of receptor-regulated Smads in the cytoplasm. Smad6 interacts with homeobox (Hox) c-8 as a transcriptional corepressor, inhibiting BMP signaling in the nucleus. Smad6, but not Smad7, interacts with both Hoxc-8 and Hoxa-9 as a heterodimer when binding to DNA. Smad6-Hoxc-8 complex inhibits interaction of Smad1 with Hoxc-8- and Smad1-induced transcription activity (Bai et al., 2000).

Metastasis-Associated Transcription Factor Binding Site

Transient transfection studies, DNA-protein binding assays, and methylation protection experiments have identified a ras-activated enhancer, distinct from known ras response elements, that appears responsible for part of the increase in Eta-1/Op transcription in cells with an activated ras (Guo et al., 1995). In electrophoretic mobility shift assays, the protein-binding motif GGAGGCAGG was found to be essential for the formation of several complexes, one of which (complex A) was generated at elevated levels by cell lines that are metastatic. Southwestern blotting and UV light cross-linking studies indicated the presence of several proteins able to interact with this sequence. The proteins that form these complexes have molecular masses estimated at approximately 16, 28, 32, 45, 80, and 100 kDa. Because the approximately 16 kDa protein was responsible for complex A formation, it was designated MATF for metastasis-associated transcription factor, a putative ETS-related transcription factor. The GGANNNAGG motif is also found in promoters other than that for Eta-1/Op, an observation which suggests that these other promoters may be similarly controlled by MATF (Guo et al., 1995).

Hormones That Regulate the Expression of Eta-1/Op

TGFs 1 and 2, the calcitropic hormones 1,25-dihydroxyvitamin D_3, dexamethasone, and leukemia inhibitory factor (Kimbro and Saavedra, 1995; Noda and Rodan, 1989a,b; Noda, Vogel, Craig, et al., 1990; Noda, Vogel, Hasson, et al., 1990; Quelo et al., 1994; Ridall et al., 1995; Veenstra et al., 1998; Wrana et al., 1991; Yoon et al., 1987) stimulate the expression of Eta-1/Op in osteoblasts and osteoblastic sarcoma cells through a pathway that is mediated, at least in part, by transcriptional events and can be blocked by actinomycin D.

In contrast, treatment with calcitropic parathyroid hormone (PTH), or with estrogens, suppresses the expression of Eta-1/Op in osteoblasts, at least in part through transcriptional inhibition exerted via a glucocorticoid-responsive consensus element (AGAACA) in the Eta-1/Op promoter region (Miyazaki et al., 1990).

Nuclear receptors for the thyroid hormone and vitamins A and D cooperate with the retinoid X receptor (RXR) in activating Eta-1/Op gene transcription (Arbelle et al., 1996; Berghofer-Hochheimer et al., 1997; Carlberg et al., 1994; Darwish and DeLuca, 1993, 1996; Gross et al., 1998; Haussler et al., 1997; Kimmel-Jehan et al., 1997; Lemon and Freedman, 1996; Nishikawa et al., 1994; Patel et al., 1997a,b; Sasaki et al., 1995; Schrader et al., 1994; Staal, Van Wijnen, Birkenhager, et al., 1996; Staal, Van Wijnen, Desai, et al., 1996; Tagami et al., 1998; Thompson et al., 1998; Yen et al., 1996). It should be pointed out that the vitamin D receptor displays DNA binding and transactivation activities as a heterodimer with the retinoid X receptor, but not with the thyroid hormone receptor (Thompson et al., 1999). However, although the thyroid hormone receptor does not heterodimerize with the vitamin D receptor, it represses vitamin D receptor-mediated transactivation (Raval-Pandya et al., 1998; Schrader et al., 1994). Although the hormone response elements for these receptors have been proposed in which spacing of the direct repeated motifs determines the specificity (so-called 3-4-5 rule), vitamin D response elements (VDREs) in the natural context consist of often imperfect direct repeats. Vitamin D receptor (VDR) alone can bind to the mouse Eta-1/Op VDRE, which contains a direct repeat separated by three nucleotides, but not to the rat osteocalcin VDRE having an inexact direct repeat (Noda, Vogel, Craig, et al., 1990; Noda, Vogel, Hasson, et al., 1990). The presence of RXR not only allows the VDR to bind to the rat osteocalcin VDRE, but also increases the binding affinity for the mouse Eta-1/Op VDRE (Colnot et al., 1995; Jaaskelainen et al., 1995; Peleg et al., 1995). The RXR/VDR heterodimer exhibits similar affinity constants for the mouse Eta-1/Op VDRE and the rat osteocalcin VDRE, despite the apparently different affinities for the two VDREs of the VDR homodimer (Zhang et al., 1994). A random oligonucleotide selection procedure revealed that the consensus sequence selected by the RXR homodimer is the direct repeat spaced by one adenine residue (Freedman and Towers, 1991; Freedman et al., 1994; Zhang et al., 1994). In contrast, the sequences preferentially selected by the VDR homodimer and the VDR/RXR heterodimer are similar, which are the direct repeats spaced by three nucleotides (Freedman and Towers, 1991; Hsieh et al., 1995; Kuno et al., 1994; Nishikawa et al., 1993, 1994; Zhang et al., 1994).

1α, 25-Dihydroxyvitamin D_3 [1,25$(OH)_2D_3$] and its metabolites act on several target tissues not related to calcium homeostasis (Berdal, 1992; Carlberg et al., 1994; Chang et al., 1994; Chatterjee, 2001; Chou et al., 1995; DeLuca, 1992; Dilworth et al., 1997; Hahn et al., 1994; Harant et al., 2000; Haussler et al., 1997; Liu and Freedman, 1994; Miyaura and Suda, 1993; Ohyama et al., 1994; Owen et al., 1991; Peleg et al., 1995; Sakoda et al., 1996; Staal, Van Wijnen, Birkenhager, et al., 1996; Staal, Van Wijnen, Desai, et al., 1996; Suda et al., 1992). 1,25$(OH)_2D_3$ receptors and their activities are apparent in diverse tissues such as brain, pancreas, pituitary, skin, muscle, placenta, immune cells, and parathyroid. The receptor hormone complex becomes localized in the nucleus and undergoes phosphorylation by reacting with a kinase (Darwish and DeLuca, 1993; Desai et al., 1995). This form of the receptor then interacts with the Vitamin D responsive element of target genes and modifies the transcription of those genes to develop the action. The modulation of gene transcription results in either the induction or repression of specific messenger RNAs, ultimately resulting in changes in protein expression needed to produce biological responses. Mice lacking the vitamin D receptor exhibit impaired bone formation, uterine hypoplasia, and growth retardation after weaning (Yoshizawa et al., 1997). Eta-1/Op's role in osteoblast-osteoclast differentiation reflects the genomic effect of Vitamin D on bones (Chen, Adar, et al., 1999; Chen, Jin, et al., 1999; Matkovits and Christakos, 1995; Whitfield et al., 1995). The genomic action of Vitamin D also encompasses the biosynthesis of oncogenes, polyamines, lymphokines, and calcium binding proteins (Chatterjee, 2001; Khoury et al., 1994). Intracellular vitamin D binding proteins facilitate vitamin D-directed transactivation of Eta-1/Op gene expression (Wu, Ren, et al., 2000). However, 1,25$(OH)_2D_3$ not only regulates Eta-1/Op at the transcriptional level but also modulates the Eta-1/Op phosphorylation state in a process that involves a short-term (less than three hours) treatment and is associated with membrane-initiated Ca^{2+} influx (Chang and Prince, 1991; Farach-Carson et al., 1993; Safran et al., 1998).

Both natural and recombinant vitamin D_3 receptors (VDR) bind to rat BSP and both mouse and porcine Eta-1/Op VDRE oligonucleotides in a concentration-dependent manner with a strong preference for dimer formation, whereas equal amounts of dimer and monomer bind to the human osteocalcin VDRE (Chang et al., 1994; Craig et al., 2001; Ferrara et al., 1994; Gross et al., 1998; Juntunen et al., 1999; Koszewski et al., 1996, 1999; Langub et al., 2001; Li et al., 1998). However, whereas a truncated VDR constituting the DNA binding domain alone bound the mouse Eta-1/Op VDRE, it failed to interact with the porcine Eta-1/Op and rat BSP VDREs. VDR binding to the BSP is sequence specific, as shown by mutagenesis analysis, and can be abolished by heat and VDR antibody. Although the nucleotide sequences of VDREs in different genes conform to a direct (hexamer) repeat, spaced by three nucleotides, the precise sequences are unique for each VDRE. The studies by Li et al. (1998) and others (Craig et al., 1999; Darwish and DeLuca, 1996; Norman et al., 2000; Staal, Van Wijnen, Birkenhager, et al., 1996; Staal, Van Wijnen, Desai, et al., 1996) therefore demonstrate that subtle differences in the nucleotide sequence of VDREs affect VDR binding, which mediates the vitamin D_3 response. The three-dimensional structure of the binding site is also crucial because DNA bending is induced by binding of vitamin D receptor-retinoid X receptor heterodimers to vitamin D response elements (Kimmel-Jehan et al., 1999).

Eta-1/Op inhibits inducible nitric oxide synthase (iNOS), which generates large amounts of nitric oxide production (Takahashi et al., 2000; Tian et al., 2000). On the other hand, nitric oxide directly up-regulates endogenous Eta-1/Op production in macrophages (RAW 264.7 cells) stimulated with lipopolysaccharide and IFN-γ (Guo et al., 2001). The latter up-regulation of endogenous Eta-1/Op may therefore represent a negative feedback system acting to reduce iNOS expression (Guo et al., 2001; Takahashi et al., 2000; Tian et al., 2000). Collagen types I or IV, hyaluronate, and rat IgGs prevent iNOS inhibition by Eta-1/Op, an observation which suggests that macrophages are sensitive to regulation by Eta-1/Op only in certain physiological contexts (Tian et al., 2000).

Peroxizome proliferator-activated receptor (PPAR)-γ is a member of the nuclear receptor family of transcription factors that regulates adipocyte differentiation (Oyama, Kurabayashi, et al., 2000). Liganded PPAR-γ not only promotes differentiation but also inhibits the activation of macrophages which, in atherosclerotic plaques, produce Eta-1/Op. PPAR-γ ligand regulates Eta-1/Op gene expression in THP-1 cells, a cell line derived from human monocytic leukemia cells which can differentiate to macrophage upon stimulation with phorbol myristate ester (PMA). Northern blot analysis showed that Eta-1/Op expression is markedly induced in response to PMA. Troglitazone, a PPAR-γ ligand, dramatically attenuated PMA-induced Eta-1/Op expression. Transient transfection assays of the human Eta-1/Op promoter/luciferase construct, which contains a 5'-flanking region between −1500 and +87 relative to the transcription start site, demonstrate that either treatment with troglitazone or cotransfection of PPAR-γ expression vector inhibits Eta-1/Op promoter activity. These data indicate that troglitazone reduces Eta-1/Op gene expression at the transcriptional level through PPAR-γ activation, and suggest the role of troglitazone in inhibiting the ability of macrophages to produce extracellular matrix, which is particularly relevant to atherosclerotic plaque formation (Oyama, Kurabayashi, et al., 2000).

Other Possible Regulatory Elements in the Promoter and Other Regions of the Eta-1/Op Gene

Stein et al. (1989) observed that the shutdown of proliferation preceding differentiation of osteoblasts or promyelomonocytic leukemic cells is associated with a decreased interaction between the promoter-binding factor (HiNF-D) and the site II regulatory element (GGTCC) within the promoter region of a histone gene. They postulated that such interactions may normally account for the up-regulation of gene expression at this stage of differentiation. Although there is a site II consensus sequence in the promoter of the Eta-1/Op gene, it is located 416 nucleotides upstream from the transcription initiation site compared to 70 in the histone gene, and it is not accompanied by a site I element. The functional significance of this sequence remains to be determined.

A study by Urusov et al. (1998) indicates that the Eta-1/Op promoter, similar to the osteocalcin gene promoter, binds specifically two proteins, NMP-1 and NMP-2 (nuclear matrix proteins 1 and 2), from cell line ROS 17/2.8. Osteocalcin in one of the proteins taking part in extracellular matrix mineralization during osteogenic differentiation, and the Eta-1/Op gene is also active at the late stages of osteogenesis. Computer analysis shows that the Eta-1/Op gene promoter region contains binding sites for NMP-1 and NMP-2, two proteins that may be part of a larger group of nuclear matrix attached osteogenic-specific transcriptional factors (Urusov et al., 1998).

Metastases from prostatic adenocarcinoma (prostate cancer) are characterized by their predilection for bone and typical osteoblastic features (Young et al., 1992). Bone-derived prostate cancer cells MDA PCa 2a and MDA PCa 2b promote differentiation of osteoblast precursors to an osteoblastic phenotype through a pathway dependent on the transcriptional factor Cbfa1. Soluble factors, such as Cbfa1, produced by prostate cancer cells can induce expression of osteoblast-specific genes, such as Eta-1/Op (Young et al., 1992).

Small 1,000 bp fragments of genomic DNA obtained from human malignant breast cancer cell lines when transfected into a benign rat mammary cell line enhance transcription of the Eta-1/Op gene and thereby cause the cells to metastasize in syngeneic rats. El-Tanani et al. (2001), through transient cotransfections of an Eta-1/Op promoter-reporter construct and fragments of one metastasis-inducing DNA (Met-DNA), identified the active components in the Met-DNA as the binding sites for the T-cell factor (Tcf) family of transcription factors. Incubation of cell extracts with active DNA fragments containing the Tcf recognition sequence CAAAG caused retardation of their mobilities on polyacrylamide gels, and Western blotting identified Tcf-4, β-catenin, and E-cadherin in the relevant DNA complexes in vitro. Permanent transfection of the benign rat mammary cell line with a 20 bp fragment from the Met-DNA containing the Tcf recognition sequence CAAAG caused an enhanced permanent production of endogenous Eta-1/Op protein in vitro and induced the cells to metastasize in syngeneic rats in vivo. The corresponding fragment without the CAAAG sequence was without either effect. Therefore, the regulatory effect of the C9-Met-DNA is exerted, at least in part, by a CAAAG sequence that can sequester the endogenous inhibitory Tcf-4 and thereby promote transcription of Eta-1/Op, the direct effector of metastasis in this system (El-Tanani et al., 2001).

Eta-1/Op expression is enhanced by a variety of toxicants, especially those that activate protein kinase C (Denhardt, Giachelli, et al.,

2001; Denhardt, Noda, et al., 2001). Bacterial lipopolysaccharide (LPS) induces Eta-1/Op gene expression in liver and splenic macrophages and may be considered an acute phase protein (Patarca et al., 1989). However, there are no apparent heat shock-inducible elements in the promoter region, and experiments using Jurkat cells failed to reveal heat shock inducibility (Patarca et al., 1993).

Evidence for Distinct Promoter and Other Transcriptional Regulatory Regions for the Eta-1/Op Gene

A DNA sequence located 5' from those just discussed has been identified and proposed to represent exon 1 of the mouse Eta-1/Op gene (Behrend et al., 1993; Craig and Denhardt, 1991). In this case, the mouse gene would have seven exons instead of only six. A sequence located upstream from this newly defined exon 1 has been shown to contain several regulatory motifs, including TATA-like and CAAT (inverse complement) boxes, positive and negative transcriptional elements, and AP-1 and AP-5 motifs (Craig and Denhardt, 1991). This upstream sequence also directs expression of a reporter gene in mouse JB6 epidermal cells and therefore has been proposed to represent the major functional promoter for the mouse Eta-1/Op gene (Craig and Denhardt, 1991). This suggestion is supported by an analysis of the porcine Eta-1/Op gene (Zhang et al., 1992), which indicates a promoter region similar to that of the mouse described by Craig and Denhardt (1991). It is possible that the sequences described by Miyazaki et al. (1990) also may play a role in the regulation of this gene because they contain several potentially important regulatory motifs and transcription initiation sites according to primer extension and S1-protection experiments (Miyazaki et al., 1990). If so, regulation of the Eta-1/Op gene may thus represent a complex process involving multiple *cis*-acting sequences that could function differentially in various cell types. Additional experimental analysis is needed to more closely define these candidates for physiological regulatory elements.

The POU transcription factor Oct-4 is expressed specifically in the germ line, pluripotent cells of the pregastrulation embryo, and stem cell lines derived from the early embryo. Eta-1/Op is secreted by cells of the preimplantation embryo and contains a GRGDS motif that can bind to specific integrin subtypes and modulate cell adhesion/migration. Oct-4 and Eta-1/Op are coexpressed in the preimplantation mouse embryo and during differentiation of embryonal cell lines (Botquin et al., 1998). Immunoprecipitation of the first intron of Eta-1/Op from covalently fixed chromatin of embryonal stem cells by Oct-4-specific antibodies indicates that Oct-4 binds to this fragment in vivo. The intron fragment functions as an enhancer in cell lines that resemble cells of the preimplantation embryo. Furthermore, it contains a palindromic Oct factor recognition element (PORE) that is composed of an inverted pair of homeodomain-binding sites separated by exactly 5 bp (ATTTG +5 CAAAT). POU proteins can homo- and heterodimerize on the PORE, and although strong transcriptional activation of the Eta-1/Op element requires an intact PORE, the canonical octamer overlapping with the downstream half of the PORE is not essential (Botquin et al., 1998). Sox-2 is a transcription factor that contains an HMG box and is coexpressed with Oct-4 in the early mouse embryo. Sox-2 represses Oct-4 mediated activation of the first intron of Eta-1/Op by way of a canonical Sox element that is located close to the PORE. Repression depends on a carboxyl-terminal region of Sox-2 that is outside of the HMG box. Expression, DNA binding, and transactivation data are consistent with the hypothesis that Eta-1/Op expression is regulated by Oct-4 and Sox-2 in preimplantation development (Botquin et al., 1998).

Clauss et al. (1993) point out that the TRE/CRE-binding basic region-leucine zipper protein hXBP-1 may play a role in regulating the expression of tissue specific genes (Eta-1/Op, tissue inhibitor of metalloproteinases, osteonectin, osteocalcin) expressed in osteoblasts. The Eta-1/Op gene promoter is stimulated through the SF-1 response element, by estrogen receptor-related (ERR)α as well as by estrogen receptor (ER)α, but not by ERβ (Vanacker et al., 1998, 1999).

Evidence for Alternative RNA Splicing of the Eta-1/Op Gene

RNA splicing allows the generation of various forms of mRNA that can be translated into distinct protein products from a single transcript. These products, which differ from one another by the inclusion or exclusion of specific sequences, may have distinct functions.

For example, alternative splicing events leading to changes in biological activities may affect the expression of the receptor for human IL-12 (Cosman et al., 1984) and mouse IL-4 (Mosely et al., 1989), and the expression of granulocyte colony-stimulating factor (GC-SF) (Kiefer et al., 1989) and IL-7 (Namen et al., 1988).

The Eta-1/Op gene also may use alternative splicing to generate several mRNA species and associated protein products with distinct functions. Two Eta-1/Op cDNAs differing in their potential to encode a 14 amino acid stretch have been isolated from human bone and osteosarcoma cells (Ferraz et al., 1999; Kiefer et al., 1989; Young et al., 1990). Polymerase chain reaction amplification of cDNA from normal bone and decidual cells has shown that both forms of mRNA are expressed in each tissue (Young et al., 1990). Although these mRNA species were originally thought to be derived from differential use of a cryptic splice acceptor site in one of the exons (Young et al., 1990), a comparison of the mouse and human sequences indicates that the sequence corresponds to exon 4 (Miyazaki et al., 1990) and therefore may reflect alternative splicing. The exon 4 peptide contains a potential O-linked glycosylation site, a phosphorylation site (residues 63 to 65), and an amphipathic α-helix (Table 4.2). The charged face, which is predominantly acidic, may provide binding sites for hydroxyapatite or other proteins, and this interaction could, in turn, be regulated by phosphorylation. Differential splicing of exon 4 also could explain the existence of highly and weakly phosphorylated forms of Eta-1/Op. According to this proposal, the exon 4 peptide would be absent from the less phosphorylated variant that normally interacts with plasma fibronectin (Nemir et al., 1989; Singh, De Vouge, et al., 1990).

STRUCTURE OF THE ETA-1/OP PROTEIN AND POTENTIAL RELATIONSHIP TO FUNCTIONAL ACTIVITY

General Features

The mouse Eta-1/Op gene product has a predicted molecular mass of 32,462 Da and was determined to be an acidic 69 kDa secreted pro-

TABLE 4.2. Potential Functional Domains in Eta-1/Op

Domain	Sequence (mouse)	Location (mouse)	Reference
Phosphorylation site	SSEE	26-28; 63-65	Pinna et al., 1979
(casein kinase II)			
Phosphorylation site	SDE	126-128; 132-134;	Pinna et al., 1979
(mammary gland casein kinase)		135-137	
Polyaspartic	DHMDDDDDDDDD	86-98	Oldberg et al., 1986
N-glycosylation site	NES	179-181	Oldberg et al., 1986
O-glycosylation	SDQ; SSQ; STQ; SFQ	121-123; 133-135; 142-147, 179-181	Oldberg et al., 1986
Integrin binding site	GRGDS	164-168	Oldberg et al., 1986
Thrombin-cleavage site	RG	165-166	Craig et al., 1989
	RS	174-175; 178-179	
Heparin binding site	YGLRSKSRSF	171-180	Prince, 1989
	DRYLKFRI	324-331	
Calcium binding site	DQDNNGKGSHES	222-233	Patarca et al., 1989;
			Prince et al., 1991

tein that has structural features associated with binding to cell adhesion receptors (Patarca et al., 1989) including macrophages (Singh, Patarca, et al., 1990), the host cells for RT. The first methionine in the Eta-1/Op open reading frame (ORF) fits the consensus for eukaryotic translation initiation signals, and the 3' noncoding sequence in the cDNA contains two potential polyadenylation signals. The product of the ORF of sequenced Eta-1/Op cDNA is extremely hydrophilic and displays several features of a secreted protein. It has a hydrophobic leader sequence similar to human and chicken transferrin and lacks an obvious membrane-anchoring region. The tripeptide sequence Arg-Gly-Asp (RGD) is present in Eta-1/Op and, although not unique, represents a major binding ligand for integrins on cellular adhesion receptors. The RGD tripeptide in Eta-1/Op is present within a longer sequence that is highly similar to that surrounding the RGD motif in fibronectin. Biochemical analysis of both the recombinant (Patarca et al., 1989) and natural (Singh, Patarca, et al., 1990) T-cell product revealed that the gene product found in supernatant fluids has the expected pI of 4.3 and displays a larger size than the one expected from its translated cDNA, most likely secondary to glycosylation at multiple sites (Goldberg and Warner, 1997).

Antibodies to different peptides in Eta-1/Op reveal complexities in the various secreted forms (Bautista et al., 1994; Devoll et al., 1997; Gorski et al., 1995; Hotta et al., 1999; Kon et al., 2000; Rittling and Feng, 1998). For instance, distinct sandwich enzyme-linked immunoabsorbent assay (ELISA) systems using different pairs of polyclonal and monoclonal antibodies against human Eta-1/Op allowed detection of various isoforms and truncated forms of recombinant Eta-1/Op, and the glycosylated form of native urinary Eta-1/Op and, differentially, tumor-derived Eta-1/Op (Bautista, Denstedt, et al., 1996; Bautista, Saad, et al., 1996; Kon et al., 2000). Fujisaki (2000) isolated Eta-1/Op from human milk, prepared antibodies specific to it, established an enzyme immunoassay (EIA) system to determine Eta-1/Op in serum, and found that serum Eta-1/Op but not milk Eta-1/Op showed paradoxical phenomena in reaction with the antibodies, i.e., no detectable reaction in immunoelectrophoresis and in EIA, but showing positive reaction in Western blot and in inhibition tests. Taking these phenomena and other circumstantial evidence into account, it was concluded that the serum Eta-1/Op had high molecular fragility, fragmenting into small peptides with a paucity of epitopes during incubation time (Fujisaki, 2000). Comparison of the primary structure of polypeptides translated from cDNAs from different species may provide insight into the structural basis of functional activity and tissue-specific differences of Eta-1/Op, and contribute to isolation procedures (Bayless et al.,

1997) and to the development of immunoassays for the differential detection of Eta-1/Op forms.

The Amino Terminus and N-Acetylation

The Eta-1/Op protein has the structural features associated with a secreted glycoprotein, including a 16 amino acid leader sequence encoded by the first exon. There is a conserved arginine residue (Arg 2) in the leader sequence of Eta-1/Op that is unlikely to lead to deficient signal peptidase cleavage because intracellular Eta-1/Op is localized within the apical endocytic vacuoles, lysosomes, and is associated with the Golgi apparatus (Mark, Butler, et al., 1988; Mark, Prince, Gay, et al., 1987; Mark, Prince, Oosawa, et al., 1987; Mark, Prince, et al., 1988). The Eta-1/Op leader sequence also lacks the conserved tripeptide motif (Ser-Lys-Leu) associated with protein sorting to peroxisomes (Gould et al., 1989).

The signal peptidase cleavage site fits the NH2-end rule and has been confirmed by protein sequencing. The amino-terminus of mouse Eta-1/Op secreted by T cells is acetylated (Singh, Patarca, et al., 1990), lacks the required terminal glycine residue and consensus sequence (Gly-Ser-Ser-Lys-Ser-Lys-Pro-Lys) for myristoylation (Towler et al., 1988), and does not include the consensus sequences (Ala-Ser-Xaa-Ser or Ala-Pro-Xaa-Arg/Ser-Ser/Leu) present in hematopoietic cytokines (Schrader et al., 1986).

Structural Domains of Eta-1/Op Associated with Cellular Adhesion and Binding to Calcium and Heparin

Eta-1/Op, in its cell signaling capacity, initiates a signal transduction cascade that includes changes in the intracellular calcium ion levels and the tyrosine phosphorylation status of several proteins including pp60src and components of focal adhesion complexes (Denhardt et al., 1995; Lopez, Davis, et al., 1995; Paniccia et al., 1993). In this respect, Eta-1/Op stimulates pp60c-src kinase activity associated with the $\alpha v\beta 3$ integrin, an association that requires the cytoplasmic tail of the αv chain (Chellaiah et al., 1996).

The protein segment encoded by exon 5 of mouse Eta-1/Op (and by the corresponding exon in human Eta-1/Op) includes a region containing up to ten consecutive aspartic residues (86 to 98), an Arg-Gly-Asp (RGD) domain (residues 165 to 167), and two consensus heparin-binding sites (residues 171 to 180 and 324 to 331) (Butler, 1995; Katagiri et al., 1995; Rafidi et al., 1994). One prominent region of dissimilarity in bovine Eta-1/Op compared to all other species is a 22-amino acid gap which may represent a loss of a potential Ca^{2+}-binding loop (Kerr et al., 1991).

The Asp-rich region has been proposed to be an attachment site for apatite crystals (Oldberg et al., 1986) or a binding site for calcium (Patarca et al., 1989; Singh et al., 1993). According to this notion, binding to the mineral phase of bone through this motif may contribute to compartmentalization of Eta-1/Op in this tissue. Ca^{2+}-binding is a general property of Eta-1/Op, regardless of its molecular mass and origin, and the phosphate moieties of Eta-1/Op may not influence the conformation or accessibility of the Ca^{2+} affinity sites of the molecule (Singh et al., 1993). The C-terminal EF hand disulfide-bonded, Ca^{2+}-binding loop of the matricellular Ca^{2+}-binding glycoprotein SPARC accounts for its counteradhesive and growth-inhibitory effects on cultured cells, and ectopic expression through microinjection into *Xenopus* embryos of SPARC, or of other Ca^{2+}-binding-domain containing proteins such as Eta-1/Op, before their normal embryonic activation produces severe anomalies (Damjanovski et al., 1997).

The RGD motif is a signature sequence for a family of extracellular proteins involved in cell attachment and migration (Bautista et al., 1994, 1995; Cachau et al., 1989; McFarland et al., 1995; Mickos et al., 1992; Miyauchi et al., 1993; Nasu et al., 1995; Paniccia et al., 1993; Pettersson et al., 1991; Ruohslahti and Pierschbacher, 1986; Xuan et al., 1994, 1995; Yamamoto, Nasu, et al., 1995) through interaction with integrins, a family of adhesion receptors that consists of at least 21 heterodimeric transmembrane proteins that differ in their tissue distribution and ligand specificity (Schnapp et al., 1995). Eta-1/Op may bind in vitro to osteoblastic tumor cells (Oldberg et al., 1986) and to macrophages (Patarca et al., 1989; Singh, Patarca, et al., 1990) through the RGD motif. In the latter instance, binding reflects a specific interaction with a homogeneous species of integrin receptor having a K_d of 10^{-10} M. Binding affinity and accessibility of the RGD motif may be affected by molecular changes induced by interactions with extracellular ions, as exemplified by the interaction of thrombospondin with calcium (Reed et al., 1988). In this regard, there is a sequence encoded by exon 6 of the murine Eta-1/Op gene that may constitute a calcium-binding site (residues 222 to 233) similar to that displayed by thrombospondin (Table 4.2) (Prince, 1989; Tufty and Kretsinger, 1975).

Although Eta-1/Op interacts with a number of integrins, namely $\alpha v\beta 1$, $\alpha v\beta 3$, $\alpha v\beta 5$, $\alpha 9\beta 1$, $\alpha 8\beta 1$, and $\alpha 4\beta 1$, the interaction may be apparent only when the integrin receptors are in a high activation state (Barry et al., 2000a,b; Caltabiano et al., 1999; Helluin et al., 2000; Hu, Hoyer, et al., 1995a,b; Hu, Lin, et al., 1995; Hultenby et al., 1995; Katagiri and Uede, 1998; Katagiri et al., 1996; Liaw, Lindner, et al., 1995; Liaw, Skinner, et al., 1995; Nasu et al., 1995; Rabb et al., 1996; Somerman et al., 1995; van Dijk et al., 1993; Wong et al., 1996; Yokasaki and Sheppard, 2000). When in a high activation state, $\alpha 5\beta 1$ selectively interacts with a glutathione-S-transferase (GST) fusion protein of the N-terminal fragment of Eta-1/Op (aa17-168), which is generated in vivo by thrombin cleavage of Eta-1/Op. Adhesion via $\alpha 5\beta 1$ is mediated by the Arg-Gly-Asp (RGD) motif of Eta-1/Op, because mutating this sequence to Arg-Ala-Asp (RAD) blocks binding of both cell types. Therefore, thrombin cleavage regulates the adhesive properties of Eta-1/Op (Barry et al., 2000a,b). Immobilized Eta-1/Op promotes concentration-dependent tumor cell migration (i.e., haptotaxis) in modified Boyden chambers (Senger and Perruzzi, 1996). In particular, cleavage of Eta-1/Op by thrombin, which likely occurs in the tumor microenvironment, results in enhancement of Eta-1/Op's haptotactic activity; and assays performed with purified preparations of the two individual Eta-1/Op thrombin-cleavage fragments demonstrated that all detectable activity was associated with the GRGDS-containing fragment and its association with the $\alpha v\beta 3$ integrin (Senger and Perruzi, 1996).

The function of RGD is further underscored and put into a bioengineering practical framework by the design of chimeric peptides of statherin and Eta-1/Op that bind hydroxyapatite and mediate cell adhesion (Gilbert et al., 2000). Salivary statherin contains a 15-amino-acid hydroxyapatite-binding domain (N15) that is loosely helical in solution. To test whether N15 can serve to orient active peptide sequences on hydroxyapatite, Gilbert et al. (2000) fused the RGD and flanking residues from Eta-1/Op to the C terminus of N15. The fusion peptides bound tightly to hydroxyapatite, and the N15-PGRGDS peptide mediated the dose-dependent adhesion of Moαv melanoma cells when immobilized on the hydroxyapatite surface. Experiments with an integrin-sorted Moαv subpopulation demonstrated that the $\alpha v\beta 3$ integrin was the primary receptor target for the fusion peptide. Solid state nuclear magnetic resonance experiments showed that the RGD portion of the hydrated fusion peptide is highly dynamic on the hydroxyapatite surface. This fusion peptide framework may thus provide a straightforward design for immobilizing bioactive sequences on hydroxyapatite for biomaterials, tissue engineering, and vaccine applications (Gilbert et al., 2000).

The context of the RGD sequence within a protein has considerable influence upon the final binding force for receptor interaction (Lehenkari and Horton, 1999). Lehenkari and Horton (1999) measured integrin binding forces in intact cells by atomic force microscopy for several RGD-containing (Arg-Gly-Asp) ligands and found them to be cell- and amino-acid-sequence specific, saturatable, and sensitive to the pH and divalent cation composition of the cellular culture medium. In contrast to short linear RGD hexapeptides, larger peptides and proteins containing the RGD sequence, such as Eta-1/Op and echistatin (a high affinity RGD sequence containing antagonist snake venom protein), showed different binding affinities.

Heparin also may affect the binding properties of Eta-1/Op (Prince, 1989). The first potential heparin-binding site (residues 171 to 180) is located adjacent to the RGD motif and is particularly interesting in view of the studies of Woods and Couchman (1988), who showed that focal adhesions of fibronectin are formed only if both a cell-binding RGD domain and a heparin-binding domain are present. Formation of focal adhesions may be a prerequisite for extracellular matrix deposition and induction of cellular mitosis (Prince, 1989; Woods and Couchman, 1988). The second potential heparin-binding site is near the carboxyl-end of Eta-1/Op (residues 324 to 331).

The integrin $\alpha 4\beta 1$ is involved in mediating exfiltration of leukocytes from the vasculature. It interacts with a number of proteins whose expression is up-regulated during the inflammatory response including VCAM-1 and the CS-1 alternatively spliced region of fibronectin. The α4β1 integrin is an adhesion receptor for Eta-1/Op, and two α4β1 binding sites are present in a 38 amino acid domain within the N-terminal thrombin fragment of Eta-1/Op (Bayless and Davis, 2001; Bayless et al., 1998). Synthetic peptides for both regions in human Eta-1/Op, ELVTDFPTDLPAT (131) and SVVYGLR (162), block α4β1-dependent adhesion (Barry et al., 2000a,b; Bayless and Davis, 2001). Barry et al. (2000a,b) showed that α4β1 expressed in J6 cells interacts with intact Eta-1/Op when the integrin is in a high activation state, and by deletion mapping, that the α4β1 binding region in Eta-1/Op lies between amino acid residues 125 and 168 (aa125-168). Although this region contains the central RGD motif of Eta-1/Op, which also interacts with integrins αvβ3, αvβ5, αvβ1, α8β1, and α5β1, mutating the RGD motif to RAD had no effect on the interaction with α4β1 (Barry et al., 2000a,b). The α4β1-binding peptide containing the leucine-aspartate-valine (LDV) sequence, but not a nonbinding peptide containing leucine-glutamate-valine (LEV), inhibits leukocyte binding to Eta-1/Op (Bayless et al., 1998).

The integrin α9β1 is expressed on epithelial cells, smooth muscle cells, skeletal muscle, and neutrophils and recognizes at least three distinct ligands: Eta-1/Op, vascular cell adhesion molecule 1 (VCAM-1), and tenascin-C (Marcinkiewicz et al., 2000; Smith and Giachelli, 1998; Smith et al., 1996; Yokosaki et al., 1999). However, there are structurally distinct requirements for interactions of the α9β1 integrin with VCAM-1 and the extracellular matrix ligands Eta-1/Op and tenascin-C (Marcinkiewicz et al., 2000). The disintegrins EC3 and EC6 were potent inhibitors of α9β1-mediated adhesion to VCAM-1 and of neutrophil migration across tumor necrosis factor-activated endothelial cells. Although a peptide containing a novel MLDG motif shared by both of these disintegrins also inhibited α9β1- and α4β1-mediated adhesion to VCAM-1, concentrations of EC3 that completely inhibited adhesion of α9-transfected cells to VCAM-1 had little or no effect on adhesion to either of the other α9β1 ligands, Eta-1/Op and tenascin-C. Furthermore, peptides AEIDGIEL and SVVYGLR, which inhibit binding of α9β1-expressing cells to tenascin-C and Eta-1/Op, respectively, had no effect on adhesion to VCAM-1 (Marcinkiewicz et al., 2000; Yokosaki et al., 1999).

Studies of mice lacking the expression of the α9 subunit of α9β1 integrin have evinced that α9 integrin is required for the normal development of the lymphatic system, including the thoracic duct, and that α9 deficiency could be one cause of congenital chylothorax (Huang et al., 2000). In this respect, mice homozygous for a null mutation in the α9 subunit gene appear normal at birth but develop respiratory failure and die between six and 12 days of age. The respiratory failure is caused by an accumulation of large volumes of pleural fluid that is rich in triglyceride, cholesterol, and lymphocytes. Edema and lymphocytic infiltration also develop in $\alpha 9^{-/-}$ mice in the chest wall that appears to originate around lymphatics. α9 protein is transiently expressed in the developing thoracic duct at embryonic day 14, but expression is rapidly lost during later stages of development (Huang et al., 2000).

The αvβ3 integrin has been shown to bind several ligands, including Eta-1/Op and vitronectin (Helluin et al., 2000; Liaw, Lindner, et al., 1995; Liaw, Skinner, et al., 1995; van Dijk et al., 1993). Highly invasive prostate cancer PC3 cells that constitutively express αvβ3 adhere and migrate on Eta-1/Op and vitronectin in an αvβ3-dependent manner (Zheng et al., 2000). However, exogenous expression of αvβ3 in noninvasive prostate cancer LNCaP (β3-LNCaP) cells mediates adhesion and migration on vitronectin but not on Eta-1/Op. Activation of αvβ3 by epidermal growth factor stimulation is required to mediate adhesion to Eta-1/Op but is not sufficient to support migration on this substrate. Activation of the phosphatidylinositol 3-kinase (PI 3-kinase)/protein kinase B (PKB/AKT) pathway is required for αvβ3-mediated cell migration because wortmannin, a PI 3-kinase inhibitor, prevents PC3 cell migration on both Eta-1/Op and vitronectin; furthermore, αvβ3 engagement by Eta-1/Op and vitronectin activates the PI 3-kinase/AKT pathway. Migration of β3-LNCaP cells on vitronectin also occurs through activation of the PI 3-kinase pathway; however, AKT phosphorylation is not increased upon engagement by Eta-1/Op. Furthermore, phosphorylation of focal adhesion kinase (FAK), known to support cell migration in β3-LNCaP cells, is detected on both substrates. Thus, in PC3 cells, αvβ3 mediates cell migration and PI 3-kinase/AKT pathway activation on vitronectin and Eta-1/Op; in β3-LNCaP cells, αvβ3 mediates cell migration and PI 3-kinase/AKT pathway activation on vitronectin, whereas adhesion to Eta-1/Op does not support αvβ3-mediated cell migration and PI 3-kinase/AKT pathway activation. Therefore, αvβ3 exists in multiple functional states that can bind either selectively vitronectin or both vitronectin and Eta-1/Op and can differentially activate cell migration and intracellular signaling pathways in a ligand-specific manner (Zheng et al., 2000). Kumar et al. (1997) identified an integrin β3 subunit, termed β3C, that in contrast to the β3A isoform fails to adhere to Eta-1/Op, an observation that suggests a potential role for the β3C integrin subunit in modulating cell-matrix interactions. Moreover, subtle changes in the amino acid composition immediately flanking the RGD or RYD motifs can have a profound effect on β3 integrin specificity, most likely because they influence the juxtaposition of the arginine and aspartate side chains within the extended RGD loop sequence (Kunicki et al., 1997).

Eta-1/Op binding to αvβ3 is supported by manganese, completely inhibited by calcium, and largely unaffected by magnesium (Kunicki et al., 1997; Zimolo et al., 1994). Eta-1/Op binding to integrin αvβ3 in osteoclasts stimulates gelsolin-associated phosphatidylinositol (PtdIns) 3-hydroxyl kinase (PI 3-kinase), leading to increased levels of gelsolin-bound PtdIns 3,4-P2, PtdIns 4,5-P2, and PtdIns 3,4,5-P3, uncapping of barbed end actin, and actin filament formation (Chellaiah et al., 1998). Inhibition of PI 3-kinase activity by wortmannin blocks Eta-1/Op stimulation of actin filament formation, an observation that suggests that activation of gelsolin-associated PI 3-kinase is an important pathway in cytoskeletal regulation. In this respect, Eta-1/Op stimulates gelsolin-associated src, leading to increased gelsolin-associated PI 3-kinase activity and PtdIns 3,4,5-P3 levels, which facilitate actin filament formation, osteoclast motility, and bone resorption (Chellaiah et al., 1998). Soluble αvβ3-integrin ligands raise $[Ca^{2+}]_i$ in rat osteoclasts and mouse-derived osteoclast-like cells (Zimolo et al., 1994).

McDevitt et al. (1999) engineered the hexapeptide sequences derived from Eta-1/Op and fibronectin that contain the RGD cell adhesion sequence into the three-dimensional scaffolding of streptavidin to convert streptavidin into a functional protein. Cell binding assays directly demonstrated that rat aortic endothelial cells and human melanoma cells adhered to surfaces coated with either of the two RGD streptavidin mutants in a dose-dependent fashion. Inhibition studies with soluble RGD peptides confirmed that the cell adhesion was RGD-mediated. Further inhibition studies with antibodies directed against $\alpha v\beta 3$ demonstrated that the RGD-streptavidin interaction was primarily mediated by this integrin with melanoma cells. This approach to introducing secondary functional activities into streptavidin may improve streptavidin's utility in existing applications or provide new technology opportunities (McDevitt et al., 1999).

There are at least four classes of $\beta 3$ ligands: Class I, represented by RGD peptides and vitronectin, reacts similarly with $\alpha IIb\beta 3$ and $\alpha v\beta 3$; Class II, represented by cHarGD, γ-chain peptides, and fibrinogen, reacts with both receptors in the presence of Mn^{2+} but only with $\alpha IIb\beta 3$ in the presence of Ca^{2+}; Class III, represented by barbourin, is $\alpha IIb\beta 3$-specific under all cation conditions; Class IV, represented by Eta-1/Op, binds primarily to $\alpha v\beta 3$ (Suehiro et al., 1996). In terms of $\beta 3$ ligand effects on T-cell function, Adler et al. (2001) point out that the determination of elimination versus survival of activated T cells by coligation of $\beta 3$-integrins may have bearing on the fundamental postthymic mechanisms that shape the T-cell repertoire (Adler et al., 2001). In this respect, although ligation of the T-cell antigen receptor (TCR) is central to the responsiveness and antigen specificity of T cells, it is insufficient to elicit a response. Engagement of the TCR leads to induction of Fas, but not to measurable IL-2 secretion or apoptosis, activation parameters that are in turn induced by costimulation through integrin $\alpha v\beta 3$. Furthermore, T-cell survival or elimination is determined by the type of ligand binding to this coreceptor with vitronectin, fibronectin, and fibrinogen efficiently inducing apoptosis and IL-2 production while Eta-1/Op and entactin mediate IL-2 secretion comparably without causing programmed cell death. Consistent with the cytokine properties of these ligands, differential costimulation depends on their presentation in soluble rather than immobilized form (Adler et al., 2001). Eta-1/Op lacks other known cell adhesion sequence motifs, such as the Val-Thr-Cys-Gly found in the malarial circumsporozoite protein, thrombospondin, and properdin (Rich et al., 1990), and the Ile-Lys-Val-Ala-Val motif found in the A chain of laminin (Tashiro et al., 1989). The conserved sequence and conformation found in the carboxyl-terminal helices of a subgroup of cytokines such as IL-2 and IL-6 (Bazan, 1990) are not present in Eta-1/Op, an observation that is consistent with the binding of the latter to an integrin-like receptor through the RGD motif (Singh, Patarca, et al., 1990).

Eta-1/Op binds to CD44 (Goodison et al., 1999). The CD44 proteins form a ubiquitously expressed family of cell surface adhesion molecules involved in cell-cell and cell-matrix interactions. The multiple protein isoforms are encoded by a single gene by alternative splicing and are further modified by a range of posttranslational modifications. CD44 proteins are single-chain molecules comprising an N-terminal extracellular domain, a membrane proximal region, a transmembrane domain, and a cytoplasmic tail. The CD44 gene has been detected only in higher organisms and the amino acid sequence of most of the molecule is highly conserved among mammalian species. The principal ligand of CD44 is hyaluronic acid, an integral component of the extracellular matrix. Other CD44 ligands include serglycin, collagens, fibronectin, and laminin. The major physiological role of CD44 is to maintain organ and tissue structure via cell-cell and cell-matrix adhesion, but certain variant isoforms can also mediate lymphocyte activation and homing, and the presentation of chemical factors and hormones. Increased interest has been directed at the characterization of this molecule since it was observed that expression of multiple CD44 isoforms is greatly up-regulated in neoplasia. CD44, particularly its variants, may be useful as a diagnostic or prognostic marker of malignancy and, in at least some human cancers, it may be a potential target for cancer therapy (Goodison et al., 1999).

Eta-1/Op and its cell surface receptor CD44 are coupled to the cell survival response elicited by interleukin-3 or granulocyte-macrophage colony-stimulating factor (Lin, Huang, et al., 2000). The receptors for IL-3 and GM-CSF share a common β subunit, the distal cytoplasmic domain of which is essential for the promotion of cell survival by these two cytokines. Eta-1/Op is one of the genes whose expression is specifically induced by signaling through the distal cytoplasmic domain of this receptor β subunit (Lin, Huang, et al., 2000). Conditioned medium from cells expressing wild-type Eta-1/Op, but not that from cells expressing a deletion mutant lacking residues 79 to 140, increased the viability of a non-Eta-1/Op-producing cell line in the presence of human granulocyte monocyte-colony stimulating factor (GM-CSF). Antibody blocking experiments revealed that Eta-1/Op produced as a result of IL-3 or GM-CSF signaling was secreted into the medium and, through binding to its cell surface receptor, CD44, contributed to the survival-promoting activities of these two cytokines. Furthermore, coupling of the Eta-1/Op-CD44 pathway to the survival response to IL-3 was also demonstrated in primary IL-3-dependent mouse bone marrow cells. These results show that induction of Eta-1/Op and consequent activation of its cell surface receptor CD44 are important for the antiapoptotic activities of IL-3 and GM-CSF (Lin, Huang, et al., 2000).

Cells of the mononuclear phagocyte lineage have the capability to adhere to and fuse with one another and to differentiate into osteoclasts and giant cells (Sterling et al., 1998). CD44 expression by macrophages is highly and transiently induced by fusogenic conditions both in vitro and in vivo. CD44 ligands, Eta-1/Op, hyaluronic acid, and chondroitin sulfate, prevent macrophage multinucleation. CD44 may therefore control the mononucleated status of macrophages in tissues by virtue of mediating cell-cell interactions (Sterling et al., 1998). Induction of Eta-1/Op and associated receptors may play a role during monocytic differentiation of HL-60 cells (Andersson and Johansson, 1996; Atkins et al., 1998). Promyelocytic leukemia HL-60 cells promoted by PMA to differentiate along the monocyte pathway adhere to tissue culture plates. PMA induces Eta-1/Op mRNA production and Eta-1/Op secretion into media of promyelocytic leukemia HL-60 cells; untreated cells express β1 and CD44 mRNA, and PMA induces αv and β3 mRNA and increases β1 and CD44 mRNA expression; PMA increases levels of αv, β3, β1, and CD44 protein on the cell surface; and retinoic acid, which promotes granulocytic differentiation of HL-60 cells, does not affect Eta-1/Op, αv, β3, β1, or CD44 mRNA or protein expression (Andersson and Johansson, 1996; Atkins et al., 1998; Krause et al., 1996).

To analyze which forms of CD44 mediate binding to Eta-1/Op, Smith et al. (1999) used the standard form of CD44 as CD44-human immunoglobulin fusion proteins and several splice variants in enzyme-linked immunosorbant assays. Multiple preparations of Eta-1/Op were used, including native Eta-1/Op derived from smooth muscle cells, human urinary Eta-1/Op, full-length recombinant Eta-1/Op, and two recombinant Eta-1/Op fragments formed following thrombin cleavage. Although the CD44-hIg fusion proteins could interact with hyaluronic acid as expected, there was no interaction between CD44H, CD44E, CD44v3, v8-v10, or CD44v3 with Eta-1/Op. These studies suggest that CD44-Eta-1/Op interactions may be limited to a specific CD44 isoform(s), and/or a particular modified form of Eta-1/Op (Smith et al., 1999).

Zohar et al. (Zohar, Lee, et al., 1997; Zohar, Sodek, et al., 1997; Zohar et al., 2000) identified an intracellular form of Eta-1/Op with a perimembranous distribution in migrating fetal fibroblasts. Eta-1/Op and CD44 expression are increased in migrating cells, and a distinct colocalization of perimembranous Eta-1/Op and cell-surface CD44 is observed in fetal fibroblasts, periodontal ligament cells, activated macrophages, and metastatic breast cancer cells (Zohar et al., 2000). The colocalization of Eta-1/Op and CD44 was prominent at the leading edge of migrating fibroblasts, where Eta-1/Op also colocalized with the ezrin/radixin/moesin (ERM) protein ezrin, as well as in cell processes and at attachment sites of hyaluronan-coated beads. The subcortical location of Eta-1/Op in these cells was verified by cell-surface biotinylation experiments in which biotinylated CD44 and nonbiotinylated Eta-1/Op were isolated from complexes formed with hyaluronan-coated beads and identified with immunoblotting. That perimembranous Eta-1/Op represents secreted protein internalized by endocytosis or phagocytosis appeared to be unlikely because exogenous Eta-1/Op that was added to cell cultures could not be detected inside the cells. A physical association with Eta-1/Op, CD44, and ERM, but not with vinculin or α-actin, was indicated by immunoadsorption and immunoblotting of cell proteins in complexes extracted from hyaluronan-coated beads. The functional significance of Eta-1/Op in this complex was demonstrated using Eta-1/Op$^{-/-}$ and CD$^{-/-}$ mouse fibroblasts, which displayed impaired migration and a reduced attachment to hyaluronan-coated beads. These studies indicate that Eta-1/Op exists as an integral component of a hyaluronan-CD44-ERM attachment complex that is involved in the migration of embryonic fibroblasts, activated macrophages, and metastatic cells (Zohar et al., 2000).

Glycosylation

Several studies suggest that the carbohydrate component of Eta-1/Op represents one N-glycoside and five or six O-glycosides (Butler, 1989). There is one conserved N-glycosylation site (residues 79 to 81) in the protein segment encoded by mouse exon 5, and 11 conserved potential O-linked glycosylation sites with the sequence Ser-Xxx-Glu (where Xxx is any amino acid) in segments encoded by exons 2, 4, 5, and 6 (Table 4.2). Sorensen, Hojrup, et al. (1995) identified three O-glycosylated threonines (Thr 115, Thr 124, and Thr 129) in a threonine- and proline-rich region of Eta-1/Op. Alignment analysis showed that all three O-glycosylation sites were conserved in other mammalian sequences (Sorensen, Hojrup, et al., 1995). Three putative N-glycosylation sites (Asn 63, Asn 85, and Asn 193) are present in bovine Eta-1/Op, but sequence and mass spectrometric analysis showed that none of these asparagines were glycosylated in bovine mammary gland Eta-1/Op (Sorensen, Hojrup, et al., 1995). Altered sialylation of Eta-1/Op prevents its receptor-mediated binding on the surface of oncogenically transformed tsB77 cells, which may exploit this feature for their invasive behavior (Shanmugam et al., 1997).

Susceptibility to Proteases

An important function of proteases appears to be not only degradation, but also cleavage of matrix proteins to generate functionally distinct fragments based on receptor binding, biological activity, or regulation of growth factors (Liaw and Crawford, 1999). Smaller unglycosylated proteins of 20 to 30 kDa are generated from the larger Eta-1/Op (Zhang et al., 1990), but pulse/chase experiments in culture have not yet provided evidence for a potential pathway of intracellular proteolysis in chicken (Gotoh, Gerstenfeld, et al., 1990; Gotoh, Pierschbacher, et al., 1990) or porcine cells (Zhang et al., 1990). The smaller derivatives of the Eta-1/Op protein reflect the action of trypsinlike proteases that cleave at Arg-Ser and Lys-Ala peptide bonds (Zhang et al., 1990). This specificity is similar to that of tPA, which digests extracellular matrix proteins in the course of tissue remodeling during morphogenesis or malignant growth (Dano et al., 1985; Saksela and Rifkin, 1988). The effects of tPA on Eta-1/Op have not been reported.

The Eta-1/Op protein is known to be susceptible to a highly specific cleavage by the protease thrombin (Senger, Perruzzi, and Papadopoulos, 1989; Senger et al., 1994, 1995; Xuan et al., 1994). There are three thrombin consensus cleavage sites in the Eta-1/Op protein: the Arg-Gly bond in the RGD tripeptide and two Arg-Ser sites at residues 174 to 175 and 178 to 179 (this last site is not present in human or pig proteins). The susceptibility of Eta-1/Op to thrombin opens the possibility that Eta-1/Op may be active at sites of blood coagulation and display functions independent of the domain containing an RGD motif. Cleavage of Eta-1/Op by thrombin is likely to be of physiological importance, because cleavage of blood plasma Eta-1/Op occurs naturally after activation of the blood coagulation pathway. Thrombin-cleaved Eta-1/Op promotes markedly greater cell attachment and spreading than uncleaved Eta-1/Op. Because the GRGDS sequence in Eta-1/Op is only six residues from the thrombin-cleavage site, thrombin cleavage may allow greater accessibility of the GRGDS domain to cell surface receptors. Several lines of evidence suggest that cleavage of Eta-1/Op by thrombin occurs in vivo, such as in tumors and at sites of tissue injury, and such cleavage is important in the regulation of Eta-1/Op function (Senger et al., 1994). A smaller variant of Eta-1/Op also is seen in human milk, where the 69 and 35 kDa moieties are detected (Senger, Perruzzi, Papadopoulos, et al., 1989).

To assess the relevance of thrombin cleavage to Eta-1/Op function, Takahashi et al. (1998) performed cell adhesion assays using glutathione S-transferase-Eta-1/Op fusion protein fragments and full-length Eta-1/Op fusion protein. The N-terminal fragment containing a RGD motif promoted enhanced adhesion of mouse and human fibroblasts by 2.9- and 2.8-fold in comparison with full-length Eta-1/Op, respectively. The enhanced adhesion of both cells mediated by the N-terminal fragment was significantly suppressed by addition of the C-terminal fragment lacking a RGD motif that has less cell adhesive property than full-length Eta-1/Op. These results suggest that the C-terminal domain may play a pivotal role in regulating Eta-1/Op functions by suppressing the RGD-dependent cell adhesion.

Expression of Eta-1/Op is often colocalized with members of the matrix metalloproteinase (MMP) family, and Eta-1/Op is a substrate for two MMPs, MMP-3 (stromelysin-1) and MMP-7 (matrilysin) (Agnihotri et al., 2001). Three cleavage sites were identified for MMP-3 in human Eta-1/Op, and two of those sites were also cleaved by MMP-7. These include hydrolysis of the human Gly(166)-Leu(167), Ala(201)-Tyr(202) (MMP-3 only), and Asp(210)-Leu(211) peptide bonds. Only the N-terminal Gly-Leu cleavage site is conserved in rat Eta-1/Op (Gly(151)-Leu(152)). These sites are distinct from the cleavage sites for the proteases thrombin or enterokinase. The MMP cleavage fragments of Eta-1/Op were reported in vitro in tumor cell lines, and in vivo in remodeling tissues such as the postpartum uterus, where Eta-1/Op and MMPs are co-expressed. Furthermore, cleavage of Eta-1/Op by MMP-3 or MMP-7 potentiated the function of Eta-1/Op as an adhesive and migratory stimulus in vitro through cell surface integrins. The interaction of MMPs with Eta-1/Op at tumor and wound healing sites in vivo may be a mechanism of regulation of Eta-1/Op bioactivity (Agnihotri et al., 2001). Conversely, Eta-1/Op, bone sialoprotein (BSP), and GRGDSP peptides, in solution, induce activation of metalloproteinase-2 (MMP-2) secreted by human GCT23 giant cell tumor cells. Activation of MMP-2 is RGD sequence dependent, possibly involves anti-$\alpha v\beta 3$ integrins, is preceded by a change from spread to rounded cell morphology, and is mimicked by the actin depolymerising agent cytochalasin B (Teti, Farina, et al., 1998; Teti, Taranta, et al., 1998).

Cathepsin K, a cysteine protease of the papain family, can cleave bone proteins such as Eta-1/Op, Type I collagen, and osteonectin (Yamashita and Dodds, 2000). Mutation of the gene expressing cathepsin K in humans results in pycnodysostosis, an autosomal recessive condition, resulting in osteoporosis and increased bone fragility. Knockout of cathepsin K in the mouse also results in retarded bone matrix degradation and osteopetrosis. Therefore, inhibition of cathepsin K should result in a diminution of osteoclast-mediated bone resorption. Several novel classes of cathepsin K inhibitors have been designed from X-ray co-crystal structures of peptide aldehydes bound to papain. The convergence of the design of novel inhibitors and the discovery of cathepsin K has created opportunities to further understand bone and cartilage biology as well as provide new therapeutic agents for the treatment of disease states, such as osteoporosis, in humans (Yamashita and Dodds, 2000).

Phosphorylation

Metabolic labeling and in vitro translation techniques have revealed that cells can synthesize several phosphorylated forms of Eta-1/Op that behave anomalously in sodium dodecyl sulphate-polyacrylannide gel electrophoresis (SDS-PAGE) (Chan et al., 1990; Saavedra et al., 1995;

Salih et al., 1995; Sorensen and Petersen, 1994, 1995). Eta-1/Op can be autophosphorylated on tyrosine residues, using adenosine triphosphate (ATP) or guanosine triphosphate (GTP) but not inorganic orthophosphate as phosphoryl donors, and can also be phosphorylated on serine and threonine residues by several protein kinases (Ashkar, Glimsher, et al., 1993; Ashkar, Teplow, et al., 1993; Saavedra, 1994). Autophosphorylation of Eta-1/Op may generate sites for specific interactions with other proteins on the cell surface and/or within the extracellular matrix. These interactions of Eta-1/Op are thought to be essential for bone mineralization and function. The polyaspartic acid motif of Eta-1/Op, in combination with neighboring sequences that include serine residues phosphorylated by protein kinases, could fold and assemble into a molecular structure that participates in the mineralization of the bone matrix and osteoclast binding (Saavedra, 1994; Salih, Ashkar, Gerstenfeld, et al., 1996; Salih, Ashkar, Zhou, et al., 1996).

Eta-1/Op contains 7.83 mol of phosphate/mol in its natural state. Thrombin digests of ^{32}P-labeled Eta-1/Op provided two radiolabeled thrombin fragments, with molecular masses of 30 kDa (N-terminal half) and 20 kDa (C-terminal half). The major phosphorylation was associated with the N-terminal half containing 7.0 mol of phosphate, and 1.9 mol of phosphate was associated with the C-terminal half (Salih, Ashkar, Gerstenfeld, et al., 1996; Salih, Ashkar, Zhou, et al., 1996). Chicken Eta-1/Op can be resolved by isoelectric focusing into three major variants, with pI values ranging from 3.7 to 3.9 according to the extent of phosphorylation (Gotoh, Gerstenfeld, et al., 1990). Mouse Eta-1/Op comprises variants with Mr 55,000 to 70,000 (Craig et al., 1989; Patarca et al., 1989; Singh, De Vouge, et al., 1990; Singh, Patarca, et al., 1990). It has been reported that the rat proteins contains 12 phosphoserines and one phosphothreonine (Prince et al., 1987), whereas bovine Eta-1/Op contains 3.5 percent of total phosphate (Franzen and Heinegard, 1985). Neame and Butler (1996) reported that rat bone Eta-1/Op, with 11 phosphorylated sites, differs from bovine milk Eta-1/Op in which 28 residues are completely phosphorylated. Sorensen, Justesen, et al. (1995; Sorensen, Hojrup, et al., 1995) identified twenty-seven phosphorylated serines in bovine milk Eta-1/Op. Nineteen of these phosphoacceptor sites are fully conserved in rat Eta-1/Op, all displaying the consensus for the Golgi apparatus casein kinase, G-CK (S-x-E/Sp), and rat Eta-1/Op is indeed phosphorylated more readily than casein itself by G-CK from either rat mammary gland or liver.

Eta-1/Op is also phosphorylated by casein kinases-1 and -2 (CK1, CK2), although less readily than casein. Eta-1/Op contains CK2-phosphorylatable sites and an acidic amino acid cluster, and microsomal CK2 modifies Eta-1/Op during transportation as part of the mineralization process of hard tissues (Wu, Ishikawa, et al., 1995; Wu, Pan, et al., 1995). However, if Eta-1/Op kinase activities are normalized in terms of casein phosphorylation, the Eta-1/Op phosphorylation rate by G-CK is 78-fold and 19-fold higher than those measured with CK2 and CK1, respectively. These data, in conjunction with the specific location of G-CK to the Golgi apparatus, where CK2 and CK1 are hardly detectable, support the view that G-CK is the main, if not the only, physiological agent committed to the phosphorylation of Eta-1/Op (Ashkar et al., 1995; Lasa et al., 1997). The *Saccharomyces cerevisiae* YGR262c gene, whose disruption causes severely defective growth, encodes a Ser/Thr protein kinase, piD261, that can phosphorylate casein and Eta-1/Op in the presence of [γ-^{32}P]ATP, but not histones, myelin basic protein, phosvitin, bovine serum albumin, and poly(Glu/Tyr) (Stocchetto et al., 1997).

Using tunicamycin, an inhibitor of N-linked glycosylation, and peptide N-glycosidase F, which removes N-linked oligosaccharide chains from glycoproteins, Singh, De Vouge, et al. (1990) showed that nonphosphorylated Eta-1/Op, but not phosphorylated Eta-1/Op, contains N-linked carbohydrates. Moreover, tunicamycin treatment does not inhibit the cell surface binding of phosphorylated Eta-1/Op; however, nonphosphorylated Eta-1/Op secreted by the treated cells fails to complex with plasma fibronectin. Phosphorylated Eta-1/Op forms a heat-stable complex with cell surface fibronectin (Singh, De Vouge, et al., 1990). Normal rat kidney cells secrete a phosphorylated as well as a nonphosphorylated form of Eta-1/Op (Nemir et al., 1989; Singh, De Vouge, et al., 1990). Phosphorylated Eta-1/Op is associated with the cell surface, whereas the nonphosphorylated form coimmunoprecipitates with soluble fibronectin. Vanadyl sulfate-treated cells, which acquire a reversible transformed phenotype, show increased levels of both phosphorylated Eta-1/Op on the cell surface and nonphosphorylated Eta-1/Op in conditioned media. Thus, the effects of phosphorylation on the tertiary structure of Eta-1/Op may account for the different binding properties of the molecule. Phosphoserine in the Mefp-5 adhesive protein derived from the foot of the common mussel occurs in sequences strikingly reminiscent of acidic mineral-binding motifs that appear in Eta-1/Op, statherin, and others, a feature that may reflect an adaptation for adhesion to the most common substrate for mussels, i.e., calcareous materials (Waite and Qin, 2001).

Phosphate is also a specific signal for induction of Eta-1/Op gene expression (Beck et al., 2000). In studies of the regulation of osteoblast differentiation, Beck et al. (2000) revealed a link between Eta-1/Op induction and the synthesis and enzymatic activity of alkaline phosphatase, which results in the generation of free phosphate. This elevation of free phosphate in the medium is sufficient to signal induction of Eta-1/Op RNA and protein. The strong and specific induction of Eta-1/Op in direct response to increased phosphate levels provides a mechanism to explain how expression of this product is normally regulated in bone and suggests how it may become up-regulated in damaged tissue. One example of phosphate regulation by bone proteins is provided by bone acidic glycoprotein (BAG)-75, which self-associates in vitro and in vivo into microfibrillar complexes, a property that could serve an organizational role in forming bone or as a barrier restricting local diffusion of phosphate ions, and that is not shared with the acidic phosphoproteins Eta-1/Op and bone sialoprotein (Gorski et al., 1997; Yang et al., 1995).

Purple acid phosphatases (PAPs) are binuclear acid metallohydrolases also referred to as tartrate-resistant acid phosphatases (TRAPs) or type 5 acid phosphatases (Ljusberg et al., 1999). The two-subunit bone PAP is considerably more active than the monomeric recombinant rat PAP toward a variety of serine-, threonine-, and tyrosine-phosphorylated substrates. Of these substrates, bovine milk Eta-1/Op is the most readily dephosphorylated substrate. Besides being implicated in the catabolism of the extracellular matrix, members of the cysteine proteinase family might also exert a regulatory role in degradative processes involving the PAP enzymes by converting the newly synthesized PAPs to enzymically active and microenvironmentally regulated species (Ljusberg et al., 1999).

Sulfation

The sulfate in Eta-1/Op in the form of tyrosine sulfate (Ecarot-Charrier et al., 1989), and the single conserved residue (Tyr 171) in Eta-1/Op is encoded by mouse exon 5 and its human homologue. Sulfation of Eta-1/Op has been observed only during bone tissue mineralization and has been proposed to mark the osteoblastic phenotype (Nagata et al., 1989).

Other Potential Functional Domains in the Eta-1/Op Protein

An additional set of potential functional domains, identified using the computer program of Inouye and Kirschner (1991) and by visual examination of Eta-1/Op sequences, is shown in Table 4.3. These domains include an incomplete ATP-binding site (Hanks et al., 1988), a serine protease active site (thrombin) (Lehninger, 1975), two incomplete GTP-binding sites (Dever et al., 1987), two recognition sites for myosin-I heavy chain kinase (Brzeska et al., 1989), a recognition site for proline-dependent protein kinase (Vulliet et al., 1989), a recognition site for multifunctional calmodulin-dependent kinase II (Pearson et al., 1985), and a phosphatase active site (Metzler, 1977). The significance of these potential functional domains of Eta-1/Op is not yet understood, although one possibility is that they may play a role in phosphate and calcium metabolism.

Eta-1/Op serves as a substrate for the incorporation of radiolabelled putrescine mediated by a commercial preparation of guinea pig liver transglutaminase, and in vivo Eta-1/Op serves as a substrate for the plasma transglutaminase, Factor XIIIa (Prince et al., 1991). Sorensen et al. (1994) reported the identification of two transglutaminase-reactive glutamines (Gln-34 and Gln-36) in bovine Eta-1/Op. Sequence alignment revealed that these glutamines are conserved in all known Eta-1/Op sequences, indicating a functional importance of this region of the protein. Furthermore, immunological analysis of bovine bone demonstrated that Eta-1/Op is present in high-molecular-mass complexes in vivo. These findings support the functional aspects of a transglutaminase-catalyzed cross-linking of Eta-1/Op in facilitating cellular attachment and tissue calcification (Sorensen et al., 1994).

TABLE 4.3. Other Potential Functional Domains in Eta-1/Op

Domain	Sequence (mouse)	Location (mouse)	Reference
ATP-binding site	VKVTDS	19-24	Hanks et al., 1988
Serine protease active site (thrombin)	DSG	23-25	Lehninger, 1975
GTP-binding site[a]	DDDG; DHAG	96-111; 112-115	Dever et al., 1987
Recognition site (myosin-I-heavy chain kinase)	HAGS; HMKS	113-116[b]; 198-201	Brzeska et al., 1989
Recognition site (proline-dependent protein kinase)	TP	153-154	Vulliet et al., 1989
Recognition site (multifunctional calmodulin-dependent kinase II)	RGDS	165-168	Pearson et al., 1985
Phosphatase active site	ESA[c]	277-279	Metzler,1977

[a] In GTP-binding proteins, three sequences are separated from one another by about 40 to 80 residues (Dever et al., 1987). The sequences found in Eta-1/Op correspond to the middle one. In species other than mouse, the sequence DGRG is found at position 163 to 166. The two flanking sequences characteristic of GTP-binding proteins were not found in any of the Eta-1/Op analyzed.

[b] In human, the sequences HVDS and HKQS are found at positions 99 to 102 and 246 to 249, respectively, and in pig the sequence HVDS is found at positions 99 to 102.

[c] In rat, two DSA sequences (268 to 270 and 277 to 279) can be found.

In this respect, transglutaminase-mediated cross-linking between Eta-1/Op and fibronectin represents one of the most likely mechanisms by which Eta-1/Op becomes covalently linked to bone matrix, urinary stone matrix, and to the extracellular matrix (Beninati et al., 1994).

Secondary and Tertiary Structure Analyses

Hydrophobicity/hydrophylicity analyses (Hopp and Woods, 1983; Kyte and Doolittle, 1982) and a secondary structure algorithm (Chou and Fasman, 1978) were used to analyze the primary sequence (without posttranslational modifications) of Eta-1/Op from various mammalian species. Rat Eta-1/Op shows 43.5 percent α-helix, 19.6 percent β-strand, and 36.9 percent β-turns and random coils, whereas mouse Eta-1/Op shows 34 percent α-helix, 23.5 percent β-strand, and 42.5 percent β-turns and random coils. These analyses are in general agreement with those of Craig et al. (1989) and Prince (1989).

There are four hydrophobic regions within the amino two-thirds of murine Eta-1/Op, which also show high propensity for β-strand conformation (β1, residues 40 to 45; β2, 148 to 153; β3, 169 to 175; β4, 213 to 219) and are flanked by hydrophilic regions, which show a high propensity for β-turns. Therefore, this portion of the protein could be organized as a globular domain with the β-strands arranged as antiparallel or parallel β-sheets. An antiparallel arrangement of β-sheets is most likely, because the segment linking β2 and β3 (residues 154 to 168) may be rather short to allow a parallel arrangement of β-sheets. This antiparallel β-sheet may form part of a relatively hydrophobic core, whereas the connecting loops may project outward to form relatively hydrophilic regions of the globular domain. According to this model of Eta-1/Op, the functional domains, such as the poly-Asp, the RGD, and multiple phosphorylation sites, would reside on the connecting loops. Therefore, these functional domains would be available to interact with one another, with domains that reside in the carboxyl portion of the molecule, with calcium ions (the poly-Asp), with cell surface receptors (the RGD), and with kinases or phosphatases (the phosphorylation sites). The sequence coded by exon 4, which can be alternatively spliced, is located between β-strands β1 and β2. Hence, the inclusion or exclusion of this sequence would have no significant effect on the protein's folding and/or stability.

Eta-1/Op, as member of the SIBLING (small integrin-binding ligand, N-linked glycoprotein) family of genetically related proteins that are clustered on human chromosome 4, is the result of duplication and subsequent divergent evolution of a single ancient gene (Fisher, Torchia, et al., 2001). One-dimensional proton nuclear magnetic resonance (NMR) and transverse relaxation times analysis revealed that the polypeptide backbone of free Eta-1/Op rapidly samples an ensemble of conformations consistent with being completely unstructured in solution. This flexibility appears to enable this relatively small glycoprotein to rapidly associate with a number of different binding partners including other proteins as well as the mineral phase of bones and teeth. Eta-1/Op often functions by bridging two proteins of fixed structures into a biologically active complex (Fisher, Torchia, et al., 2001).

Chapter 5

Biological Activities of the Eta-1/Op Protein in Nonimmunological Bodily Systems and Pathologies

The realization that soluble immune mediators, termed cytokines, elaborated by cells of the immune system can interact with nonimmunological cells has led to new insights into the role of the immune system in regulating cell growth and differentiation of other organ systems. In many instances, these cytokines are produced by different organ systems sometimes as variants of a common form that are particularly suited for the specialized organs' functions. Dysregulation of the production of cytokines, whether as a consequence of alterations in the interactions between the immune and other systems or as a result of pathologies intrinsic to particular organs, can lead to a variety of clinical disorders. The role of cytokines in nonimmunological disease has come to light relatively recently. For example, immunological cells have been implicated in the etiology of gastric ulcer disease in studies that show that the target of the histamine-receptor blocker class of antiulcer drugs is macrophages of the lamina propria (rather than parietal cells, as had been generally believed) (Mezey and Palkovits, 1992). However, the soluble mediators released by macrophages that may act on gastrointestinal cells have not been precisely defined. In other cases, soluble mediators responsible for the regulatory effects of the immune system have been well defined, but their precise role in diseases awaits clarification. For example, the angiogenic activity of interleukin-8 has been well established, but the role of this mediator in angiogenesis-dependent disorders, such as rheumatoid arthritis and tumor growth, is not yet defined (Koch et al., 1992).

Studies of Eta-1/Op, which as described is involved in immune resistance to certain bacterial and viral pathogens, have revealed that it may also represent a molecular message that links the immune system with several somatic organ systems, and that it is also produced by different organ systems, serving in each a variety of functions (Denhardt, Giachelli, et al., 2001). Expression of Eta-1/Op in several cell types and the presence of multiple functionally distinct motifs found on the protein suggest that this product mediates more than one function. The presence of motifs that are potentially amenable to modification by tissue-specific enzymes provides a possible mechanism by which the protein could play different roles in various tissues. Likewise, isoforms of Eta-1/Op mRNA generated by alternative splicing also could mediate different biological activities.

The following sections provide a synopsis of our current knowledge regarding the function of Eta-1/Op in different organ systems.

OSSEOUS SYSTEM

Bone cells, such as mesenchymal-derived osteoblasts and osteocytes and hematopoietic-derived osteoclasts, predominantly modulate bone modeling and remodeling as well as systemic calcium homeostasis (Ozawa and Amizuka, 1994). Osteoblasts are classified into preosteoblasts, mature osteoblasts, and bone lining cells (BLCs) based on their cell structures and biological functions. Preosteoblasts appear to regulate the activities of mature osteoblasts and osteoclasts, and they differentiate into mature osteoblasts. Cuboidal mature osteoblasts show a well-developed Golgi apparatus and rough endoplasmic reticulum, and actively synthesize major bone matrix proteins including type I collagen, Eta-1/Op, osteonectin, and osteocalcin (Zhu et al., 2001). Unlike mature osteoblasts, BLCs display flattened cell bodies and few cell organelles, an indication of fewer activities. These osteoblasts communicate through gap junctions with one another or with osteocytes, consequently forming a three-dimensional cellular network in bone tissues (Lecanda et al., 1998; Li et al., 1999; Schiller et al., 2001). In contrast, osteocytes, the compacted cells embedded in the bone matrix, provide a cellular environment in the bone matrix by means of their numerous cytoplasmic processes. It is likely that they participate in calcium transport from bone matrix to tissue fluid, which is called osteocytic osteolysis. Osteoclasts, multinucleated giant cells with ruffled borders and clear zones, are responsible for bone resorption, although probably the surrounding osteoblast phenotype controls them. Active osteoclasts secrete H^+ and proteolytic enzymes, such as cathepsin and ACPase, toward resorption pits through ruffled borders (Ozawa and Amizuka, 1994; Sasano et al., 2000).

Bone matrix proteins can be divided into several groups according to their function: structural proteins, cell adhesive molecules, growth factors, proteinases, and others. For example, (1) Type I collagen is a major structural protein; (2) Eta-1/Op and bone sialoprotein (BSP) are RGD-containing cell adhesive proteins. Cadherins, OSF-2, and MGP also act as cell adhesive molecules in cell-to-cell or cell-to-matrix signal transition systems; (3) bone morphogenetic proteins (BMPs), tumor growth factor (TGF)-β, insulin growth factors (IGFs), fibroblast growth factors (FGFs), and platelet-derived growth factor (PDGF) are bone growth factors associated to bone matrix that also modulate Eta-1/Op expression; and (4) collagenases and cathepsins are well-known organic bone matrix degrading enzymes (Aeschlimann et al., 1996; Ahrens et al., 1993; Alberius and Gordh, 1996, 1998; Alberius and Johnell, 1990, 1991; Alberius et al., 1996a,b; Arai et al., 1995; Ayukawa et al., 1998; Barone et al., 1991, 1993, 1994; Benayahu, Fried, et al., 1994; Benayahu, Gurevitz, et al., 1994; Bhalerao et al., 1995; Binkert et al., 1999; Bliziotes et al., 1996; Boskey et al., 1993; Butler et al., 1992; Carlson et al., 1993; Carter et al., 1998; Chackalaparampil et al., 1996; Cheifetz et al., 1996; Chen et al., 1991; Chen, Bal, et al., 1992; Chen, Harris, et al., 1997; Chen, Ke, et al., 1997; Chen, Shapiro, et al., 1992; Chen, Singh, et al., 1993, 1994; Cheng, Lai, et al., 2000; Cheng, Lai, et al., 2001; Cheng, Lou, et al., 2001; Cheng, Shin, et al., 2000; Chenu and Delmas, 1992; Daculsi et al., 1999; De Bri et al., 1996; Denhardt and Guo, 1993; Derkx et al., 1998; Doherty et al., 1998; Dorheim et al., 1993; Einhorn, 1998; El-Ghannam et al., 1997; Fagenholz et al., 2001; Farach-Carson et al., 1992; Faucheux et al., 1998; Feuerbach et al., 1997; Filippini et al., 2001; Flores et al., 1996; Franzen et al., 1989; Fujisawa and Kuboki,

1998; Gerstenfeld et al., 1994, 1995; Gerstenfeld, Uporova, et al., 1996; Gerstenfeld, Zurakowski, et al., 1996; Giannobile et al., 2001; Goldberg and Hunter, 1995; Gorski, 1992, 1998; Gorski et al., 1990, 1996; Gotoh, Gerstenfeld, et al., 1990; Gotoh, Pierschbacher, et al., 1990; Gronthos et al., 1999; Guidon et al., 1993; Harada et al., 1999; Hayami et al., 2000; Heinegard, 1995; Heinegard, Hultenby, et al., 1989; Heinegard, Andersson, and Reinholt, 1995; Hirota et al., 1994; Huang et al., 1997; Hulth et al., 1993; Hunter and Goldberg, 1993; Hunter et al., 1994, 1996; Ikeda et al., 1992; Ikenoue et al., 1999; Inoue et al., 1995; Ishizeki et al., 1999; Kasahara et al., 1992; Kasugai, Todescan, et al., 1991; Kasugai, Zhang, et al., 1991; Kasugai et al., 1992; Katayama et al., 1997; Kim et al., 1997, 1999; Klein-Nulend et al., 1997; Knopov et al., 1995a,b, 1997; Kockx et al., 1994; Kremer et al., 1998; Lai et al., 2001; Landis et al., 1992; Lavelin et al., 1998; Lecanda et al., 1997; Lee et al., 1992; Lee, Lowe, et al., 1999; Lee, Shin, et al., 1999; Lefebvre et al., 1995; Li et al., 1996; Liang et al., 1992; Liu, Malaval, et al., 1997; Liu, Uemura, et al., 1997; Liu, Wantanabe, et al., 1997; Loeser, 1993; MacDougall et al., 1996; Mackie et al., 2001; Mahmoodian et al., 1996; Majeska et al., 1993; Mark, Prince, Gay, et al., 1987; Mark, Prince, Oosawa, et al., 1987; Mathieu et al., 1994; Maxian et al., 1998; McKee and Nanci, 1995a,b, 1996a-d; McKee et al., 1991, 1993; Midura et al., 1990; Miles et al., 1998; Monsonego et al., 1997; Moore et al., 1991; Morriss-Kay et al., 2001; Moursi et al., 1996; Mukherjee et al., 1995; Nakase et al., 1994; Nomura et al., 1989; Nordahl et al., 1995; Ohtsuki et al., 1998; Omigbodun et al., 1995; O'Neal et al., 1992; Otawara-Hamamoto, 1990, 1994; Pacifici et al., 1991; Padrines et al., 2000; Palmer et al., 1999; Panheleux et al., 1999; Pinero et al., 1995; Pines et al., 1995, 1998; Pockwinse et al., 1992, 1993; Pounds et al., 1991; Puleo et al., 1993; Qiu et al., 1998; Quarto et al., 1995; Rifas et al., 1997; Riminucci et al., 1997; Ritchie et al., 1994; Ritter et al., 1992; Roach, 1992, 1994; Roach and Erenpreisa, 1996; Rosati et al., 1994; Rowatt et al., 1997; Sammons et al., 1994; Sasaguri et al., 1998; Sasaki et al., 2000; Sato et al., 1990; Sato, Morii, et al., 1998; Sato, Yasui, et al., 1998; Sauk, Van Kampen, Norris, Foster, et al., 1990; Sauk, Van Kampen, Norris, Moehring, et al., 1990; Shalhoub, Bettencourt, et al., 1994; Shalhoub, Bortell, et al., 1994; Shukunami et al., 1998; Silbermann et al., 1990; Sodek, Ganss, et al., 2000; Sodek, Tupy, et al., 2000; Sommer et al., 1996; Strauss et al., 1990; Strayhorn et al., 1999; Suva et al., 1993; Suzuki et al., 1996; Tanaka and Liang, 1995; Termine, 1988; Thayer et al., 1995; Tokunaga et al., 1996; Toma, Ashkar, et al., 1997; Toma, Schaffer, et al., 1997; Vary et al., 2000; Wang et al., 1993; Wang, Glimcher, et al., 1998; Wang, Louden, et al., 1998; Weinreb et al., 1990; Winn et al., 1999; Woitge and Kream, 2000; Woitge and Seibel, 2001; Yabe et al., 1997; Yamagiwa et al., 1999; Yao et al., 1994; Young et al., 1992).

Eta-1/Op is abundant in bone matrix, and is synthesized by preosteoblasts, osteoblasts, and osteocytes, is secreted into osteoid tissue, and is incorporated into bone (Aarden, Nijweide, et al., 1996; Aarden, Wassenaar, et al., 1996; Anselme et al., 2000; Attawia et al., 1999; Atkins et al., 1997; Aubin, 1999; Aubin et al., 1995; Barak-Shalom et al., 1995; Beck et al., 1998; Berry et al., 1995; Boskey, 1995; Butler, 1989; Byers et al., 1999; Carvalho et al., 1998; Cheng, Lai, et al., 2001; Cheng, Lou, et al., 2001; Cooper et al., 1998; Cowles et al., 1998; Culbert et al., 1996; Davey et al., 2000; Davies, 1996; Denhardt and Noda, 1998; Ecarot-Charrier et al., 1989; Effah Kaufmann et al., 2000; Evans et al., 2000; Frank et al., 1993; Frick and Bushinsky, 1998, 1999; Fried et al., 1996; Ghilzon et al., 1999; Giachelli and Steitz, 2000; Goldberg et al., 1996; Gruber et al., 2001; Grzesik and Robey, 1994; Harris, Bonewald, et al., 1994; Harris, Sabatini, et al., 1994; Harris et al., 1995; Hay et al., 1999; Heath et al., 1989a,b; Heinegard and Oldberg, 1989; Hirakawa et al., 1994; Hoshi et al., 1999, 2001; Hruska et al., 1995a,b; Ibaraki et al., 1992; Ikedo et al., 1999; Ikenoue et al., 1999; Irie et al., 1998; Isogai et al., 2000; Jin et al., 1990; Johansson et al., 1999; Johnson-Pais and Leach, 1995; Kaji et al., 1996; Kato et al., 1997; Keeting et al., 1992; Kido, Nishikawa, et al., 1997; Kido, Yamauchi, et al., 1997; Lanske et al., 1998; Lawton et al., 1999; Liao et al., 1999; Lisignoli et al., 2001; Liu et al., 1994; Liu, Malavel, et al., 1997; Liu, Watanabe, et al., 1997; Liu, Uemura, et al., 1997; Luan et al., 2000; Malaval et al., 1994, 1999; Mark, Butler, et al., 1988; Mark, Prince, et al., 1988; Masuda et al., 2000; Matsumura et al., 1998; McCabe et al., 1994; Meleti etal., 2000; Motomura et al., 1996; Mueller et al., 1999; Nagata et al., 1989, 1991; Nakase et al., 1998; Nanci et al., 1996; Nemoto and Uemura, 1999; Nishio, Hatanaka, et al., 2000; Nishio, Iseda, et al., 2000; Nishio, Neo, et al., 2000; Nishio et al., 2001; Noble and Reeve,

2000; Noda and Denhardt, 1995; Ohmura, 1993; Ohsawa et al., 2000, 2001; Onyia et al., 1999; Owen et al., 1990; Oyajobi et al., 1999; Ozawa and Kasugai, 1996; Park et al., 2001; Phillips et al., 2001; Puleo and Nanci, 1999; Raynal et al., 1996; Rickard et al., 1996; Rodan and Noda, 1991; Roser et al., 2000; Roth et al., 1999; Sakamoto et al., 1999; Salih, Ashkar, et al., 1996; Salih, Ashkar, Zhou, et al, 1996; Salih, Zhou, et al., 1996; Salih et al. 1997; Sato, Morii, et al., 1998; Sato, Yasui, et al., 1998; Schulz et al., 1998; Schulze et al., 1999; Seitz et al., 1995; Shah et al., 1999; Shelly and Laborde, 1992; Shibata et al., 2000; Snyder et al., 1997; Sodek et al., 1995; St-Arnaud et al., 1995; Stein et al., 1989, 1990; Stubbs, 1996; Sun et al., 1997; Tavassoli et al., 2001; Thalmeier et al., 2001; Traianedes et al., 1995; Uemura et al., 1999; Wennberg et al., 2000; Winnard et al., 1995; Wong et al., 2000; Wu, Ikezawa, et al., 1996; Wu, Ishikawa, et al., 1995; Wu, Pan, et al., 1995; Wu, Shimizu, et al., 1996; Yamagiwa et al., 2001; Yamate, Mocharla, et al., 1997; Yamate, Umekawa, et al., 1997; Yang et al., 2001; Yoon et al., 1987; Zayzafoon et al., 2000; Zhang et al., 1995a,b; Zhou et al., 1993, 1994; Zhu et al., 1997; Zohar, Cheifetz, et al., 1998; Zohar, Lee, et al., 1997; Zohar, McCulloch, et al., 1998; Zohar, Sodek, et al., 1997; Zreiqat and Howlett, 1999; Zreiqat, Evans, et al., 1999; Zreiqat, McFarland, et al., 1999; Zreiqat et al., 1996).

Although Eta-1/Op is expressed in osteoclasts, and Eta-1/Op facilitates angiogenesis, accumulation of osteoclasts, and resorption in ectopic bone, Eta-1/Op deficiency does not suppress osteoclastogenesis (Arai et al., 1993; Asou et al., 2001; Chenu et al., 1994; Connor et al., 1995; Dodds et al., 1995; Duong and Rodan, 1998; Duong et al., 1998; Ek-Rylander et al., 1994; Flores et al., 1992; Grano et al., 1994; Halasy-Nagy and Hofstetter, 1998; Hall and Chambers, 1996; Heymann et al., 1998; Higuchi et al., 1999; Hultenby et al., 1991, 1994; James et al., 1996; Katayama et al., 1998; Maeda et al., 1994; Marusic et al., 2000; Matsumoto et al., 1995; Merry et al., 1993; Reinholt et al., 1990, 1999; Rittling et al., 1998; Sato et al., 1992; Takeshita et al., 2000; Tani-Ishii et al., 1997; Teti, Farina, et al., 1998; Teti, Taranta, et al., 1998; Tong et al., 1994; Wesolowski et al., 1995). However, enhancement of osteoclastic bone resorption and suppression of osteoblastic bone formation in response to reduced mechanical stress do not occur in the absence of

Eta-1/Op (Ishijima et al., 1998). Moreover, Eta-1/Op-integrin αvβ3 binding plays a more important role than collagen type I-α2β1 binding in the regulation of osteoclast activity (Chellaiah and Hruska, 1996; Chellaiah, Kizer, et al., 2000; Chellaiah, Soga, et al., 2000; Duong et al., 2000; Faccio et al., 1998; Grzesik, 1997; Helfrich et al., 1992; Horton et al., 1995; Hruska, Rifas, et al., 1995; Hruska, Rolnick, et al., 1995a,b; Miyauchi et al., 1991; Rodan and Rodan, 1997; Ross et al., 1993; Tezuka et al., 1992; Uemura et al., 2000; Wozniak et al., 2000). Indeed, peptidomimetic antagonists of αvβ3 inhibit bone resorption by inhibiting osteoclast bone resorptive activity, not osteoclast adhesion to bone (Carron et al., 2000).

Eta-1/Op, as well as other factors such as transcription factors (cfos, cbfa1, and msx-2), matrix molecules (bone sialoprotein and osteocalcin), and hormones (PTH-rP), are differentially expressed in subpopulations of osteoblasts, preosteoblasts, and osteocytes based on cell maturational status, environment (ectocranial versus endocranial surfaces), and microenvironment (adjacent osteoblasts) and through different transcriptional and translational mechanisms (Ber et al., 1991; Candeliere et al., 2001; Daiter et al., 1996; Fragale et al., 1999; Ingram et al., 1993; Komori et al., 1997; Liu, Malaval, et al., 1997; Liu, Uemura, et al., 1997; Liu, Watanabe, et al., 1997; Marzia et al., 2000; Ohta et al., 1991; Tsuji et al., 1998; Zohar, Cheifetz, et al., 1998; Zohar, Lee, et al., 1997; Zohar, McCulloch, et al., 1998; Zohar, Sodek, et al., 1997). Eta-1/Op gene expression is up-regulated by oscillatory fluid flow via intracellular calcium mobilization and activation of mitogen-activated protein kinase in MC3T3-E1 osteoblasts (Hillsley and Frangos, 1997; You et al., 2000, 2001). Extraneous stimuli also play a role. For instance, Eta-1/Op and L-type calcium-channel expression are up-regulated in bone cells in response to mechanical strain (Kubota et al., 1990, 1993; Meazzini et al., 1998; Nomura and Takano-Yamamoto, 2000; Owan et al., 1997; Raab-Cullen et al., 1994; Terai et al., 1999; Toma, Ashkar, et al., 1997; Toma, Schaffer, et al., 1997; Walker et al., 2000; Yamauchi, 1990).

Exogenous administration or up-regulation of fibroblast-growth factor (FGF) expression are also accompanied by Eta-1 expression up-regulation in the developing skull vault (Amizuka et al., 1998; Chen, Adar, et al., 1999; Chen, Jin, et al., 1999; Iseki et al., 1997, 1999; Lemonnier et al., 2000; Morriss-Kay et al., 2001; Rodan et al.,

1989; Tanaka et al., 1999). FGF-1 treatment renders osteoblast precursors resistant to the cytotoxic effects of the apoptosis-inducer peroxinitrite, an observation that suggests that FGF-1 promotes the progression of bone repair mechanisms by increasing the population of osteoblasts and imparting protection to the cell line from the hostile inflammatory environment (Reiff et al., 2001; Tang et al., 1996). Eta-1/Op is localized in bone and cartilage during endochondral ossification in the chicken tibia (McKee et al., 1992). Endothelin-1 (ET-1) enhances approximately twofold the mRNA expression of both Eta-1/Op and osteocalcin genes in rat osteoblastic osteosarcoma ROS17/2.8 cells in a dose- and time-dependent manner. ET-1 modulation of the expression of the two phenotype-related gene products of osteoblasts suggests that endothelin is one of the cytokines which modulates osteoblastic functions and that this molecule may play a role in the regulation of bone metabolism (Kitano et al., 1998; Shioide and Noda, 1993; Stern, Glimcher, et al., 1995; Stern, Tatrai, et al., 1995). Collagen type I, with involvement of the $\alpha 2\beta 1$ integrin, also stimulates Eta-1/Op expression in osteoblasts during differentiation from bone marrow cell precursors (Celic et al., 1998; Chimal-Monroy et al., 1998; Kinoshita et al., 1999; Lynch et al., 1995; Mizuno and Kuboki, 2001; Mizuno et al., 2000; Roehlecke et al., 2001; Shi et al., 1996; Sugimoto et al., 1998; Traianedes et al., 1996). On the other hand, a dominant negative cadherin inhibits osteoblast differentiation and Eta-1/Op expression (Cheng, Lai, et al., 2000; Cheng, Shin, et al., 2000; Lin et al., 1999).

Eta-1/Op plays a role in dental root formation (Arzate et al., 1996; Bosshardt and Nanci, 1997, 1998; Bowers et al., 1989; Chen, McCulloch, et al., 1993; D'Errico et al., 1995, 1997; Fujita, 1993; Helder et al., 1993; Kido et al., 1995; Kido, Nishikawa, et al., 1997; Kido, Yamauchi, et al., 1997; Nakajima et al., 1996; Shigeyama et al., 1996; Shyng et al., 1999; Sodek, Ganss, et al., 2000; Sodek, Tupy, et al., 2000; Somerman et al., 1988, 1992; Sun et al., 1998; Yamada, 1990; Zhang, Fan, et al., 2000; Zhang, Zhang, et al., 2000). In this respect, Eta-1/Op is expressed in the dental follicle region of molars obtained from three-day-old CD-1 mice, but was not expressed in the odontoblast layer (Somerman et al., 1992). In contrast by day 8, positive staining was noted in the odontoblast layer, as well as in the area of Hertwig's epithelial root sheath. However, at this same time point no positive labeling for Eta-1/Op is observed in the enamel organ or in the dental papillae cells. By day 15, positive staining for Eta-1/Op is seen in the area of the periodontal ligament, as well as the region of primary deposition of extracellular matrix onto dentin (Boskey et al., 2000; Narayanan et al., 2001; Qin et al., 2001; Somerman et al., 1992). Eta-1/Op is localized in fibroblasts of periodontal structures from humans and other species (yielding a stronger signal in the periodontal ligament compared to the gingiva) and in the cementum and bone (Chien et al., 1999a,b; Hakki et al., 2001; Harle et al., 2001; Hou et al., 1999; Ivanovski et al., 2000, 2001; Kadono et al., 1999; Kikukawa, 1996; Lekic et al., 1996a,b, 1997, 2001a,b; Li et al., 2001; Lin et al., 1999; Lin, Huang, et al., 2000; Lin, Kenny, et al., 2000; MacNeil, Berry, D'Errico, Strayhorn, Piotrowski, et al., 1995; MacNeil, Berry, D'Errico, Strayhorn, and Somerman, 1995; Nanci, 1999; Nguyen et al., 1997; Nohutcu et al., 1996, 1997; Parkar et al., 1999; Rajshankar et al., 1998; Somerman, Shroff, et al., 1990; Somerman, Young, et al., 1990; Takano-Yamamoto et al., 1994).

Eta-1/Op is localized in cellular and acellular cementum (Amar et al., 1997; Arzate et al., 1998; BarKana et al., 2000; Beertsen et al., 1998; Bosshardt et al., 1998; Bronckers et al., 1989, 1994; Hashimoto et al., 2001; Hou et al., 2000; MacNeil et al., 1998; McKee et al., 1996; Sasano et al., 2000; Somerman et al., 1989; Somerman, Shroff, et al., 1990; Somerman, Young, et al., 1990; VandenBos et al., 1999; Wu, Ikezawa, et al., 1996; Wu, Shimizu, et al., 1996), and PDGF and growth hormone stimulate Eta-1/Op expression in dental cementoblasts (D'Errico et al., 1999, 2000; Giannobile et al., 2001; Li et al., 2001; Saygin et al., 2000; Tokiyasu et al., 2000). Clonal dental pulp cells (RDP4-1, RPC-C2A) synthesize and secrete Eta-1/Op (Nagata, Kaho, et al., 1994; Nagata, Yokota, et al., 1994; Nagata et al., 1995; Yokota et al., 1992). Dental pulp cells in vivo produce Eta-1/Op, which has been localized in their peripheral area of dental pulp stones (Ninomiya et al., 2001; Pramanik et al., 1996). Dental pulp cells play an important role in maintaining dental mineralized tissue throughout life and supplementary mineralization such as reparative dentin and pulp stone that frequently occurs after primary dentin formation (Butler, 1991; Butler and Ritchie, 1995; Fujisawa et al., 1993; MacDougall, 1998; Ohishi et al., 1999; Ohma et al., 2000; Salih et al., 1998; Takata et al., 1998; Yokota et al., 1992).

It was originally proposed that the poly-Asp motif of Eta-1/Op binds to the mineral phase of bone and the RGD motif binds to the osteoblastic cell surface (Oldberg et al., 1986). According to this notion, Eta-1/Op would serve as a bridge between the mineral phase and the cell surface. This hypothesis, however, is inconsistent with the fact that the distance between the mineral phase and the osteoblast surface is too large to be covered by a protein the size of Eta-1/Op (Glimcher, 1989). The putative functional domains and tissue distribution of Eta-1/Op also suggest that this protein may play a role in the overall metabolism of phosphate and calcium. According to this notion, mobilization of phosphate from the extracellular milieu may occur if cells internalize the protein upon phosphorylation in the extracellular matrix. Similarly, the protein may serve as a reservoir and/or carrier of calcium. In this respect, secreted phosphoproteins are found in the extracellular matrix of all mineralized vertebrate tissues (Gotoh et al., 1995). This observation and the stereochemical configuration of apatite crystals have led to the proposals that phosphoprotein(s) may play a role in the initiation and/or spatial distribution of mineral (Glimcher, 1976, 1989) and that Eta-1/Op alone or in combination with other protein(s) may play such a role in bone (Glimcher, 1989). Support for this hypothesis comes from the observations that phosphorylated Ser and Thr residues as well as calcium-binding motifs are present on Eta-1/Op (Oldberg et al., 1986; Prince, 1989). Eta-1/Op secreted by osteoblasts also may play a role in bone readsorption by mediating attachment of osteoclasts (Reinholt et al., 1990). A hallmark of Eta-1/Op expression in pathologically mineralizing tissue, and in other soft tissues experiencing a more generalized type of necrotic injury, is the production of Eta-1/Op by macrophages at the lesion site (McKee and Nanci, 1996a-d). Eta-1/Op secreted by macrophages may serve as a macrophage adhesion protein, and where concentrated at the surface of small particulate, mineralized tissue debris may act as an opsonin, thereby facilitating cell adhesion and phagocytosis by macrophages, a process likely mediated by integrin-binding, signal transduction, and cytoskeletal restructuring (McKee and Nanci, 1996a-d). Several Eta-1/Op receptors may participate in bone remodeling, and Eta-1/Op, rather than hyaluronic acid, is the major ligand for CD44 on bone cells in the remodeling phase of healing of fractures (Yamazaki et al., 1999).

The synthesis of Eta-1/Op by bone cells is regulated by glucocorticoids and growth factors, which promote bone formation, and by the osteotropic hormone calcitriol (1,25-dihydroxycholecalciferol) and retinoic acid, which mediate bone resorption, indicating a bifunctional role for this protein in bone remodeling (Bellows et al., 1999; Benayahu, Fried, et al., 1994; Benayahu, Gurevitz, et al., 1994; Benayahu, Kompier, et al., 1994; Ben-Bassat et al., 1999; Beresford et al., 1994; Bidder et al., 1998; Bonnelye et al., 1997; Breen et al., 1994; Broess et al., 1995; Chang et al., 1995; Chen et al., 1996; Cheng et al., 1994, 1996; Choong et al., 1993; Dieudonne et al., 1998; Donahue et al., 1997; Farach-Carson and Ridall, 1998; Fromigue et al., 1997; Gerstenfeld, 1999; Gerstenfeld, Uporova, et al., 1996; Gerstenfeld, Zurakawski, et al., 1996; Harada et al., 1995; Harter et al., 1995; Haussler et al., 1995; Heath et al., 1989a,b; Higashi et al., 1996; Iba et al., 1995, 1996; Ikeda et al., 1995, 1996; Ingram et al., 1994, 1996; Iwamoto et al., 1993, 1994; Jakob et al., 1997; Jenis et al., 1993, 1994; Jin et al., 1992; Kaji et al., 1994, 1995; Kondo et al., 1997; Kraichely and MacDonald, 1998; Kubota et al., 1989; Lafage-Proust et al., 1999; Leboy et al., 1991; Lian et al., 1997; Liang et al., 1992; Majeska et al., 1994; Malaval et al., 1995; Manji et al., 1998; Maor et al., 1989; Marks et al., 1989; Mathieu and Merregaert, 1994; Matsue et al., 1997; Miyamoto et al., 1995; Mocetti et al., 2000; Monsonego et al., 1995; Mundy, 1996; Nagata, Kaho, et al., 1994; Nagata, Yokota, et al., 1994; Noda, Vogel, Craig, et al., 1990; Noda, Vogel, Hasson, et al., 1990; Ohishi et al., 1994, 1995; Ongphiphadhanakul et al., 1993; Park et al., 1997; Partridge et al., 1994; Pavlin et al., 1994; Pockwinse et al., 1995; Prince and Butler, 1987; Qu et al., 1998; Rickard et al., 1994; Ringbom-Anderson et al., 1995; Roth et al., 1999; Seto et al., 1999; Shalhoub et al., 1992; Shalhoub, Bettencourt, et al., 1994; Shalhoub, Bortell, et al., 1994; Staal et al., 1994, 1997; Suwanwalaikorn et al., 1996; Takeshita et al., 1998; Tanaka et al., 1994, 1996; Termine, 1990; Thiebaud et al., 1994; Thomas et al., 2000; Traianedes et al., 1993; Turner et al., 1990; Wakisaka et al., 1998; Waterhouse et al., 1992; Watson et al., 1994; Williams et al., 1999; Williams, Halpert, et al., 1995; Williams, Bland, et al., 1995; Willing et al., 1998; Wisner-Lynch et al., 1995; Woodard et al., 1997; Yanaka et al., 1998; Yeh et al., 1999; Zhang et al., 1992; Zhou et al., 1991). Vitamin D_3 and its analogs stimulate Eta-1/Op expression in osteoblasts (Farach-Carson, 2001), and zinc increases the activity of vitamin D-dependent promoters in osteoblasts (Lutz et al., 2000). The orphan nuclear estrogen receptor-related receptor (ERR)α is expressed by many cell types, but is very highly expressed by osteoblastic cells throughout their differentiation and regulates bone formation partly through transactivation of Eta-1/Op expression (Bonnelye et al., 2001). Parathyroid hormone-induced bone resorption does not occur in the absence of Eta-1/Op, as evinced in Eta-1/Op-deficient mice (Ihara et al., 2001).

A novel osteotropic prodrug of estradiol conjugated with L-Asp-hexapeptide enhances the expression of Eta-1/Op mRNAs and those of other bone matrix proteins, thereby ameliorating bone loss (Yokogawa et al., 2001). Although tamoxifen attenuates glucocorticoid actions on bone formation in vitro, it does not affect Eta-1/Op expression (Sukhu et al., 1997). Eta-1/Op is essential for postmenopausal osteoporosis, Eta-1/Op-deficient mice are resistant to ovariectomy-induced bone resorption (Yoshitake et al., 1999). In vivo nicotine exposure, likely through the nicotinic receptor α4 subunit that has been shown to be present in human primary bone cells, up-regulates c-fos and Eta-1/Op expression in human-derived osteoblast-like cells and human trabecular bone organ culture, a feature that may underlie the link between smoking and osteoporosis (Singh et al., 2000; Walker et al., 2001). A combination of subtherapeutic doses of chemically modified doxycycline (CMT-8) and a bisphosphonate (clodronate) inhibits bone loss in the ovariectomized rat, as evinced by decreased collagenase and Eta-1/Op mRNA, an observation that points to the utility of this approach in the treatment of osteoporosis (Binkert et al., 1999; Duncan et al., 1999; Ramamurthy et al., 2001; Stanford et al., 2000). Biphosphonates also help in wound healing of periodontal ligament cells (Lekic et al., 1996a,b, 1997); the bisphosphonate etidronate (ethane-1-hydroxy-1,1-bisphosphonate) promotes osteoblast differentiation and wound closure in rat calvaria by increasing Eta-1/Op expression and osteoid/mineralized tissue formation and by reducing the proliferation of precursor cells (D'Aoust et al., 2000).

JOINTS AND TENDONS

Endochondral bone formation is one of the most extensively examined developmental sequences within vertebrates (Gerstenfeld and Shapiro, 1996). This process involves the coordinated temporal/spatial differentiation of three separate tissues (cartilage, bone, and the vasculature) into a variety of complex structures. In the embryonic growth plate, Eta-1/Op expression is found in bone-forming cells and in hypertrophic chondrocytes (Inada et al., 1999; Pullig et al., 2000; Stern, Glimcher, et al., 1995; Stern, Tatrai, et al., 1995; Sun and Kandel, 1999; Yoshida et al., 2001). The differentiation of chondrocytes during this process is characterized by a progressive morphological change associated with the eventual hypertrophy of these cells. These cellular morphological changes are coordinated with proliferation, a columnar orientation of the cells, and the expression of unique phenotypic properties including type X collagen, high levels of bone, liver, and kidney alkaline phosphatase, and mineralization of the cartilage matrix. Several studies indicate that hypertrophic chondrocytes express Eta-1/Op, osteocalcin, and bone sialoprotein. The calcitropic hormones, morphogenic steroids, and local tissue factors regulate hypertrophic chondrocytes. These considerations are based on the regulation by 1,25 $(OH)_2D_3$ and retinoids of the cartilage specific genes as well as Eta-1/Op and osteocalcin expression in hypertrophic chondrocytes, cells that are functionally coupled during endochondral bone formation to functions influenced or mediated by Eta-1/Op, such as the recruitment of osteoblasts, vascular cells, and osteoclasts (Akazawa et al., 2000; Gerstenfeld and Shapiro, 1996).

Binette et al. (1998) studied chondrocytes that were isolated from adult human articular cartilage and changed phenotype during monolayer tissue culture, as characterized by a fibroblastic morphology and cellular proliferation. Increased proliferation was accompanied by down-regulation of the cartilage-specific extracellular matrix proteoglycan, aggrecan, by cessation of type-II collagen expression, and by up-regulation of type-I collagen and versican. This phenomenon observed in monolayer was reversible after the transfer of cells to a suspension culture system. The transfer of chondrocytes to suspension culture in alginate beads resulted in the rapid up-regulation of aggrecan and type-II collagen and the down-regulation of expression of versican and type-I collagen. Type-X collagen and Eta-1/Op, markers of chondrocyte hypertrophy and commitment to endochondral ossification, were not expressed by adult articular chondrocytes cultured in alginate, even after five months. In contrast, type-X collagen was expressed within two weeks in a population of cells derived from a fetal growth plate. The inability of adult articular chondrocytes to express markers of chondrocyte hypertrophy has underscored the fundamental distinction between the differentiation pathways that lead to articular cartilage or to bone. Adult articular chondrocytes expressed only hyaline articular cartilage markers without evidence of hypertrophy (Binette et al., 1998).

Castagnola et al. (1991) reported that Eta-1/Op mRNA was detected in sternal resting chondrocytes at higher levels than in hypertrophic chondrocytes; therefore Eta-1/Op gene transcription occurs in chondrocytes at many stages of differentiation. The steady state level of Eta-1/Op mRNA was enhanced by trypsin treatment of cultured cells. Castagnola et al. (1991) also observed an increased level of Eta-1/Op mRNA in quail chondrocytes constitutively expressing the v-myc oncogene. In contrast to the absence of expression in normal cartilage, Eta-1/Op is overexpressed in osteoarthritic cartilage (Attur et al., 2000, 2001; Martin et al., 2001; Pullig et al., 2000), and, in a qualitative analysis, Pullig et al. (2000) documented that Eta-1/Op protein deposition and mRNA expression increase with the severity of the osteoarthritic lesions and the disintegration of the cartilaginous matrix. Eta-1/Op expression in the cartilage is limited to the chondrocytes of the upper deep zone, showing cellular and territorial deposition, and in clusters of proliferating chondrocytes from samples with severe osteoarthritic lesions. These data suggest that chondrocyte differentiation and the expression of differentiation markers in osteoarthritic cartilage resembles that of epiphyseal growth plate chondrocytes (Pullig et al., 2000). Eta-1/Op and hyaluronan, and their CD44 receptor, are also found in the synovial membranelike interface tissue around loosened total hip prostheses, a synovial membrane similar to that found in osteoarthritis (Konttinen et al., 2001).

Although interleukin-1β induces Eta-1/Op expression in human articular chondrocytes (Margerie et al., 1997), Attur et al. (2001) point out that one of the functions of intraarticular Eta-1/Op, which is overexpressed in osteoarthritic cartilage (Attur et al., 2000, 2001; Martin et al., 2001; Pullig et al., 2000), is to act as an innate inhibitor of inflammation by inhibiting the spontaneous and interleukin-1β-induced production of nitric oxide and prostaglandin E2 production. These findings suggest that the production of pleiotropic mediators of inflammation which influence cartilage homeostasis, such as nitric oxide and prostaglandin E2, is regulated by the interaction of chondrocytes with differentially expressed proteins, such as Eta-1/Op, within the extracellular matrix (Attur et al., 2001). The extracellular matrix is an "information-rich" environment and interactions between the chondrocyte and extracellular matrix regulate many biological processes important to cartilage homeostasis and repair including cell attachment, growth, differentiation, and survival. The integrin family of cell surface receptors appears to play a major role in mediating cell-matrix interactions that are important in regulating these processes. Chondrocytes have been found to express several members of the integrin family, which can serve as receptors for fibronectin (α5β1), types II and VI collagen (α1β1, α2β1, α10β1), laminin (α6β1), and vitronectin and Eta-1/Op (αvβ3) (Attur et al., 2000). Integrin expression can be regulated by growth factors including IGF-I and TGF-β. By providing a link between the extracellular matrix (ECM) and the cytoskeleton, integrins may be important transducers of mechanical stimuli. Integrin binding stimulates intracellular signaling, which in turn can affect gene expression and regulate chondrocyte function (Loeser, 2000).

Functional genomic analysis shows that the engagement of the integrin receptors α5β1 and αvβ3 of fibronectin and Eta-1/Op, respectively, have profound effects on chondrocyte functions. Ligation of α5β1 using activating mAb JBS5 (which acts as agonist similar to fibronectin N-terminal fragment) up-regulates the inflammatory mediators such as nitric oxide and PGE2 as well as the cytokines, IL-6 and IL-8. Furthermore, up-regulation of these proinflammatory mediators by α5β1 integrin ligation is mediated via induction and autocrine production of IL-1β, because type II soluble IL-1 decoy receptor inhibits their production. In contrast, αvβ3 complex-specific function-blocking mAb (LM609), which acts as an agonist similar to Eta-1/Op, attenuates the production of IL-1β, NO, and PGE2 (triggered by α5β1, IL-1β, IL-18, or IL-1β plus LPS, TNF-α, plus LPS) in a dominant negative fashion by osteoarthritis-affected cartilage and activated bovine chondrocytes. These data demonstrate a cross-talk in signaling mechanisms among integrins and show that integrin-mediated "outside in" and "inside out" signaling very likely influences cartilage homeostasis, and its deregulation may play a role in the pathogenesis of osteoarthritis (Attur et al., 2000).

As another mechanism for Eta-1/Op-associated involvement in arthritic pathologies, Sakata et al. (2001) reported that almost 10 percent of patients with osteoarthritis and 15 percent of patients with rheumatoid arthritis studied display autoimmunity against Eta-1/Op. The anti-Eta-1/Op-positive rheumatoid arthritis patients showed high serum levels of rheumatoid factor and C-reactive protein and accelerated erythrocyte sedimentation rate compared to the anti-Eta-1/Op-negative group, although the differences did not achieve statistical significance. These observations are relevant because Eta-1/Op, secreted mainly from chondrocytes, is involved in ossification and remodeling of bone (Nishida et al., 2000). Cell types other than chondrocytes also influence and are influenced by Eta-1/Op expression in normal and arthritic bone and cartilage. In situ hybridization and immunocytochemical analysis of Eta-1/Op localization in Meckel's cartilage cells, which bipotentially expressed cartilage and bone phenotypes during cellular transformation in vitro, revealed that Eta-1/Op was synthesized by cells that were autonomously undergoing a change from chondrocytes to bone-forming cells at the top of nodules (Ishizeki et al., 1999). Double immunofluorescence staining of two-week-old cultures revealed that chondrocytic cells at the top of nodules first synthesized Eta-1/Op. After further time in culture, the distribution of Eta-1/Op expanded from the central toward the peripheral regions of the nodules. Electron probe microanalysis revealed that the localization of Eta-1/Op was associated with matrices of calcified cartilage and osteoid nodules that contained calcium and phosphorus. Immunoperoxidase electron microscopy revealed that, in addition to the intracellular immunoreactivity in chondrocytes and small round cells that were undergoing transformation, matrix foci of calcospherites and matrix vesicles, in particular, included growing crystals that were immunopositive for Eta-1/Op. An intense signal due to mRNA for Eta-1/Op in three-week-old cultures was detected in nodule-forming round cells, while fibroblastic cells, spreading in a monolayer over the periphery of nodules, were only weakly labeled. These findings indicate that Eta-1/Op might be expressed sequentially by chondrocytes and by cells which are transdifferentiating further and which exhibit an osteocytic phenotype—and moreover, that expression of Eta-1/Op is closely associated with calcifying foci in the extracellular matrix (Ishizeki et al., 1999).

Chenoufi et al. (2001) showed that in vitro differentiated primary human osteoblasts from osteoarthritic and rheumatoid arthritic bone, in contrast to those from nonarthritic bone, constitutively secreted high levels of intelerleukin-6, the maximal expression of which corresponded to the mineralization stage reflected by decreasing Eta-1/Op, collagen I (α_1), bone sialoprotein, and alkaline phosphatase mRNA levels, and by increasing osteocalcin mRNA levels. The latter inherent property suggests that osteoblasts, independent of local inflammatory parameters, can also contribute to enhanced recruitment of osteoclast progenitors and thereby bone resorption. Eta-1/Op produced by synovial fibroblasts in the synovial lining layer and at sites of cartilage invasion not only mediates attachment of these cells to cartilage but also contributes to matrix degradation in rheumatoid arthritis by stimulating the secretion of collagenase 1 in articular chondrocytes (Petrow et al., 2000). Eta-1/Op is involved in the interactions between tumor cells and host matrix, including those involved in the invasion and spread of tumor cells, and similarly joint destruction in rheumatoid arthritis is mediated by the invasive growth of synovial tissue through its attachment to cartilage (Petrow et al., 2000). Eta-1/Op is expressed in the synovial lining and sublining layer and at the interface of cartilage and invading synovium (Petrow et al., 2000). Double labeling revealed that the majority of Eta-1/Op-expressing cells are positive for the fibroblast-specific enzyme prolyl 4-hydroxylase and negative for the macrophage marker CD68, while only a few, single Eta-1/Op-expressing cells were positive for CD68 at sites of synovial invasion into cartilage. Eta-1/Op staining was not observed in lymphocytic infiltrates or leukocyte common antigen (CD45)-positive cells. Three of three cultures of human articular chondrocytes secreted detectable basal amounts of collagenase, with a dose-dependent increase upon Eta-1/Op stimulation, while synovial fibroblast cultures produced much lower levels of collagenase, with only two of four fibroblast cultures responding in a dose-dependent manner (Petrow et al., 2000).

Calcifying tendinitis of rotator cuff tendons is a common and painful condition caused by ectopic calcification in humans. Eta-1/Op is involved in the process of calcification of rotator cuff tendons and it is produced in two cell types surrounding, but not away from, the calcified area: fibroblast-like cells negative for CD68 and tartrate-resistant acid phosphatase (TRAP) and multinucleated macrophages positive for CD68 and TRAP (Takeuchi et al., 2001). Two forms of Eta-1/Op (67 and 61 kDa) are also synthesized during development of mineralized nodules by rat periodontal ligament cells in vitro (Ramakrishnan et al., 1995).

SKIN

Eta-1/Op is one of several matrix molecules associated with elastin in normal skin fiber (Pasquali-Ronchetti and Baccarani-Contri, 1997). Elastin molecules aggregate in the extracellular space where they are cross-linked by stable desmosine bridges. The resulting polymer is structurally organized as branched fibers and lamellae, which, in skin, are wider (a few microns) in the deep dermis and become progressively thinner (fraction of a micron) toward the papillary dermis. Several general and local factors seem to regulate elastin gene expression, deposition, and degradation. In skin, the volume density of the elastin network increases from birth up to maturity, when it accounts for about 3 to 4 percent of the tissue. However, its amount and distribution depend on dermis areas, which are different among subjects and change with age. Several matrix molecules (glycosaminoglycans, decorin, biglycan, and Eta-1/Op) have been found to be associated with elastin in normal fiber, and several others have been recognized within pathologic elastic fiber (osteonectin, vitronectin, alkaline phosphatase in PXE). With age, and in some pathologic conditions, skin elastin may undergo irreversible structural and compositional changes, which seem to progress from localized deposition of osmiophilic materials to the substitution of the great majority of the amorphous elastin with interwoven filaments negative for elastin-specific antibodies (Pasquali-Ronchetti and Baccarani-Contri, 1997). Eta-1/Op and other matrix proteins with high affinity for calcium ions are associated with mineralization within the elastic fibers of pseudoxanthoma elasticum dermis (Contri et al., 1996).

Eta-1/Op is an in vitro and in vivo substrate of tissue transglutaminase which catalyzes formation of cross-linked protein aggregates. Transglutaminase treatment significantly increases the binding of Eta-1/Op to collagen, an interaction that is calcium- and Eta-1/Op-conformation-dependent. Circular dichroism analysis of monomeric and polymeric Eta-1/Op indicates that transglutaminase treatment induces a conformational change in Eta-1/Op, probably exposing motives relevant to its interactions with other extracellular molecules. This altered collagen binding property of Eta-1/Op may have relevance to its biological functions in tissue repair, bone remodeling, and collagen fibrillogenesis (Kaartinen et al., 1999). Transglutaminase-catalyzed cross-linking of Eta-1/Op is inhibited by osteocalcin (Kaartinen et al., 1997), the most abundant noncollagenous protein of bone matrix that inhibits bone growth. Using a set of synthetic peptides, Kaartinen et al. (1997) found that the inhibitory activity resides within the first 13 N-terminal amino acid residues of osteocalcin, and the N-terminal peptide also inhibits cross-linking of another tissue transglutaminase substrate, β-casein. Since the N terminus of osteocalcin exhibits homology to the substrate recognition site sequences of two transglutaminases, the inhibitory effect is most likely secondary to competition with the enzyme for the transglutaminase-binding region of the substrates, Eta-1/Op and β-casein, which prevents access of the enzyme to them to perform its function.

Studies in Eta-1/Op null mutant mice, generated by targeted mutagenesis in embryonic stem cells, have evinced a role for Eta-1/Op in tissue remodeling in vivo, and suggest physiological functions during matrix reorganization after injury (Liaw et al., 1998). In Eta-1/Op mutant mice, embryogenesis occurs normally and mice are fertile, an observation that points to the presence of proteins similar to Eta-1/Op that can compensate for its absence. However, although Eta-1/Op expression is up-regulated as early as six hours after skin wounding by incisions, and the tensile properties of the wounds are unchanged, ultrastructural analysis shows a significantly decreased level of debridement, greater disorganization of matrix, and an alteration of collagen fibrillogenesis leading to small diameter collagen fibrils in the Eta-1/Op mutant mice (Liaw et al., 1998).

Chitosan is a copolymer of β(1→4) glucosamine and N-acetyl-D-glucosamine, which accelerates the infiltration of polymorphonuclear leukocytes (PMN) in the early phase of wound healing. In the granulation tissue treated with chitosan in canine experimental wound, Eta-1/Op was strongly positive in PMN immunohistochemically (Ueno et al., 2001). Moreover, PMN stimulated with granulocyte-colony stimulating factor (G-CSF) and chitosan accumulated Eta-1/Op mRNA, and released

Eta-1/Op into their culture supernatant fluids. These findings suggest that Eta-1/Op is synthesized by migrating PMN, an activity which regulates the evolution of wound healing with chitosan treatment at the early phase of healing (Ueno et al., 2001).

Giachelli et al. (1998) investigated the role of Eta-1/Op in intradermal macrophage infiltration using immunohistochemistry and neutralizing antibodies. Purified Eta-1/Op induced macrophage accumulation after injection in rat dermis and facilitated adhesion and migration of cultured macrophage-like cells in vitro. Intradermal injection of N-formyl-met-leu-phe (FMLP), a potent macrophage chemotactic peptide, induced a macrophage-rich infiltrate at the site of injection. Most of these macrophages expressed high levels of Eta-1/Op as shown by immunochemical analysis. FMLP-induced macrophage accumulation was largely inhibited (>60 percent) by anti-Eta-1/Op antibody treatment compared with rats receiving nonimmune antibody. These data indicate that Eta-1/Op may be a critical mediator of inflammation in specific disease and injury states, potentially by promoting macrophage adhesion and migration (Giachelli et al., 1998).

RENAL SYSTEM

In the kidney, Eta-1/Op is expressed in the renal tubules and collecting ducts and is excreted into the urine (Crivello and Delvin, 1992; Denda, 1999; Gang et al., 2001; Koka et al., 2000; Lopez et al., 1993; Maslamani et al., 2000; Nemir et al., 1989; Worcester et al., 1995). Singh et al. (1992) confirmed the identity of normal rat kidney (NRK) cell-secreted 69 kDa major phosphoprotein as Eta-1/Op (Nemir et al., 1989). Eta-1/Op is expressed in the human embryonic renal tubular epithelium beginning on approximately day 75 to 80 of gestation (Hudkins et al., 1999). In the fetal kidney, Eta-1/Op can also be seen occasionally expressed in the ureteric buds and in some interstitial cells. Eta-1/Op is a ligand for the integrin $\alpha8\beta1$, an interaction that is involved in kidney development and other morphogenetic processes based on the observations that epithelio-mesenchymal interactions during kidney organogenesis are disrupted in integrin $\alpha8\beta1$-deficient mice and that anti-Eta-1/Op antibodies disrupt kidney morphogenesis (Denda et al., 1998). Eta-1/Op plays an important antiapoptotic role during the process of metanephric blastema condensation that is a prerequisite for the formation of nephrons in vivo (Rogers et al., 1997). As localized at the protein and mRNA level, the tubular expression of Eta-1/Op increases with increasing gestational age and persists into adulthood. Eta-1/Op is present in the filamentous glycocalyx, small apical cytoplasmic smooth membrane-bound vesicles, large membrane-bound cytoplasmic granules, and in portions of the Golgi complex in gallbladder columnar epithelial cells (Qu-Hong et al., 1994). These findings suggest that newly synthesized Eta-1/Op is packaged in Golgi-derived granules that release their contents by classical exocytosis from the cell surface. At least a portion of secreted Eta-1/Op remains on the cell surface, where it becomes integrated into the filamentous glycocalyx coating the luminal surface of gallbladder epithelial cells (Qu-Hong et al., 1994).

In the normal adult kidney, Eta-1/Op is localized primarily to the distal nephron and is strongly expressed by the thick ascending limb of the loops of Henle (Lopez et al., 1993; Madsen et al., 1997; Muller and Strutz, 1995). Eta-1/Op expression can also be observed in some collecting duct epithelium (Hudkins et al., 1999). High salt concentration or salt crystal enhances Eta-1/Op expression in intact kidney or cultured renal cells. Cha et al. (2000) showed that in rats fed a normal sodium diet, Eta-1/Op mRNA and protein were expressed only in the descending thin limbs of Henle's loop (DTL) and in the papillary and pelvic surface epithelium (PSE), while in rats fed a sodium-deficient diet or in those injected with lipopolysaccharide, there was a marked decrease in Eta-1/Op immunoreactivity (but not in mRNA levels) in the DTL, but no changes in the PSE (Cha et al., 2000; Madsen et al., 1997). These results suggest that dietary sodium may be involved in the regulation of Eta-1/Op expression in the DTL of the rat kidney (Cha et al., 2000).

Eta-1/Op isolated from human urine is a potent inhibitor of calcium oxalate (CaOx) monohydrate (COM) crystallization (Hedgepeth et al., 2001; Honda et al., 1997; Hoyer, 1994; Hoyer et al., 1995, 2001; Jiang et al., 1998; Khan and Thamilselvan, 2000; Kleinman, Beshensky, et al., 1995; Kleinman, Worcester, et al., 1995; Min et al., 1998; Nishio, Hatanaka, et al., 2000; Nishio, Iseda, et al., 2000; Nishio, Neo, et al., 2000; Ryall, 1996; Scheid et al., 2000; Shiraga et al., 1992; Sorensen, Hojrup, et al., 1995; Sorensen, Justesen, et al., 1995; Suzuki, 1999; Umekawa, 1999; Worcester, 1994; Worcester and

Beshensky, 1995; Worcester et al., 1992; Yagisawa et al., 1998), and oxalate exposure up-regulates Eta-1/Op expression in renal cells (Jonassen et al., 1999; Lieske, Hammes, et al., 1997; Lieske, Norris, et al., 1997). Urine from patients with a high frequency of kidney stones contains serine proteases that contribute to proteolytic cleavage of Eta-1/Op (Bautista, Denstedt, et al., 1996; Bautista, Saad, et al., 1996). Min et al. (1998) reported that Eta-1/Op concentration varies inversely with urine volume, a feature that favors protection from urinary crystallization of calcium oxalate by Eta-1/Op. The natural defense against nephrolithiasis may include impeding crystal attachment by an effect of macromolecular inhibitors, such as Eta-1/Op, on the preferred CaOx crystal structure that forms in urine (Wesson et al., 1998). In a study with Eta-1/Op-derived peptides, Hoyer et al. (2001) reported that growth of COM crystals was inhibited by approximately 50 percent by two unmodified Eta-1/Op peptides with the closest clustering of aspartic acid residues, while growth was not inhibited by two other unmodified peptides, with aspartic residues more evenly distributed within their sequences. Phosphorylation of peptides markedly increased inhibition of COM crystal growth but did not cause changes in secondary structure that would favor interaction with COM crystal surfaces. Therefore, the inhibition of crystal growth induced by phosphorylation appears to result from altered local patterns of charge density (Hoyer et al., 2001).

Studies in rats have revealed that testosterone appears to promote stone formation by suppressing Eta-1/Op expression in the kidneys and increasing urinary oxalate excretion, while estrogen appears to inhibit stone formation by increasing Eta-1/Op expression in the kidneys and decreasing urinary oxalate excretion (Iguchi et al., 1999; Umekawa, Kohri, et al., 1995; Umekawa, Yamate, et al., 1995; Yagisawa et al., 1998). Increased risk of renal stone formation during space flight has been linked primarily to increased calcium excretion from bone demineralization induced by space flight, and to increased urinary calcium oxalate supersaturation, while urinary citrate, magnesium, and volume are all decreased. Although Hoyer et al. (1999) failed to observe a compensatory increase in urinary Eta-1/Op excretion during space flight, the Eta-1/Op excretion of a majority of astronauts was increased during the period after space flight and was maximal at two weeks after landing.

Yamate et al. (2000) investigated hereditary predisposing factors for urolithiasis, by assessing changes in Eta-1/Op DNA within a family with familial urolithiasis, controls, and patients with recurrent urinary calculi. Eta-1/Op DNA nucleotide sequencing revealed a mutation of GCC to GCT, encoding amino acid position 250 (Ala-250). On examining the frequency of this mutation, the ratio of normal homozygous GCC was 11/36 in the control group, 1/25 in familial urolithiasis, and 1/40 in recurrent urolithiasis. The gene frequency of the normal codon GCC was 0.528 in the control group, 0.3 in familial urolithiasis and 0.35 in recurrent urolithiasis, showing a significantly higher incidence in the control group. On the other hand, the gene frequency of mutated GCT was 0.472 in control group, 0.7 in familial urolithiasis, and 0.65 in recurrent urolithiasis, showing a significantly higher incidence in urolithiasis patients. On investigating the inheritance of Ala-250 in five families in which both parent and offspring demonstrated urolithiasis, the nucleotide substitution in Ala-250 in parents with urolithiasis was inherited by their offspring. In all five families the offspring developed urinary calculus. This study showed that there is no difference in Eta-1/Op structure between the control group and urolithiasis patients. However, it was predicted that because of the frequency of normally coded GCC being high in the control group a difference in the amount of Eta-1/Op might be caused by a difference in transcription velocity between the two groups. Therefore, examining the inheritance of Ala-250 within a family may be a diagnostic method for identifying the predisposing hereditary factors for urolithiasis patients (Yamate et al., 2000).

In contrast to the studies mentioned, Eta-1/Op in the extracellular matrix was found to be the main cause of CaOx crystal deposition on the surface of Madin-Darby canine kidney cell membranes (Losch and Koch-Brandt, 1995; Ullrich et al., 1991; Yamate et al., 1996, 1998, 1999), which have stone-forming potential when inoculated in nude mice (Sakakura et al., 1999). Eta-1/Op and calprotectin play roles as the matrix in the structure of urinary calcium stones (Atmani et al., 1996, 1998, 1999; De Bruijn et al., 1996, 1997; Gokhale et al., 1996; Ito, 1996; Kajikawa, 1998; Khan, 1997; Kohri et al., 1992, 1993; Lieske, Hammes, et al., 1997; Lieske, Norris, et al., 1997; McKee et al., 1995; Tawada et al., 1999; Umekawa, Kohri, et al., 1995; Umekawa, Yamate, et al., 1995; Yamate, Mocharla, et al.,

1997; Yamate, Umekawa, et al., 1997). Administration to rats of the oxalate precursor ethylene glycol increased calcium oxalate stone formation and Eta-1/Op expression (Yasui, Fujita, Sasaki, et al., 1999), an effect that was decreased by takusha, a kampo medicine that decreases renal stone formation and Eta-1/Op expression (Yasui, Fujita, Sato, et al., 1999). In another rat urolithiasis model, citrate prevented renal stone formation by acting against not only the calcium oxalate crystal aggregation and growth of calcium oxalate but also by inhibiting Eta-1/Op expression (Yasui, Sato, Fujita, Tozawa, et al., 2001). Likewise, allopurinol prevents renal calcium oxalate stone formation by acting against not only the control of oxalate but also by reducing Eta-1/Op expression (Yasui, Sato, Fujita, Ito, et al., 2001). Eta-1/Op expression is enhanced in the distal tubular cells of hypercalcemic rats and is decreased by alendronate, a biphosphonate derivative that inhibits bone resorption and may also act as inhibitor of stone formation in the urinary tract (Yasui et al., 1998). Moreover, low urinary concentrations of Eta-1/Op and prothrombin F1 but not α2-HS-glycoprotein are associated with calcium phosphate stone formation (Nishio et al., 1999; Nishio, Hatanaka, et al., 2000; Nishio, Iseda, et al., 2000; Nishio, Neo, et al., 2000). Yasui, Fujita, Sato, et al. (1999) suggest that urinary Eta-1/Op levels are decreased in these cases because of Eta-1/Op incorporation by kidney stones.

Eta-1/Op expression is induced in both proximal and distal tubular cells during rat toxic acute renal failure induced by mercuric chloride or gentamicin administration; the distinct subcellular localization in proximal (perinuclear vesicular staining) versus distal (apical cell membrane) tubular cells indicates differences in Eta-1/Op processing and/or handling (Verstrepen et al., 2001). The latter Eta-1/Op staining pattern was also seen in renal ischemia/reperfusion injury in rats (Padanilam, 1996; Persy et al., 1999). Interestingly, Eta-1/Op expression up-regulation is involved in both the injury and the recovery from gentamicin-induced acute tubular necrosis (Xie, Nishi, et al., 2001; Xie, Pimental, et al., 2001), and in early interstitial macrophage influx and interstitial fibrosis in unilateral ureteral obstruction and as a survival factor for renal tubulointerstitial cells (Ophascharoensuk et al., 1998, 1999). Two distinct epithelial responses may compensate for the ureteral obstruction in the early and late phases of unilateral ureteral obstruction-treated rat: cellular proliferation in acute phase and Eta-1/Op expression in chronic phase (Sakai et al., 1997). Eta-1/Op expression also is up-regulated in a murine model of experimentally induced protein-overload proteinuria (Nagasawa et al., 1991). Chronic hypokalemia has been associated with renal hypertrophy, interstitial disease, and hypertension in both adult animals and humans (Ray et al., 2001). Chronically potassium-depleted animals have significant growth retardation and increased renin-angiotensin system activity, manifested by high plasma renin activity, recruitment of renin-producing cells along the afferent arterioles, and down-regulation of angiotensin II receptors in renal glomeruli and ascending vasa rectae. Potassium-depleted kidneys also show tubulointerstitial injury with tubular cell proliferation, Eta-1/Op expression, macrophage infiltration, and early fibrosis (Ray et al., 2001).

Up-regulation of Eta-1/Op expression by proximal tubular epithelium has been demonstrated in both human and rodent models of renal injury in association with macrophage influx (Abbate et al., 1998; Baud, 1996; Couser and Johnson, 1994; Diamond et al., 1995; Eddy, 1994, 1996; Eddy and Giachelli, 1995; Floege et al., 1997; Hartner et al., 2001; Hudkins et al., 2000; Kleinman, Beshensky, et al., 1995; Kleinman, Worcester, et al., 1995; Lan et al., 1998; Malyankar et al., 1997; Nagasaki et al., 1997; Narita et al., 1997; Okada, Moriwaki, Kalluri, et al., 2000; Okada, Moriwaki, Konishi, et al., 2000; Pichler et al., 1994; Pichler, Franceschini, et al., 1995; Pichler, Giachelli, et al., 1995; Prols, Heidgress, et al., 1998; Young et al., 1995). Eta-1/Op is up-regulated in chronic puromycin aminonucleoside nephrosis (Magil et al., 1997). Glomerular Eta-1/Op expression and macrophage infiltration occur in chronic hypertensive glomerulosclerosis and in glomerulosclerosis of deoxycorticosterone acetate (DOCA)-salt rats (Hartner et al., 2001), as well as in salt-sensitive hypertension (Johnson, Burghardt, et al., 1999; Johnson, Gordon, et al., 1999; Johnson, Spencer, et al., 1999; Thomas, Lombardi, et al., 1998). Progressive glomerular macrophage infiltration parallels development of DOCA hypertension and the degree of glomerulosclerosis, and glomeruli staining positive for Eta-1/Op contains more macrophages than Eta-1/Op-negative glomeruli (Hartner et al., 2001). IL-1β induces MCP-1, CINC, RANTES, and ICAM-1 gene expression in a time-dependent manner in cultured rat mesangial cells (Lee et al., 1998). IL-1β-induced MCP-1, CINC, and ICAM-1 mRNA amounts are maximal at three hours exposure around 14.5, 15.7, and 2.2 folds increase, and IL-1β-induced RANTES mRNA at 24 hours around 2.0 folds. TNF-α and LPS also induce MCP-1 and ICAM-1 gene expression. TNF-α induces RANTES gene expression, but LPS does not. On the other hand, IL-1β, TNF-α, and LPS had little effect on Eta-1/Op gene expression but fetal calf serum could increase Eta-1/Op mRNA. Dexamethasone suppressed the IL-1β-induced MCP-1 and CINC mRNA. These results suggest that, through these gene expressions, mesangial cells are able to communicate directly or indirectly with macrophages or neutrophils, which may lead to glomerulosclerosis (Lan et al., 1998; Lee et al., 1998). IL-1 also up-regulates Eta-1/Op expression in rat antiglomerular basement membrane glomerulonephritis, and inhibition of Eta-1/Op expression is one mechanism by which IL-1 receptor antagonist treatment suppresses macrophage-mediated renal injury (Yu et al., 1998, 1999).

There is significant expression of the angiotensin type II receptor (AT2R) in the adult kidney, and AT2R has a role in mediating angiotensin II-induced proliferation and apoptosis in proximal tubular epithelial cells and up-regulation of Eta-1/Op expression (Cao et al., 2000; Diamond, Kreisberg, et al., 1998; Diamond, Ricardo, et al., 1998). Angiotensin II plays a pivotal role in the progression of renal diseases, including obstructive nephropathy (Giachelli, 1994; Klahr, 2001; Klahr and Morrissey, 2000; Pichler, Franceschini, et al., 1995; Pichler, Giachelli, et al., 1995; Truong et al., 1998), and increasing levels of angiotensin II in obstructive nephropathy up-regulate the expression of Eta-1/Op and other factors: transforming growth factor (TGF)-β1, tumor necrosis factor(TNF)-α, platelet-derived growth factor (PDGF), insulin-like growth factor (IGF-1), vascular cell adhesion molecule-1 (VCAM-1), nuclear factor-kappaB (NF-kappaB), monocyte chemoattractant peptide-1 (MCP-1), intercellular adhesion molecule-1 (ICAM-1), and CD14, among others (Diamond, Kreisberg, et al., 1998; Diamond, Ricardo, et al., 1998; Giachelli, 1994; Kaneto et al., 1998; Klahr and Morrissey, 2000; Lombardi et al., 2001: Ricardo et al., 2000; Truong et al., 1998). Local production of TGF-β, by intrinsic renal cells or by macrophages invading the kidney, is a key mediator of renal fibrosis. Activation of TGF-β stimulates endothelin production; endothelin, in turn, is a potent stimulus for fibrogenesis and also stimulates Eta-1/Op expression (Benigni and Remuzzi, 1996; Nambi et al., 1997). Antisense oligonucleotide inhibition of angiotensinogen and angiotensin II receptor translation in rat proximal tubules results in down-regulation of Eta-1/Op expression induced by cell stretch (Ricardo et al., 2000). Therefore stretch-induced up-regulation of Eta-1/Op mRNA expression is mediated, in part, via production of angiotensin II, and Eta-1/Op up-regulation leads to macrophage infiltration in the tubulointerstitium in experimental hydronephrosis (Ricardo et al., 2000). Up-regulation of Eta-1/Op expression in renal cortex of streptozotocin-induced diabetic nephropathy in Wistar rats is mediated by bradykinin (Fischer et al., 1998; Patel et al., 1996, 1997a,b). A number of pharmacologic interventions that ameliorate the increased expansion of the interstitial volume, decrease the expression of TGF-β, and down-regulate the production of extracellular matrix, such as Eta-1/Op, and the infiltration of the interstitium by macrophages include ACE inhibitors, administration of arginine, administration of osteogenic protein-1, and Pirferidone, among others (Klahr, 2001; Klahr and Morrissey, 2000).

CD44-ligand interactions are involved in the regenerating proximal tubule during recovery after ischemic injury (Lewington et al., 2000) and in leukocyte infiltration in crescentic glomerulonephritis (Lan et al., 1998) and interstitial nephritis (Sibalic et al., 1997). Eta-1/Op, not normally expressed in the renal proximal tubule, is expressed in regenerating tubules by three days after induction of acute ischemic injury (Pawar et al., 1995). Immunoreactive Eta-1/Op peptide continues to be localized in those tubules still undergoing repair for as long as seven days after the injury. Although no expression is detectable in nonischemic kidneys, several mRNAs for CD44 are present within one day after injury: CD44 mRNA is expressed in proximal tubules undergoing repair, and CD44 peptide is present in basal and lateral cell membranes (Lewington et al., 2000).

Patients with primary glomerular diseases show differential excretion of Eta-1/Op: a reduction, compared to normal controls, of urinary excretion of intact and thrombin-cleaved Eta-1/Op is seen in patients with immunoglobulin (Ig) A nephropathy, but not in those with minimal change nephrotic syndrome or with membranous nephropathy (Gang et al., 2001). However, Okada, Moriwaki, Kalluri, et al. (2000) and Okada, Moriwaki, Konishi, et al. (2000) reported that Eta-1/Op expression was up-regulated in the cytoplasm of proximal and distal tubular epithelium parallel to the degree of interstitial mononuclear cell infiltration in patients with IgA nephropathy, results that are congruent with those of Hudkins et al. (2000). Bonvini et al. (2000), using Eta-1/Op knockout mice, also showed up-regulation of Eta-1/Op in murine antiglomerular basement membrane nephritis but concluded that it does not significantly contribute to the glomerular and tubulointerstitial mononuclear cell infiltration in this model (Bonvini et al., 2000). In contrast to the latter observation, Okada, Moriwaki, Kalluri, et al. (2000) and Okada, Moriwaki, Konishi, et al. (2000) injected Eta-1/Op antisense to Goodpasture syndrome (GPS) rats every second day between days 27 and 35, the time when renal Eta-1/Op expression increases and interstitial monocyte infiltration is aggravated. In parallel to blockade of tubular Eta-1/Op expression, this treatment significantly attenuated monocyte infiltration and preserved renal plasma flow in GPS rats at day 37, compared with sense Eta-1/Op-treated and untreated GPS rats. Therefore, Eta-1/Op expressed by tubular epithelium appears to play a pivotal role in mediating peritubular monocyte infiltration consequent to glomerular disease (Abbate et al., 1998; Okada, Moriwaki, Kalluri, et al., 2000; Okada, Moriwaki, Konishi, et al., 2000).

Progressive autosomal dominant polycystic kidney disease, in which tubule cells proliferate, causing segmental dilation in association with the abnormal deposition of extracellular matrix proteins, is associated with the cellular expression of chemokines (Eta-1/Op, MCP-1), proto-oncogenes (fos, myc, ras, erb), growth factors (EGF, HGF, acid and basic FGF), metalloproteinases, and apoptotic markers, and the interstitial accumulation of Types I and IV collagen, laminin, fibronectin, macrophages, and fibroblasts, the magnitudes of which increase with age (Grantham, 1997). Endogenous iNOS-derived nitric oxide has a protective role against tubulointerstitial injury and production of cytokines, such as Eta-1/Op, in adriamycin nephropathy (Rangan et al., 2001). Inhibition of Eta-1/Op binding to αv integrin decreases TNF-α-induced nitric oxide synthesis in rat mesangial cells (Nagasaki et al., 1999). Tubular expression of Eta-1/Op, which is an inhibitor of nitric oxide synthase 2 (Hwang, Lopez, et al., 1994; Hwang, Wilson, et al., 1994), correlated with the systolic blood pressure in individual Dahl-salt sensitive rats (Johnson, Gordon, et al., 2000; Johnson, Spencer, et al., 2000). Inhibition of intrarenal nitric oxide production and activation of the renin-angiotensin system appear to be associated with the hyperuricemia that exacerbates chronic cyclosporine nephropathy in rats (Bennett, 1996; Mazzali et al., 1994). Enalapril and verapamil attenuate the cyclosporine nephrotoxicity by significantly blunting cyclosporine-induced Eta-1/Op and TGF-β gene expressions (Bennett, 1996; Lee, Lowe, et al., 1999; Lee, Park, et al., 1999; Lee, Shin, et al., 1999; Pichler, Franceschini, et al., 1995; Pichler, Giachelli, et al., 1995; Young et al., 1995). An up-regulation of Eta-1/Op expression may play a role in progressive renal injury following nephrectomy, and inhibition of Eta-1/Op expression may be one of the mechanisms by which angiotensin II blockade attenuates renal injury after renal ablation (Narita et al., 1997; Sawaya et al., 1997; Yu et al., 2000).

The remnant kidney model of progressive renal failure (renal injury after renal ablation) is associated with impaired angiogenesis and decreased vascular endothelial growth factor (VEGF) expression, and VEGF administration reduces renal fibrosis and stabilizes renal function, as shown by normalized nitric oxide and Eta-1/Op levels (Kang, Hughes, et al., 2001; Yu et al., 2000). As mentioned, cyclosporine-associated renal microvascular and tubulointerstitial injury results in the development of salt-sensitive hypertension, an effect that is also reduced by treatment with VEGF (Kang, Kim, et al., 2001) and vitamin E (Jenkins et al., 2001). The use of angiogenic factors may therefore represent an approach to the treatment of kidney disease (Kang, Hughes, et al., 2001; Kang, Kim, et al., 2001). Moreover, glomerular and peritubular capillary loss in the aging kidney also correlate with alterations in VEGF and thrombospondin-1 expression and with the development of glomerulosclerosis and tubulointerstitial fibrosis. In the latter setting, tubular VEGF expression correlates directly with peritubular capillary density and inversely with tubular Eta-1/Op and macrophage infiltration. These findings therefore suggest that impaired angiogenesis associated with progressive loss in renal microvasculature also may have a pivotal role in age-related nephropathy (Kang, Anderson, et al., 2001). Tubulointerstitial injury in aging, an active process associated with interstitial inflammation, fibroblast activation, and apoptotic cell losses in fibrotic areas, may be the consequence of ischemia secondary to peritubular capillary injury and altered iNOS and Eta-1/Op expression (Hwang, Lopez, et al., 1994; Hwang, Wilson, et al., 1994; Liang and Barnes, 1995; Thomas,

Anderson, et al., 1998). Manzano et al. (1999) pointed out that tretinoin, through inhibition of Eta-1/Op and TNF-β1, prevents age-related renal changes and stimulates antioxidant defenses in cultured renal mesangial cells.

Glomerular inflammation is characterized by a consecutive infiltration of immunoreactive cells (Rovin and Phan, 1998), and a coculture of platelets and renal mesangial cells is used to mimic the early phase of glomerular injury (Goppelt-Struebe et al., 2000). Cyclooxygenase (Cox)-2 and Eta-1/Op are independently up-regulated upon interaction of platelets with mesangial cells. The inhibition of the signaling pathways of platelet-derived growth factor (PDGF) and epidermal growth factor (EGF) or interference with G_i-protein signaling partially inhibited platelet-induced Cox-2 expression. Down-regulation of protein kinase C (PKC), which is a common signaling module in many pathways leading to Cox-2 induction, almost completely abrogated platelet-induced Cox-2 expression. The up-regulation of Eta-1/Op expression was dependent on de novo protein synthesis and was induced by high levels of exogenous prostaglandin E2 (PGE2; 10 μM/L). Endogenous PGE2, however, proved not to be essential for Eta-1/Op mRNA expression, because inhibition of Cox activity did not change Eta-1/Op mRNA levels. Dexamethasone inhibited Cox-2 mRNA induction but increased Eta-1/Op mRNA and protein expression (Goppelt-Struebe et al., 2000). Mycophenolic acid inhibits PDGF-induced Eta-1/Op expression in rat mesangial cells (Wang et al., 1999).

Human mesangial cells might be a target for the treatment of inflammatory glomerulopathies with 9-*cis* retinoic acid, an activator of both retinoic acid receptors and retinoid X receptors, because it inhibits Eta-1/Op expression (Manzano et al., 2000). Hypoxia in high glucose medium produces exaggerated rat mesangial cell growth and type IV collagen synthesis, a process that is mediated by Eta-1/Op and its β3-integrin receptor (Sodhi et al., 2001a,b). Eta-1/Op, but not endothelin or platelet-derived growth factor, expression mediates hypoxia-induced proliferation of mesangial cells. Hypoxia causes an activation of p38 mitogen-activated protein (MAP) kinase in a calcium- and PKC-dependent manner, activation that, in turn, appears to be involved in the stimulation of both Eta-1/Op and mesangial cell proliferation induced by hypoxia (Sahai et al., 1999; Sodhi et al., 2000).

The lack of detectable pathological manifestations in kidneys of mice with the targeted disruption of the Eta-1/Op gene (Eta-1/Op$^{-/-}$) makes them an excellent model for studies of pathophysiological processes that are accompanied by changes in renal Eta-1/Op expression. Indeed, comparative analysis of functional and morphological sequelae of acute renal ischemia in Eta-1/Op$^{+/+}$ and Eta-1/Op$^{-/-}$ mice provides strong evidence of the renoprotective action of Eta-1/Op in acute ischemia (Noiri et al., 1999). Control Eta-1/Op$^{+/+}$ mice showed a significant retention of blood urea nitrogen and creatinine, which is indicative of the development of ischemic acute renal dysfunction. This was accompanied by a 2.7-fold increase in the immunodetectable Eta-1/Op compared with sham-operated control. Animals with the disrupted Eta-1/Op gene exhibited ischemia-induced renal dysfunction, which was twice as pronounced as that observed in mice with the intact Eta-1/Op response to stress. In addition, the structural damage to the ischemic kidneys obtained from Eta-1/Op$^{-/-}$ mice was more pronounced than that observed in similarly treated wild-type mice. This was associated with the augmented expression of inducible nitric oxide synthase and the prevalence of nitrotyrosine residues in kidneys from Eta-1/Op$^{-/-}$ mice versus wild-type counterparts. In vitro studies with proximal tubular cells subjected to hypoxia in the presence of Eta-1/Op, but not Eta-1/Op with deleted arginine-glycine-aspartic acid (RGD) domain, resulted in cytoprotection (Noiri et al., 1999).

Patients with severe proteinuria and progressive idiopathic membranous nephropathy have an overexpression in tubular epithelial cells of the chemokines Eta-1/Op, MCP-1, and RANTES, and the profibrogenic cytokines PDGF-BB and TGF-β, a feature that points to their use as predictors of disease progression (Mezzano et al., 2000). Eta-1/Op and chemokines are differentially expressed in glomeruli and tubules in a rat model of antiglomerular basement membrane glomerulonephritis. Chemokines play a primary role in the glomeruli, whereas Eta-1/Op has a predominant role in tubulointerstitial monocyte/macrophage recruitment. The roles of chemokines and Eta-1/Op may thus be dependent on the renal compartment and on the disease model (Panzer et al., 2001). This is perhaps illustrated by the observation that Eta-1/Op expression alone is insufficient to serve as the principal mediator of intrarenal monocyte/macrophage influx in the transplant setting because strong Eta-1/Op protein and mRNA expression by tubular epithelium is observed in pretransplant donor biopsies and in biopsies with cyclosporine toxicity without an inflammatory cell infiltration (Hudkins et al., 2001).

Eta-1/Op also may be relevant to complement-mediated renal disease. Generation of complement activation products from filtered complement components in urine with nonselective proteinuria leads to tubulointerstitial disease, resulting in progressive loss of renal function (Nangaku et al., 1999). Complement membrane attack complex (C5b-9) formation resulting from proteinuria contributes to the loss of nephron function by damaging the tubulointerstitium, and prevention of C5b-9 formation in tubules can slow the deterioration of renal function in nephrotic syndrome (Nangaku et al., 1999). Eta-1/Op binds to the human plasma protein factor H, which is a multifunctional, multidomain protein that acts as a central regulator of the complement system; is involved in hemolytic-uremic syndrome; acts as an extracellular matrix component; binds to cellular receptors of the integrin type; and, in addition to Eta-1/Op, interacts with a wide selection of ligands, such as the C-reactive protein, thrombospondin, bone sialoprotein, and heparin (Zipfel, 2001).

CARDIOVASCULAR SYSTEM

The presence of Eta-1/Op in the normal artery wall and its increased expression after injury suggests a role for this molecule in the vascular system (Baccarini-Contri et al., 1995; Bonin et al., 1999; Demer, 1995; Gadeau et al., 1993; Giachelli et al., 1991, 1995; Green et al., 1995; Hao et al., 1995; Hultgardh-Nilsson et al., 1997; Lemire et al., 1994; Liaw et al., 1994, 1997; Newman, Bruun, Mistry, et al., 1995; Newman, Bruun, Porter, et al., 1995; Shanahan et al., 1993; Singh et al., 1995; Thyberg et al., 1995; Weintraub et al., 1996; Weissberg et al., 1995; Yamamoto et al., 1997). Eta-1/Op mRNA is expressed in normal rat aorta and carotid arteries at levels 50- to 60-fold greater than heart, and about three to four times the levels found in adult rat kidney on a per micrograms of total RNA basis (Giachelli et al., 1991). Eta-1/Op mRNA levels in both carotid and aortic artery increase with age, and are elevated approximately fivefold in the carotid artery 48 hours after balloon angioplasty (Wang et al., 1996). The bHLH-leucine zipper transcription factor upstream stimulatory factor-1 (USF1) is induced in vivo within 24 hours of balloon angioplasty of rat carotids coordinately with Eta-1/Op induction, to which promoter it binds (Malyankar et al., 1999). Neointima formation is associated with up-regulation of Eta-1/Op expression and of its receptor integrins αvβ3 and αvβ5 (Bennett, Chan, et al., 1997; Bennett, Lindner, et al., 1997; Corjay et al., 1999; Giachelli et al., 1993; Liaw et al., 1994, 1997; Panda et al., 1997; Veinot et al., 1999). Eta-1/Op is expressed in spontaneous neointimal plaque formation in fowl *(Gallus gallus)* abdominal aorta (Kuykindoll et al., 2000), a process that resembles injury from balloon angioplasty. cGMP-dependent protein kinase I reduces Eta-1/Op expression (Dey et al., 1998), and cGMP-dependent protein kinase I expression is transiently reduced in response to balloon catheter injury in the population of coronary arterial smooth muscle cells that are actively proliferating and producing Eta-1/Op (Remy-Martin et al., 1999), a reduction that is also correlated temporally with increases in inflammatory activity in the injured vessels as assessed by increased iNOS expression (Lincoln et al., 1998; Anderson et al., 2000). Eta-1/Op inhibits inducible nitric oxide synthase activity in rat vascular tissue (Scott et al., 1998).

Endothelial cell migration is stimulated by vascular permeability factor/vascular endothelial growth factor through cooperative mechanisms involving Eta-1/Op, the αvβ3 integrin, and thrombin (Liaw, Lindner, et al., 1995; Liaw, Skinner, et al., 1995; Senger et al., 1996; Yue et al., 1994). Tolbert and Oparil (2001) used the rat carotid injury model to show that estrogen inhibits neointima formation through an estrogen receptor (ER)-dependent mechanism operative in the early period after vascular injury. Activation of vascular smooth muscle cells and subsequent release of soluble factors including Eta-1/Op stimulate the migration of adventitial fibroblasts in a luminal direction to eventually take up residence in the neointima, and the production, release, or posttranslational processing of these factors are inhibited by estrogen through an ER-dependent mechanism (Tolbert and Oparil, 2001). Estrogen attenuates integrin-β3-dependent adventitial fibroblast migration after inhibition of Eta-1/Op production in vascular smooth muscle cells (Li et al., 2000).

Reckless et al. (2001) found a common phenotype, namely similar amounts of Eta-1/Op per lesion, active tumor growth factor-β, and plasminogen activator inhibitor-I, associated with atherogenesis in diverse mouse models of vascular lipid lesions and regardless of the genetic basis of susceptibility (Reckless et al., 2001). Eta-1/Op and c-Ha-ras are critical molecular targets during oxidant-induced atherogenesis (Ramos, 1999), and Eta-1/Op is overexpressed in vascular smooth muscle cells transfected with the c-Ha-rasEJ oncogene (Parrish et al., 1997). Differential processing of Eta-1/Op characterizes the proliferative vascular smooth muscle cell phenotype following chemical injury by allylamine (Parrish and Ramos, 1995, 1997). Pure atmospheric pressure promotes Eta-1/Op expression in human aortic smooth muscle cells, an observation which suggests that high blood pressure-mediated mechanical compression is involved in the process of atherosclerosis and remodeling via Eta-1/Op expression (Iizuka et al., 2001). Pulse pressure on cultured cells has a similar effect on Eta-1/Op expression (Cappadona et al., 1999).

Hypoxia stimulates Eta-1/Op expression and proliferation of cultured rat aortic vascular smooth muscle cells in a process that involves protein kinase C and p38 mitogen-activated protein (MAP) kinase; is potentiated by high glucose; and is relevant to the development of diabetic atherosclerosis (Mori and Saito, 2000; Simon, 1997; Sodhi et al., 2000; Takemoto, Tada, et al., 1999; Takemoto, Yokote, et al., 1999; Takemoto, Yokote, Nishimura, et al., 2000; Takemoto, Yokote, Yamazaki, et al., 2000). Indeed, Takemoto et al. (2000) found by immunohistochemistry that medial layers of the carotid arteries of streptozotocin-induced diabetic rats and the forearm arteries of diabetic patients stained positively for Eta-1/Op antibodies, whereas the staining from arteries of control rats and nondiabetic patients was negative. High fat diet-induced diabetes activates Eta-1/Op gene expression in the aortas of low density lipoprotein receptor-deficient mice (Towler et al., 1998). Tamoxifen elevates transforming growth factor-β and suppresses diet-induced formation of lipid lesions in mouse aorta (Grainger et al., 1995). NK-104, a 3-hydroxy-3-methylglutaryl coenzyme A reductase inhibitor, reduces Eta-1/Op expression by cultured rat aortic smooth muscle cells, an inhibitory effect that is almost completely reversed by mevalonate, suggesting that mevalonate or its metabolites play important roles in the regulation of Eta-1/Op expression (Takemoto et al., 2001). Furthermore, oral administration of NK-104 (3 mg·kg^{-1} per day for seven days) effectively suppressed abnormally up-regulated expression of Eta-1/Op mRNA in the aorta and kidney of streptozotocin-induced diabetic rats, an observation that suggests that NK-104 is a suitable drug for the treatment of diabetic patients with hypercholesterolemia (Takemoto et al., 2001).

Platelet adherence to Eta-1/Op mediated by activated αvβ3 could play a role in anchoring platelets to disrupted atherosclerotic plaques and the walls of injured arteries (Bennett, Chan, et al., 1997; Bennett, Lindner, et al., 1997). By inhibiting αvβ3 function, it may be possible to inhibit platelet-mediated vascular occlusion with a minimal effect on primary hemostasis (Bennett, Chan, et al., 1997; Bennett, Lindner, et al., 1997), one of the possible mechanisms of action of abciximab (Coller, 1999). Eta-1/Op participates in αvβ3-mediated platelet adhesion. Although the polymorphism responsible for the Pl(A2) alloantigen on the β3-component of β3-containing integrins is a risk factor for coronary thrombosis, no differences were detected in the ability of β3-integrins to interact with ligands, such as Eta-1/Op, based on the presence or absence of the Pl(A2) polymorphism, an observation which suggests that factors unrelated to β3-integrin function may account for the reported association of the Pl(A2) allele with coronary thrombosis (Bennett et al., 2001).

Galectin 1, a β-galactoside-binding lectin that interacts with Eta-1/Op, is involved in vascular smooth muscle cell proliferation (Moiseeva et al., 2000). Eta-1/Op and platelet-derived growth factor-BB increase, via αvβ3 integrin, smooth muscle cell matrix metalloproteinase-9 production (Bendeck et al., 2000), which in turn induces expression of proteins such as tenascin-C associated with progression of pathologies such as pulmonary hypertension (Cowan et al., 2000). On the other hand, Eta-1/Op protects endothelial cells from apoptosis induced by growth factor withdrawal, an interaction that is mediated by the αvβ3 integrin and is NF-kappaB-dependent (Scatena et al., 1998) through the induction of osteoprotegerin, a member of the tumor necrosis factor receptor superfamily (Malyankar et al., 2000). The chimeric c7E3 Fab (abciximab) inhibits vascular smooth muscle cell adhesion on Eta-1/Op and migration to Eta-1/Op via the αvβ3 integrin, observations that suggest a possible mechanism for its effects on reducing restenosis after coronary angioplasty (Baron et al., 2000). Selective

$\alpha v \beta 3$ integrin blockade of Eta-1/Op binding potently limits neointimal hyperplasia and lumen stenosis following deep coronary arterial stent injury (Srivatsa, Fitzpatrick, et al., 1997; Srivatsa, Harrity, et al., 1997).

Macrophages, mast cells, and smooth muscle cells are the primary cells implicated in arterial calcification and Eta-1/Op is one of the proteins that regulates this process (Boot et al., 1999; Frangogiannis et al., 1998; Gadeau et al., 1993, 2001; Jono et al., 1998; Maeda et al., 1996; Proudfoot, Shanahan, et al., 1998; Proudfoot, Skepper, et al., 1998; Shioi et al., 1995; Taooka et al., 1999; Tintut et al., 1998; Wallin et al., 2001). Eta-1/Op is localized in calcified coronary atherosclerotic plaques (Bini et al., 1999; Canver et al., 2000; Demer and Tintut, 1999; Farrington et al., 1998; Fitzpatrick, 1996; Fitzpatrick et al., 1994; Giachelli et al., 1993; Hirota et al., 1993; Ikeda et al., 1993; Kennedy et al., 2000; Liaw et al., 1994; O'Brien et al., 1994; Severson et al., 1995; Shanahan et al., 1993, 1994), and soluble Eta-1/Op released near the sites of vascular calcification may represent an adaptive mechanism aimed at regulating the process of vascular calcification (Kwon et al., 2000). Takemoto, Yokote, et al. (1999) and Takemoto, Tada, et al. (1999) reported a negative relationship between plasma Eta-1/Op level and serum levels of total cholesterol and low-density lipoprotein (LDL) cholesterol, an observation which suggests that hypercholesterolemia facilitates vascular calcification by suppressing Eta-1/Op synthesis. On the other hand, in nondiabetic and normotensive cases, there is a positive relationship between the plasma Eta-1/Op level and age, which may reflect a defense mechanism against age-related increase of vascular calcification (Takemoto, Yokote, et al., 1999; Takemoto, Tada, et al., 1999).

Eta-1/Op is a potent inhibitor of ectopic calcification, a common response to soft tissue injury and systemic mineral imbalance that can lead to devastating clinical consequences when present in heart valves or blood vessels (Arai et al., 1998; Barros and Gimeno, 2000; Giachelli, 2001; Lavelin et al., 2000; Wada et al., 1999). Phosphorylation of Eta-1/Op is required for inhibition of vascular smooth muscle cell calcification; hence, regulation of Eta-1/Op phosphorylation represents one way in which mineralization may be controlled by cells (Jono et al., 2000). Mesenchymal and inflammatory cells normally maintain the balance between procalcific and anticalcific regulatory proteins in soft tissues such that ectopic deposition of apatite is avoided. Alterations in this balance induced by injury or disease induces ectopic apatite deposition (Giachelli, 2001; Yamagishi et al., 1999). Hyperphosphatemia and increased Eta-1/Op expression by vascular smooth muscle cells are associated with hyperphosphatemia and calciphylaxis or calcific uremic arteriolopathy (CUA), which is a fatal disease in dialysis patients due to calcification of cutaneous blood vessels, the pathogenesis of which had been attributed to elevated parathyroid hormone levels (Ahmed et al., 2001; Vaskuring and Vaskuring, 2001). However, in agreement with the observations in calciphylactic patients, studies evaluating vascular calcification in nondialysis patients have found that the smooth muscle cells play an active role, including production of Eta-1/Op (Ahmed et al., 2001). Eta-1/Op and osteocalcin also are among the most abundant proteins expressed in calcified native human valves, porcine valve bioprostheses in humans, and animal models of valvular calcification (Gura et al., 1997; Mohler et al., 1997; O'Brien et al., 1995; Shen et al., 1997, 2001; Srivatsa, Fitzpatrick, et al., 1997; Srivatsa, Harrity, et al., 1997). Unlike the vascular calcification processes described above, calcification of the media of peripheral arteries, referred to as Monckeberg's sclerosis and occurring commonly in aged and diabetic individuals, is associated with little Eta-1/Op mRNA expression (Shanahan et al., 1999).

Eta-1/Op deficiency in rat vascular smooth muscle cells is associated with an $\alpha 1\beta 1$-mediated inability to adhere to collagen and an increased propensity for apoptosis (Weintraub et al., 2000). Exaggerated left ventricular dilation and reduced collagen Iα deposition after myocardial infarction have been observed in mice lacking Eta-1/Op (Trueblood et al., 2001).

Myocardial Eta-1/Op expression is associated with left ventricular hypertrophy (Graf et al., 1997). In the hamster, Eta-1/Op is expressed in heritably cardiomyopathic hearts under conditions of chronic injury and repair, and the source of Eta-1/Op message appears to be macrophage-like cells in foci of inflammation (Williams, Bland, et al., 1995; Williams, Halpert, et al., 1995). Eta-1/Op from infiltrating macrophages also appears to participate during repair of myocardial necrosis (Murry et al., 1994). Using spontaneously hypertensive and aortic-banded rats, Singh et al. (1999), Xie, Nishi, et al. (2001), and Xie, Pimental, et al. (2001) showed that expression of myocardial Eta-1/Op coincides with the development of heart failure and is inhibited by captopril, suggesting a role for angiotensin II. Angiotensin

II plays a critical role in cardiac remodeling (Hsueh et al., 1998; Nunohiro et al., 1997). This peptide promotes cardiac myocyte hypertrophy and cardiac fibroblast interstitial fibrotic changes associated with left ventricular hypertrophy, post myocardial infarction remodeling, and congestive heart failure (Schnee and Hsueh, 2000). Angiotensin II induces Eta-1/Op expression in cardiac microvascular endothelial cells (Hu et al., 2000; Wiener et al., 1996), a process that is mediated via activation of mitogen-activated protein kinases (p42/44 MAPK) and that involves reactive oxygen species (Xie, Nishi, et al., 2001; Xie, Pimental, et al., 2001). Angiotensin II directly increases transforming growth factor β1 and Eta-1/Op expression and indirectly, through the latter mediators, affects collagen mRNA expression in the human heart (Ashizawa et al., 1996; DeBlois et al., 1996; Kawano et al., 2000; Kupfahl et al., 2000). Angiotensin II also enhances αv, β1, β3, and β5 integrins, and α-actinin mRNA and protein levels in cardiac fibroblasts (Kawano et al., 2000), and promotes Eta-1/Op-induced and β3 integrin-mediated collagen gel contraction by adult rat cardiac fibroblasts (Nunohiro et al., 1999).

GASTROINTESTINAL SYSTEM

Stomach

Eta-1/Op is present in mucous and chief cells of the epithelial layer and in macrophages in the lamina propria of the human stomach (Qu-Hong et al., 1997). Parietal and endocrine cells of the epithelial layer and mast cells and plasma cells in the lamina propria do not contain Eta-1/Op. Subcellular localizations of Eta-1/Op include secretory granules and synthetic organelles in mucous and chief cells and phagolysosomes in macrophages. Extracellular concentrations of Eta-1/Op are present in the glycocalyx and in an electron-lucent band between epithelial surface cells and the gastric lumen, while paracellular edema between the epithelium of the same cells was devoid of Eta-1/Op. The subcellular distribution of Eta-1/Op in human gastric mucosa suggests possible roles for this glycoprotein in barrier function, host defense, and/or secretion (Qu-Hong et al., 1997).

Intestine

Eta-1/Op immunoreactivity is localized to phagolysosomes of macrophages, fibroblasts, absorptive epithelial cells of the small intestine, and Paneth cells (Qu-Hong and Dvorak, 1997). The mucigen secretory granules and Golgi structures of mucous epithelial cells of the small intestinal epithelium contain Eta-1/Op, but secretory granules of numerous other cells, including Paneth cells, do not. Extracellular and phagocytosed *Tropheryma whippelii* within macrophage phagolysosomes also bind Eta-1/Op. These localizations are supportive of a role for Eta-1/Op in phagocytic and some secretory cell functions in the human intestine (Qu-Hong and Dvorak, 1997).

Liver

Whereas Eta-1/Op mRNA expression in the rat liver is minimal and there is no detectable Eta-1/Op mRNA in Kupffer cells from normal rats (Kawashima et al., 1999; Wang, Mochida, et al., 2000), there is increased Eta-1/Op expression in activated Kupffer cells and hepatic macrophages during macrophage migration and granuloma formation in rats given heat-killed *Propionibacterium acnes* (Wang, Mochida, et al., 2000). Eta-1/Op derived from Kupffer cells and hepatic macrophages may contribute to the infiltration of monocytes and macrophages into the liver cooperatively with the actions of monocyte chemotactic protein-1 (MCP-1) and macrophage inflammatory protein-1 (MIP-1) α in *Propionibacterium acnes*-treated rats (Itoh and Okanoue, 2000; Wang, Mochida, et al., 2000).

The role of Eta-1/Op in liver pathology is underscored by another model, namely that of liver necrosis induced by carbon tetrachloride intoxication. When rats receive carbon tetrachloride, liver necrosis develops between one and three days following the intoxication. In these rats, hepatic Eta-1/Op mRNA expression is also increased following the intoxication: Kupffer cells, hepatic macrophages, and hepatic stellate cells isolated from such livers show marked expression of Eta-1/Op mRNA (Kawashima et al., 1999). Immunohistochemical examination also discloses the presence of Eta-1/Op in macrophages, including Kupffer cells and stellate cells, in the necrotic areas. On electron microscopy, Eta-1/Op stains are present in the Golgi apparatus in these cells. Recombinant human Eta-1/Op promotes migration of Kupffer cells isolated from normal rats and cultured in a Transwell cell culture chamber in a dose-related manner (Kawashima et al., 1999). Cholesterol feeding also up-regulates Eta-1/Op expression in Kupffer cells, an observation that suggests that Eta-1/Op may also be involved in the pathogenesis of atherosclerosis in association with increased levels of cellular cholesterol (Remaley et al., 1995).

PULMONARY SYSTEM

Eta-1/Op is expressed by alveolar macrophages (Miyazaki et al., 1995). Eta-1/Op is relevant to the development of pulmonary fibrosis, which is initiated by migration, adhesion, and proliferation of fibroblasts, induced by both alveolar macrophages and T cells (Nakama et al., 1998). In this respect, Eta-1/Op gene expression is significantly increased in the lungs of transgenic mice expressing TNF-α in type II pneumocytes, a condition leading to pulmonary alveolitis and progressive fibrosis (Miyazaki et al., 1995). One study found that Eta-1/Op mRNA is mostly localized in alveolar macrophages, a finding that is consistent with the increased expression of Eta-1/Op mRNA in a macrophage cell line after treatment with TNF-α (Miyazaki et al., 1995). Another study found that lymphocytes, particularly γδ T cells and B1 cells, also play a role in the development of pulmonary fibrosis in this transgenic model (Nakama et al., 1998). In another model, that of bleomycin-induced pulmonary fibrosis, Eta-1/Op was found to be strongly expressed in alveolar macrophages accumulating in the fibrotic area of the lung. The development of the fibrotic process was also associated with an increase in the expression of Eta-1/Op mRNA and protein (Takahashi et al., 2001). Nakama et al. (1998) also provided evidence for the involvement of αβ T cells through antigen-driven mechanisms in the development of bleomycin-induced pulmonary fibrosis. Eta-1/Op produced by alveolar macrophages and T cells therefore functions as a fibrogenic cytokine that promotes, through interaction with αv integrin, the migration, adhesion, and proliferation of fibroblasts in the development of pulmonary fibrosis (Takahashi et al., 2001).

Eta-1/Op is associated with T cells in sarcoid granulomas (O'Regan et al., 1999). Sarcoidosis is a systemic disease characterized by the accumulation of activated T cells and widespread granuloma formation. In addition, individual genetic predisposition appears to be important in this disease. Eta-1/Op expression correlates with granuloma maturity, and Eta-1/Op induces T-cell chemotaxis, supports T-cell adhesion (an effect enhanced by thrombin cleavage of Eta-1/Op), and costimulates T-cell proliferation (O'Regan et al., 1999). Carlson et al. (1997) reported strong expression of Eta-1/Op mRNA and protein in the epithelioid histiocytes and multinucleate histiocytic giant cells in granulomas from 22 cases of granulomatous inflammation including cases of sarcoidosis, granulomatous temporal arteritis, histoplasmosis, rheumatoid nodule, granuloma annulare, erythema nodosum, granulomatous gastritis, foreign body giant-cell granulomatous reactions, and lipogranulomas. Increased Eta-1/Op expression is also associated with silicosis, another granulomatous disease (Nau et al., 1997).

NERVOUS SYSTEM

Eta-1/Op is expressed in the nervous system, and Eta-1/Op-immunoreactive primary sensory neurons are found in the rat spinal and trigeminal nervous systems (Ichikawa et al., 2000; Shin et al., 1999). An examination of the distribution of Eta-1/Op mRNA in the rat brain revealed its presence in likely neurons in the olfactory bulb and the brainstem (with higher levels in the pons and the medulla than in the midbrain), but not in the telencephalon and the diencephalon. In the brainstem, Eta-1/Op mRNA is found in functionally diverse areas including motor-related areas, sensory system, and reticular formation (Shin et al., 1999). Eta-1/Op is immunohistochemically localized in the white matter of the chick central nervous system, particularly in myelin (Kang et al., 1999). The fact that Eta-1/Op expression also has been identified in the retina and that Eta-1/Op-like immunoreactivity is present in a number of ganglion cells suggests that Eta-1/Op may be also important in retinal homeostasis (Ju et al., 2000).

Eta-1/Op expression is apparent in the early notochord and rostral hindbrain during formation of the rat neuraxis. Both of these sites are known to have important organizing capacities associated with the expression of a number of transcription factors and secreted signaling molecules. Eta-1/Op could play a role in the patterning of the neuraxis. Although notochord expression of Eta-1/Op is not conserved between rat and chick, expression is clearly present in the primitive neuroepithelia of the chick caudal hindbrain and restricted to rhombomeres 5 and 6 and to a subpopulation of neural crest cells that arise from these segments (Kang et al., 1999; Thayer and Schoenwolf, 1998). The latter localized expression suggests that Eta-1/Op may have a role in patterning of postotic neural crest cells that arise from particular segments of the hindbrain.

Eta-1/Op is involved in the process of ischemic axonal death in periventricular leukomalacia (PVL), and Eta-1/Op immunoreactivity parallels the number of ionized calcium binding adaptor molecule 1 (Iba1; microglia/macrophage marker)-positive foam cells, a finding that suggests the production of Eta-1/Op protein by these foam cells (Tanaka et al., 2000). Eta-1/Op immunoreactivity is absent in either normal white matter or acute PVL lesions, but is detectable at the subacute and chronic stages in swollen and calcified axons bordering the ischemic zone. The latter findings suggest that Eta-1/Op is closely associated with the death of swollen axons at the periphery of the ischemic zone, regulating the presence or absence of calcification (Tanaka et al., 2000).

Eta-1/Op and its integrin receptor $\alpha v\beta 3$ are key molecular components of the matrix remodeling process after focal ischemia (Ellison et al., 1998, 1999). Focal brain ischemia induces inflammation, extracellular matrix remodeling, gliosis, and neovascularization (Wang, Louden, et al., 1998). Following an ischemic insult to the central nervous system a reorganization of cells and tissue takes place as the surrounding cells attempt to limit the injury, repair the damage, and restore the normal architecture of the brain. This tissue remodeling requires de novo synthesis of genes and proteins that enables cells to actively change their relationship with the existing extracellular matrix and with other cells to reorganize the damaged tissue. Microglia and astrocytes in the peri-infarct region are activated in response to focal stroke. A critical function of activated glia is formation of a protective barrier that ultimately forms a new glial-limiting membrane. Eta-1/Op is initially expressed by activated macrophages and microglia in the periinfarct region (24 to 48 hours) and at later times (5 to

15 days) in the core infarct. After focal stroke, the αvβ3 integrin is up-regulated by astrocytes in the periinfarct region. Eta-1/Op derived from microglia at the infarct border zone (and possible macrophages in the infarct core) may therefore serve as an astrocyte chemoattractant to organize the astrocyte scar after focal stroke (Ellison et al., 1998, 1999). Indeed, Wang, Louden, et al. (1998) demonstrated a dose-dependent chemotactic activity of Eta-1/Op in C6 astroglia cells and normal human astrocytes. The de novo expression and interaction of the Eta-1/Op ligand with its receptor integrin αvβ3 therefore suggests a role in wound healing after focal stroke (Ellison et al., 1998, 1999).

Lee, Shin, et al. (1999) reported that, following global forebrain ischemia in rats, the hippocampus and the striatum up-regulate Eta-1/Op mRNA in different spatiotemporal profiles: transient induction of Eta-1/Op mRNA occurred earlier in the striatum than in the hippocampus; it was pronounced in the dorsomedial striatum close to the lateral ventricle and in the CA1 subfield and the subiculum of the hippocampus before microglial cells became more reactive; and it also could be detected in the dentate hilus and to a marginal extent in the CA3 (Lee, Shin, et al., 1999).

REPRODUCTIVE SYSTEM

Siiteri and Hamilton (1995) and Siiteri et al. (1995) identified Eta-1/Op mRNA and protein in rat epididymis and epididymal sperm. Eta-1/Op is a bull fertility-associated factor, and Eta-1/Op gene expression in the Holstein bull reproductive tract was localized to the epithelial cells of the ampulla, seminal vesicle, caput, corpus, and cauda epididymis, and in the testes to developing germ cells (Cancel et al., 1997, 1999; Rodriguez et al., 2000). Eta-1/Op expression is high in decidua cells as well as in the endometrial glands of the nonpregnant secretory-phase human and baboon uterus (Fazleabas et al., 1997; Young et al., 1990). In mammals, Eta-1/Op, among other molecules, has been implicated in the initial attachment between the trophectoderm, the outer layer of the blastocyst and precursor of the placenta, and the luminal epithelium lining the uterus, an interaction that initiates implantation of the embryo (Kimber, 2000). Eta-1/Op mRNA levels increase in the endometrial glandular epithelium of early-pregnant ewes, a process that is induced by progesterone, and Eta-1/Op protein is secreted into the uterine lumen (Johnson, Spencer, et al., 2000). Secreted Eta-1/Op is then available as a ligand for αvβ3 integrin heterodimer on trophectoderm and uterus to stimulate changes in morphology of conceptus trophectoderm, and induce adhesion between luminal epithelium and trophectoderm essential for implantation and placentation (Johnson, Spencer, et al., 1999). Eta-1/Op is also involved in cytotrophoblast invasion of the maternal vasculature/extracellular matrix during non-preeclamptic placentation (Omigbodun et al., 1997), and Eta-1/Op may serve as a marker for placental bed remodeling, which fails in preeclampsia (Gabinskaya et al., 1998).

An Eta-1/Op-like protein is expressed in the trout ovary during ovulation (Bobe and Goetz, 2001). Eta-1/Op has been localized to ovary, and in the skin and ventral fatty tissue of pregnant and lactating mice (Craig and Denhardt, 1991), and the latter induction of Eta-1/Op mRNA is partially mimicked by painting β-estradiol or progesterone on the skin of nonpregnant females (Craig and Denhardt, 1991). Eta-1/Op is present in bovine and human milk (Dhanireddy et al., 1993; Sorensen and Petersen, 1993). Targeted inhibition of Eta-1/Op expression in the mammary gland causes abnormal morphogenesis and lactation deficiency (Nemir et al., 2000). The pregnant Eta-1/Op-deficient mice displayed a lack of mammary alveolar structures, a drastic reduction in the synthesis of β-casein, whey acidic milk protein, and lactation deficiency. The mechanism of Eta-1/Op effect on these processes involves down-regulation of metalloproteinase (MMP)-2 (Nemir et al., 2000).

Rittling and Novick (1997) examined the expression pattern of Eta-1/Op in mouse mammary glands at different stages of postnatal development. Whereas Eta-1/Op is expressed at low-to-moderate levels in mammary glands from virgin and pregnant mice, the levels of Eta-1/Op mRNA are extremely high in the lactating gland, consistent with the presence of the protein in milk. Expression is highest at two days of lactation and declines thereafter, but it remains high through involution. Eta-1/Op expression is restricted to small nests or groups of cells at nine days of involution. These results suggest that Eta-1/Op may play a specific role in the process of involution that may be distinct from its role during lactation (Baik et al., 1998; Lee et al., 2000; Rittling and Novick, 1997). Eta-1/Op expression by gonadotropes in the rat anterior pituitary is down-regulated in lactating rats, is higher in male than in female rats, and increases after gonadectomy (Ehrchen et al., 2001).

AUDITORY SYSTEM

Eta-1/Op is expressed in the inner ear (Davis et al., 1995; Ichimiya et al., 1994; Sakagami et al., 1994; Swanson et al., 1989). Eta-1/Op is widely distributed within the membranous labyrinth of adult mammalian cochleae, and Eta-1/Op immunoreaction product and mRNA are found within the stria vascularis, VIIIth cranial nerve, spiral ligament, and limbus (Lopez, Olson, et al., 1995). Only specific cell types within these regions contain abundant Eta-1/Op mRNA or protein, the main cell type being Type I fibrocytes that populate the spiral limbus and spiral ligament (Ichimiya et al., 1994). Epithelial cells that line the luminal surface of the stria vascularis (marginal cells) and neurons that compose the vestibular and auditory ganglia also show high Eta-1/Op expression. Eta-1/Op epitopes are also detectable in cochlear fluids withdrawn from the scalae media and tympani of the cochlea. The Eta-1/Op protein species in cochlear fluid differ from those present in cerebrospinal fluid, an observation that underscores the notion that Eta-1/Op exists in tissue-specific isoforms with particular cellular functions (Lopez, Olson, et al., 1995; Stark et al., 2001).

Eta-1/Op is also a matrix protein of otoconia, which consist of calcium bicarbonate and organic materials (Takemura et al., 1994), and Eta-1/Op can be used as a marker of otoconial genesis in otolithic maculae (Uno et al., 2000). Eta-1/Op mRNA is present in the sensory hair cells that are involved in the production of otoconia (Sakagami et al., 1994; Takemura et al., 1994). A one-week exposure to hypergravity does not affect Eta-1/Op expression in rat otolith organs, a finding which suggests that changes in neurotransmission at the synapses of the peripheral and/or central vestibular system rather than changes in otoconial morphology and synthesis may be involved in adaptive mechanisms to an altered gravitational environment (Uno et al., 2000). Eta-1/Op also participates in pathological calcification of the middle ear, and Eta-1/Op secreted by exudate macrophages may be an important mediator of tympanosclerosis, a condition leading to a calcification process in the middle ear that often develops after chronic inflammation (Makiishi-Shimobayashi et al., 1996).

NEOPLASIA

The expression of Eta-1/Op in metastatic neoplastic cells (Craig et al., 1989, 1990; Oates et al., 1997; Senger, Perruzzi, and Papadopoulos, 1989; Smith and Denhardt, 1987), activated T lymphocytes (Patarca et al., 1989), and possibly macrophages (Miyazaki et al., 1990) is consistent with the notion that expression of this protein may be associated with cell motility. This potential function of Eta-1/Op may reflect binding of its RGD sequence to cellular integrins (Miyachi et al., 1991, 1993; Oldberg et al., 1986), such as the vitronectin receptor, because antibodies to the vitronectin receptor may block the attachment of cells to surfaces coated with Eta-1/Op (Oldberg et al., 1988). There are thrombin cleavage sites located in the RGD segment and eight to 11 residues from this sequence toward the amino terminus (Prince, 1989). The location of these thrombin sites suggest a possible mechanism by which neoplastic cells may become detached from local stromal tissue and mobilized into circulation (Senger et al., 1989). Thus, cleavage of Eta1-1/Op by thrombin at the tumor/host interface may result in disruption of the RGD-mediated attachment and detachment. A similar mechanism could apply to the activation and mobilization of lymphocytes and macrophages during an acute immune response (Miyazaki et al., 1990; Patarca et al., 1989).

Phorbol dibutyrate, teleocidin, and aplysiatoxin, which activate protein kinase C and are also tumor promoters, induce Eta-1/Op to the same extent as the tumor promoter 12-O-tetradecanoylphorbol-13-acetate (TPA) in confluent and subconfluent cultures. The increased expression by TPA was prevented by cycloheximide and by H7, a specific inhibitor of protein kinase C. Epidermal growth factor, platelet-derived growth factor, and the nonphorbol promoter diethylhexylphthalate were more effective inducers in confluent than in subconfluent cultures. All-trans retinoic acid, dexamethasone, and fluocinolone acetonide, inhibitors of tumor promotion, diminished

Eta-1/Op induction in both confluent and subconfluent cells. In TPA-treated subconfluent cultures indomethacin produced a slight inhibition, whereas difluoromethyl ornithine potentiated the induction. In TPA-treated confluent cultures, in contrast, indomethacin enhanced Eta-1/Op mRNA levels and difluoromethyl ornithine was inhibitory. Therefore, different pathways in subconfluent and confluent cultures control the protein kinase C-mediated induction of Eta-1/Op expression, indicative of apparent changes in the regulation of gene expression as proliferating cells become quiescent (Smith and Denhardt, 1989).

Eta-1/Op is expressed in a variety of tumors. For instance, Eta-1/Op was one of nine genes, including thymosin β4, secreted protein acidic and rich in cysteine (SPARC), Cap43, ceruloplasmin, serum amyloid A, heat shock protein 90 (HSP90), LOT1, and casein kinase I, identified as highly expressed in the cancerous region compared with the noncancerous region of human renal cell carcinoma (Nishio et al., 2001). Eta-1/Op is expressed in murine osteoma cell lines (Goralczyk et al., 1998), and is prominently expressed by a murine osteosarcoma cell lines with a potential to develop ossification upon transplantation and distant metastatasis (Fisher et al., 2000; Fisher, Mackie, et al., 2001; Grigoriadis et al., 1993; Hara et al., 1996; Khanna et al., 2000; Koistinen et al., 1999; Kusumi et al., 2001; Noda et al., 1988; Ogawa et al., 1998; Rochet et al., 1999; Siggelkow et al., 1998; Sturm et al., 1990). Fibrous dusts almost exclusively induce human malignant mesotheliomas, and a study in rats of asbestos-induced carcinogenesis demonstrated up-regulated expression of Eta-1/Op and of zyxin and integrin-linked kinase (intracellular proteins associated with the focal adhesion contact) (Sandhu et al., 2000). Eta-1/Op is expressed in the stroma of the myxoid and hyaline areas of salivary pleomorphic adenomas but not in normal salivary glands (Kusafuka et al., 1999). Moreover, Eta-1/Op is expressed in premalignant and malignant lesions (normal epithelium, epithelial hyperplasia, epithelial dysplasia, carcinoma in situ and squamous cell carcinoma) of oral epithelium, and in cell lines derived from squamous cell carcinoma of the oral cavity (Devoll et al., 1999; Sato et al., 1997). Transcripts of Eta-1/Op, osteonectin, and matrix Gla protein are expressed by some Shionogi carcinoma SC115-derived cells, an androgen-dependent medullary carcinoma, during the events along the connective tissue differentiation pathway that occur after androgen removal (Nagoshi et al., 1994).

Tianiakos et al. (1998) reported that Eta-1/Op expression was weak or absent in 93 percent of ovarian adenocarcinomas or their metastases. In contrast, 81.5 percent of the borderline tumors (low malignant potential, LMPs) and 50 percent of omental and lymph node implants were Eta-1/Op positive. However, histological type, grade, or clinical stage did not correlate with Eta-1/Op expression. Expression of Eta-1/Op primarily by ovarian neoplasms with favorable prognosis is of potential importance in the pathogenesis of ovarian LMPs (Poliard et al., 1993; Tiniakos et al., 1998). Likewise, Chambers et al. (1996) reported that Eta-1/Op levels in lung tumors have the potential to provide clinically important predictive information on patient outcome, and that Eta-1/Op may play a role in the biology of lung cancer. In some cases of lung cancer, Eta-1/Op is present in tumor cells, while in the majority of cases Eta-1/Op is detected primarily in tumor-infiltrating macrophages and necrotic areas. Overexpression of Eta-1/Op RNA or protein generally is not related to clinicopathological findings in lung cancer; however, there is a statistically significant association between Eta-1/Op-immunopositivity in the tumor and patient survival (Chambers et al., 1996).

Transformation of preneoplastic epidermal JB6 cells with tumor promoter 12-O-tetradecanoyl-phorbol-13-acetate (TPA) is an in vitro model of late-stage tumor promotion. Eta-1/Op is highly expressed in JB6 cells with TPA treatment, and its expression persists for at least four days, which is the time required for subsequent expression of transformed phenotype (Chang and Prince, 1993). Expression of antisense Eta-1/Op RNA inhibits tumor promoter-induced neoplastic transformation of mouse JB6 epidermal cells (Su et al., 1995). These observations suggest that Eta-1/Op may play a role in promoting JB6 cell transformation. TPA-treated JB6 cells had significantly increased adherence to Eta-1/Op compared with dimethylsulfoxide-treated control cells. Enhanced attachment of JB6 cells to Eta-1/Op was also observed after treatment with another tumor promoter phorbol dibutyrate but not with nontumor promoters (phorbol and 1α, 25-dihydroxyvitamin D_3), suggesting that tumor promoters specifically modulate attachment to Eta-1/Op. Calcitriol enhances TPA-induced JB6 tumorigenic transformation through vitamin D receptor-dependent and -independent pathways (Chang et al., 1997). Calphostin C, a specific protein kinase C (PKC) inhibitor, decreased TPA-treated JB6 cell adhesion to Eta-1/Op by 50 percent, an observation which suggests that TPA increases integrin affinity or avidity for Eta-1/Op through a PKC-mediated pathway (Chang and Chambers, 2000).

Eta-1/Op deficiency reduces experimental tumor cell metastasis to bone and soft tissues in Eta-1/Op knockout mice (Nemoto et al., 2001). Expression of antisense Eta-1/Op RNA in metastatic mouse fibroblasts is associated with reduced malignancy (Behrend et al., 1995; Gardner et al., 1994). Using a cDNA probe, Craig et al. (1990) found that Eta-1/Op mRNA, which is barely detectable in normal mouse epidermis, was expressed at moderate-to-high levels in two of three epidermal papillomas and at consistently high levels in seven of seven squamous-cell carcinomas induced by an initiation-promotion regimen. This contrasts with the transient induction observed after a single application of the tumor promoter 12-O-tetradecanoylphorbol-13-acetate (TPA) (Hashimoto et al., 1990; Smith and Denhardt, 1987). In a set of five independently isolated T24-H-ras-transfected mouse C3H 10T1/2 cell lines, the levels of Eta-1/Op mRNA correlated well with ras mRNA levels and with both experimental and spontaneous metastatic ability (Chambers, 1995; Chambers and Tuck, 1993; Chambers et al., 1992, 1993; Krook et al., 1993; Marshall-Heyman et al., 1994; Nose et al., 1990; Su et al., 1993; Tuck et al., 1991). Eta-1/Op mRNA expression was also elevated in a derivative of mouse LTA cells transfected with genomic DNA from B16F1 melanoma cells and selected for increased experimental metastatic ability in the chick embryo. This apparent association of Eta-1/Op expression with invasion, progression, and metastasis suggests that Eta-1/Op may act as an autocrine adhesion factor for tumor cells (Craig et al., 1990).

Qualitative increases in Eta-1/Op blood levels have been reported in a small number of patients with metastatic tumors of various kinds (Brown et al., 1994; Singhal et al., 1997). Eta-1/Op is an autocrine mediator of hepatocyte growth factor (HGF)-induced invasive growth (Medico et al., 2001). HGF induces cell migration of several mammary epithelial cell (MEC) lines, via activation of its cognate receptor (Met). Eta-1/Op-induced, integrin ($\alpha v\beta 5$ or $\alpha v\beta 3$)-dependent migration of human mammary epithelial cells involves activation of the hepatocyte growth factor receptor (Met) (Tuck et al., 2000). In epithelial cells, HGF activates a genetic program involving cell-cell dissociation ("scattering"), growth, and invasiveness (Medico et al., 2001). The full program is not elicited by other growth factors such as epidermal growth factor, and is aberrantly activated during cancer progression to the invasive-metastatic phenotype. Eta-1/Op is a major HGF transcriptional target, and the wave of Eta-1/Op induction is maximal at six hours, in concomitance with the initiation of scattering, and is specific. HGF, but not epidermal growth factor, promotes cell adhesion to Eta-1/Op via the CD44 receptor. Antibodies against Eta-1/Op and CD44 significantly impair scattering; conversely, constitutive Eta-1/Op overexpression dramatically increases the motile and invasive responses to HGF, leading to disruption of the ordered morphogenetic program triggered by this ligand (Medico et al., 2001). Eta-1/Op and thrombospondin bind to insulin-like growth factor (IGF)-binding protein-5, leading to an alteration in IGF-I-stimulated cell growth (Nam et al., 2000).

Weber et al. (1997) found that two events occurring in some neoplastic processes, namely secretion of Eta-1/Op and expression of CD44v, are linked in such a way that they may cause migration of tumor cells to specific sites of metastasis formation. Eta-1/Op binds to naturally expressed and stably transfected CD44 in a manner that is specific, dose-dependent, inhibitable by anti-CD44 antibodies, insensitive to competition by Gly-Arg-Gly-Asp-Ser, and sensitive to competition by hyaluronate. The receptor-ligand interaction mediates chemotaxis or attachment, depending on presentation of Eta-1/Op in soluble or immobilized form. In contrast, binding of CD44 to hyaluronate mediates aggregation or attachment but not chemotaxis (Weber et al., 1996, 1997). Co-expression of Eta-1/Op and CD44v9 in gastric tumor cells correlates well with the degree of lymphatic vessel invasion or long distant lymph node metastasis in diffuse type gastric carcinoma, indicating that mutual interaction between Eta-1/Op and CD44v9 on the tumor cells is implicated in lymphogenous metastasis (Tahara et al., 2000; Ue et al., 1998). On the other hand, IL-8 produced by gastric cancer cells is used for sustained angiogenesis and tissue invasion and metastasis via autocrine/paracrine manners (Tahara, 2000). In another model, introduction of antisense CD44 cDNAs down-regulates expression of overall CD44 isoforms and inhibits tumor growth and metastasis in highly metastatic colon carcinoma cells

(Harada et al., 2001). In vitro studies showed a significantly reduced ability of the stable antisense transfectants to bind Eta-1/Op and hyaluronate, ligands for CD44. These cells developed tumors more slowly than controls when the cells were subcutaneously injected into SCID mice. The latter observations open the possibility of application of antisense CD44s to the treatment of colorectal carcinoma (Harada et al., 2001; Katagiri et al., 1999), and maybe other cancers because CD44, but not Eta-1/Op, is also involved in matrix metalloproteinase-2 regulation in human melanoma cells (Takahashi et al., 1999).

Malignant gliomas are the most common primary intracranial neoplasms in adults and are largely refractory to postsurgical therapy despite intensive therapeutic efforts. Using a number of different brain tumor-derived cell lines, Tucker et al. (1998) demonstrated that the Eta-1/Op mRNA, which is substantially overexpressed by some tumors in comparison with normal tissues, is preferentially expressed in high grade and metastatic brain tumors compared to low grade brain tumors. Saitoh et al. (1995) also demonstrated Eta-1/Op expression in human gliomas, and showed a positive correlation between Eta-1/Op levels and malignancy. TPA mediates regulation of Eta-1/Op expression in human malignant glioma cells (Tucker et al., 1998). Markert et al. (2001) also showed that Eta-1/Op, along with other genes, such as nicotinamide N-methyltransferase, murine double minute 2 (MDM2), and epithelin (granulin) are up-regulated in glioblastoma multiforme tumors; however, the cells in which this up-regulation is apparent are tumor-associated macrophages. Gliosarcoma tumors derived from rat C6 cell implants into rat brain exhibit similar morphological characteristics and degree of vascularization to human glioblastomas, and genes expressed at increased levels in C6 cells are associated with cell surface interactions, migration, or metastasis formation and proliferation, including Eta-1/Op, the receptor for hyaluronan-mediated motility (RHAMM), S-100 related protein 42A, galectin I, preproenkephalin, autocrine motility factor, α-tubulin, ad1 antigen, and cofilin (Gunnersen et al., 2000). Expression of Eta-1/Op is not universal to all brain tumors as exemplified by the study of Gladson et al. (1997), who reported absence of Eta-1/Op expression in five of five ganglioneuroblastomas.

The homing receptor CD44 is frequently expressed on primary brain tumors and brain metastases as well as other cancers (Naot et al., 1997; Rudzki and Jothy, 1997). Its engagement by Eta-1/Op physiologically induces macrophage chemotaxis, a mechanism that may be utilized by metastatic brain tumors in the process of dissemination (Gladson, 1999; Weber and Ashkar, 2000). In host defense, Eta-1/Op and its receptors, CD44 and integrin $\alpha v\beta 3$, play key roles in mediating delayed type hypersensitivity responses by activating macrophages to induce Th1 cytokines while inhibiting Th2 cytokines. Other metastasis associated gene products similarly contribute to host defenses. Hence, cancer spread is regulated by a set of developmentally nonessential genes, which physiologically mediate stress responses, inflammation, wound healing, and neovascularization. The functions of the relevant gene products are extensively modified posttranscriptionally and their dysregulation in cancer occurs at the levels of expression and splicing. Consistent patterns of organ preference by malignancies of particular tissue origin suggest a necessary connection between loss of growth control and senescence genes and expression of genes mediating the dissemination of tumor cells (Weber and Ashkar, 2000).

Eta-1/Op has distinct roles in host defense activity and tumor survival during squamous cell carcinoma progression in vivo (Crawford et al., 1998). In this respect, Eta-1/Op null animals exhibit accelerated tumor growth and progression and have a greater number of metastases per animal compared with wild-type animals (Crawford et al., 1998). However, metastases in the Eta-1/Op null animals were significantly smaller than in controls. When injected into nude mice, the growth of Eta-1/Op null tumor lines and the same lines engineered to reexpress Eta-1/Op recapitulate the growth differences observed in the progression study. These differences in tumor growth inversely correlated with the degree of macrophage infiltration. Slower-growing, Eta-1/Op-producing tumors contain significantly more macrophages, although a higher proportion are mannose receptor positive, a characteristic of differentiated resting macrophages. In vitro, Eta-1/Op null cell lines display decreased survival at clonal density compared with Eta-1/Op-producing lines, an observation consistent with the smaller metastases of the Eta-1/Op null mice. Therefore, Eta-1/Op acts as a macrophage chemoattractant, whereas tumor-derived Eta-1/Op is able to inhibit macrophage function and enhances the growth or survival of metastases (Crawford et al., 1998).

When stimulated with the inflammatory mediators lipopolysaccharide and interferon-γ, mouse macrophages secrete nitric oxide (NO) as a cytotoxic agent effective against microbial invaders and tumor cells (Rollo and Denhardt, 1996). Eta-1/Op-induced inhibition of nitric oxide production and cytotoxicity by activated RAW64.7 macrophages suggests that tumor-cell-derived Eta-1/Op functions to protect tumor cells from macrophage-mediated destruction (Denhardt and Chambers, 1994; Feng et al., 1995; Rollo et al., 1996). Rollo and Denhardt (1996) documented that thioglycollate-elicited peritoneal macrophages, activated with the inflammatory mediators, produced less nitric oxide and exhibited reduced cytotoxicity toward target cells when they were obtained from old animals than when they were obtained from young animals; and that Eta-1/Op was able to inhibit both the induced nitric oxide synthesis and cytotoxicity, but more effectively in macrophages from the young animals than those from the old animals. This may be secondary to the observed higher level of Eta-1/Op expression in macrophages from old animals (Rollo and Denhardt, 1996).

Metastatic cancer cells, like trophoblasts of the developing placenta, are invasive and must escape immune surveillance to survive. Complement has long been thought to play a significant role in the tumor surveillance mechanism. Eta-1/Op and bone sialoprotein (BSP) are expressed by trophoblasts and are strongly up-regulated by many tumors. Indeed, BSP has been shown to be a positive indicator of the invasive potential of some tumors (Fedarko et al., 2000). Eta-1/Op and BSP form rapid and tight complexes with complement Factor H. Besides its key role in regulating complement-mediated cell lysis, Factor H also appears to play a role when "hijacked" by invading organisms in enabling cellular evasion of complement. Recombinant Eta-1/Op and BSP can protect murine erythroleukemia cells from attack by human complement as well as human MCF-7 breast cancer cells and U-266 myeloma cells from attack by guinea pig complement. The expression of Eta-1/Op and BSP in tumor cells provides a selective advantage for survival via initial binding to αvβ3 integrin (both) or CD44 (Eta-1/Op) on the cell surface, followed by sequestration of Factor H to the cell surface and inhibition of complement-mediated cell lysis (Fedarko et al., 2000).

Eta-1/Op is expressed in prostate adenocarcinoma and benign prostatic hyperplasia and is an indicator of cell differentiation; however, it cannot be used as a marker of malignancy in prostate cancer (Elgavish et al., 1998; Koeneman et al., 1999; Thalmann et al., 1999; Tozawa et al., 1999). The study of Tozawa et al. (1999) showed positive staining of Eta-1/Op in prostate adenocarcinoma cells and macrophages in 52.9 percent of the primary prostate cancers and 14.5 percent of the prostate cancers after hormonal therapy. In benign prostatic hyperplasia specimens, 66.7 percent of the cases displayed positive staining of Eta-1/Op. The staining level of Eta-1/Op showed no correlation with serum prostate-specific antigen, but did correlate with stage, differentiation, and Gleason's score (Tozawa et al., 1999). However, Eta-1/Op plays a role in the growth and progression of metastatic prostate cancer (Koeneman et al., 1999; Lecrone et al., 2000). Cancer of the prostate commonly metastasizes to bony sites where cells acquire an aggressive, rapidly proliferating, androgen-independent osteomimetic phenotype, an observation that has also been made in breast cancer bone metastases (Bellahcene and Castronovo, 1997; Sung et al., 1998; Van der Pluijm et al., 1997). The interaction between bone and prostate thus becomes a key factor in disease progression (Koeneman et al., 1999). Fluctuations in intracellular ionized calcium $[Ca^{2+}]_i$ are rapid, regulated signal transduction events often associated with cell proliferation. Hence, Ca^{2+} signals provide a convenient measure of early events in cancer cell growth. Lecrone et al. (2000) found that two bone fractions that contained a number of non-collagenous matrix proteins, such as Eta-1/Op, osteonectin, as well as prothrombin, triggered Ca^{2+} signals in prostate cancer cells derived from bone (PC-3), but not brain (DU-145) metastases of prostate cancer. Lymph node derived LNCaP cells also did not produce a Ca^{2+} signal in response to addition of soluble bone matrix. No other bone fractions produced a Ca^{2+} signal in PC-3 cells. An antibody that recognizes the $\alpha v\beta 3$ integrin, blocks the ability of Eta-1/Op to trigger a Ca^{2+} transient flux in PC-3 cells.

Tumor cells frequently have pronounced effects on the skeleton including bone destruction, bone pain, hypercalcemia, and depletion of bone marrow cells. The disruption of bone homeostasis by tumor cells is secondary in part to the ability of tumor cells to up-regulate Eta-1/Op mRNA in osteoblasts. Secretory products from PC-3 and MCF-7 tumor cell lines that elicit osteolytic responses, but not from LNCaP that elicits osteoblastic responses, up-regulate Eta-1/Op, while inhibiting osteoblast proliferation and differentiation, in the osteoblastic precursor cell line MC3T3-E1 cells (Hullinger et al., 2000). The latter regulation of Eta-1/Op was dependent on both protein kinase C (PKC) and the mitogen-activated protein (MAP) kinase cascade. These results suggest that the up-regulation of Eta-1/Op may play a key role in the development of osteolytic lesions. Furthermore, these results suggest that drugs which prevent activation of the MAP kinase pathway may be efficacious in the treatment of osteolytic metastases (Hullinger et al., 2000).

In contrast to the situations just described, Choi et al. (2000) found that activated leukocyte cell adhesion molecule (ALCAM) and annexin II, but not Eta-1/Op, are involved in the metastatic progression of tumor cells after chemotherapy with adriamycin. However, tumor growth and metastasis are angiogenesis-dependent and tumor angiogenesis is a result of a complex interplay of positive and negative regulators (Shijubo et al., 2000). Vascular endothelial growth factor (VEGF) occupies a particular place among the positive regulators of angiogenesis due to its potency and specificity for endothelial cells. VEGF up-regulates several molecules such as growth factors, adhesion molecules, proteases, and protease receptors, and VEGF induces microvascular hyperpermeability, resulting in activation of thrombin from prothrombin. Eta-1/Op contains a predicted thrombin cleavage site, it is up-regulated in human carcinomas, and it induces endothelial cell migration and up-regulates endothelial cell migration induced by VEGF. Therefore, both VEGF and Eta-1/Op have functional roles in angiogenesis and have clinical significance in tumor biology (Prols, Loser, et al., 1998; Shijubo et al., 2000). For instance, Eta-1/Op, tissue factor, and $\alpha v\beta 3$ integrin expression in microvasculature of gliomas is associated with vascular endothelial growth factor expression (Takano et al., 2000). Microvascular expression of these molecules could be an effective antiangiogenesis target for human gliomas (Takano et al., 2000).

Other studies point to the relevance of Eta-1/Op in tumor-associated angiogenesis. Cooperation of Eta-1/Op is important in VEGF-mediated tumor angiogenesis in stage I lung adenocarcinoma (Shijubo et al., 1999). Shijubo et al. (1999) found that in lung adenocarcinoma, microvessel counts of VEGF-positive and Eta-1/Op-positive tumors were significantly higher than VEGF-negative and Eta-1/Op-negative tumors, respectively, whereas in squamous cell carcinoma they were not. More important, patients with VEGF- and Eta-1/Op-positive stage I lung adenocarcinoma had significantly worse prognoses as compared with other groups (Shijubo et al., 1999). Jin et al. (2000) reported a case of a fifty-two-year-old Japanese man with a benign bronchial granular cell tumor with Eta-1/Op and osteonectin expression. Eta-1/Op-positive tumor cells were randomly distributed in the tumor tissue, but few stromal cells were positive. In contrast, osteonectin was mainly expressed in the peripheral tumor cells and was also distributed in the stromal cells. Blood vessels at the tumor border in which osteonectin-positive tumor cells were distributed proliferated moderately. These observations suggest that Eta-1/Op and osteonectin may play a role in the progression of granular cell tumors and in the interaction between the tumor and host or angiogenesis around the tumor, respectively (Jin et al., 2000).

Some human breast cancer cells express Eta-1/Op (Bellahcene and Castranovo, 1995; Gillespie et al., 1997; Kim et al., 1998; Rittling and Novick, 1997; Sharp et al., 1999), and Eta-1/Op induces increased invasiveness and plasminogen activator expression of human mammary epithelial cells (Barraclough et al., 1998; Chen, Ke, et al., 1997; Morris et al., 1993; Oates et al., 1996; Tuck et al., 1999). In a pilot study, Tuck et al. (1998) also concluded that the ability of breast cancer cells to either synthesize Eta-1/Op or to bind and sequester Eta-1/Op from the microenvironment may be associated with tumor aggressiveness and poor prognosis. However, several studies argue against a role of Eta-1/Op in primary breast cancer. Transgenic mice expressing c-myc and v-Ha-ras specifically in the mammary gland under the control of the mammary-specific promoter of the mouse mammary tumor virus (MMTV) develop unifocal mammary tumors with a half time of about 46 days, and these tumors express high levels of Eta-1/Op mRNA and protein (Feng and Rittling, 2000). Crosses of transgenic mice expressing these two oncogenes with mice with a targeted disruption of the Eta-1/Op gene yielded litter-mates expressing both myc and ras, and with either wild-type or disrupted Eta-1/Op alleles. Tumor incidence and growth rate were unaffected by a lack of Eta-1/Op in the whole animal. Ras and myc expression level, measured at the level of mRNA, was not different in tumors of the two genotypes. Macrophage accumulation, while extremely variable among different tumors, did not correlate with the Eta-1/Op status of the animals. These observations indicate that despite its high level of expression, Eta-1/Op is either not required for mammary primary tumor formation and growth in this system, or can be replaced by other molecules in mice that totally lack Eta-1/Op (Feng and Rittling, 2000). It should be noted, however, that the observations described are not applicable to all tumor types because Eta-1/Op is required for full expression of the transformed phenotype by the ras oncogene in 3T3 cells (Behrend et al., 1994; Wu, Denhardt, et al., 2000). Experiments with 3T3 cells derived from wild-type and Eta-1/Op-deficient mice and transformed by transfection with oncogenic ras evinced that maximal transformation by ras requires Eta-1/Op expression, and implicate increased Eta-1/Op expression as an important effector of the transforming activity of the ras oncogene (Feinleib and Krauss, 1996; Wu, Denhardt, et al., 2000). The latter conclusion is underscored by the study of Casson et al. (1997), who reported that the ras-regulated gene Eta-1/Op was overexpressed in 100 percent of squamous-cell carcinomas and in 58 percent of adenocarcinomas relative to matched normal esophageal mucosa. Patterns of immunoreactivity for Eta-1/Op protein also varied between squamous-cell carcinomas (tumor cell staining) and adenocarcinomas (predominantly tumor-infiltrating macrophages) (Casson et al., 1997).

Also undermining a possible involvement of Eta-1/Op in primary breast cancer tumor growth and formation are the observations of Arihiro et al. (2000), who reported that although α9β1, an integrin that binds to Eta-1/Op, was expressed in the cytoplasm of breast carcinoma cells in 23 of 90 cases (26 percent) and αvβ6 in the membrane of breast carcinoma cells in 16 of 90 cases (18 percent), the presence of α9β1 and αvβ6 did not correlate with any clinicopathological factors including the patients' age, tumor size, histological type of carcinoma, location of carcinoma cells, and hormone receptor status. With regard to the histological grade of carcinoma, αvβ6 and α9β1 expression did not statistically correlate, although no expression of αvβ6 was observed in 14 cases of Grade I (Arihiro et al., 2000). Kim et al. (1998)

and Jang and Hill (1997) also failed to find prognostic significance for Eta-1/Op expression in primary breast tumors.

In contrast to Eta-1/Op's apparent lack of association with primary breast tumor growth, Eta-1/Op may be involved in microcalcifications associated with breast tumors because Eta-1/Op-positive histiocytes infiltrate Kossa-positive (type II microcalcification) cribriform and comedo-type breast carcinomas, and calcified atypical cystic lobules of the breast, an early stage of low-grade ductal carcinoma in situ (Bellahcene and Castronovo, 1995, 1997; Castronovo and Bellahcene, 1998; Hirota, Ito, et al., 1995; Hirota, Nakajima, et al., 1995; Oyama, Iijima, et al., 2000). Besides breast cancer-associated microcalcifications, Eta-1/Op produced and promptly secreted by macrophages and subsequently translocated to psammoma bodies may be causally related with the calcium phosphate deposition in the psammoma bodies of ovarian serous papillary cystadenocarcinomas (Maki et al., 2000), papillary carcinoma of the thyroid (Tunio et al., 1998), and meningiomas (Hirota, Ito, et al., 1995; Hirota, Nakajima, et al., 1995). Eta-1/Op is also involved in deposition of calcium phosphate in the shadow cell nests of human pilomatricomas, benign epidermal appendage tumors composed of hair matrix-like basaloid cells and keratinized remnant cells (Hirota, Asada, et al., 1995; Hirota, Ito, et al., 1995; Hirota, Nakajima, et al., 1995). Eta-1/Op was detected in the mesenchymal cells of an ameloblastic fibro-odontoma arising from a calcifying odontogenic cyst (Matsuzaka et al., 2001).

Tuck et al. (1997) reported an association between Eta-1/Op and p53 expression with tumor progression in a case of synchronous, bilateral, invasive mammary carcinomas. Moreover, a study by Noti (2000) indicated that breast cancer cells, which have metastasized to bone, may have a survival advantage resulting from interaction of αvβ3 on these cells with the bone protein Eta-1/Op. In this respect, overexpression of protein kinase C-α in MCF-7 breast cancer cells (MCF-7-PKC-α cells) results in anchorage-independent growth and increased tumorigenicity of these cells in nude mice (Carey et al., 1999; Noti, 2000). MCF-7-PKC-α cells, unlike their parental MCF-7 cells, are sensitized to apoptosis by phorbol esters; however, when adhered to Eta-1/Op, MCF-7-PKC-α cells were resistant to phorbol ester mediated apoptosis. Fluorescence-activated cell sorting revealed that Eta-1/Op receptors, αvβ3 and αvβ5, are expressed on MCF-7-

PKC-α cells and that both are used to adhere to Eta-1/Op. Addition of an RGD-containing peptide inhibited survival of MCF-7-PKC-α cells exposed to phorbol ester and adhered to Eta-1/Op. This indicated that an integrin was involved in the cell death suppression signal. Whereas anti-αvβ5 antibody did not reduce survival of MCF-7-PKC-α cells adhered to Eta-1/Op, anti-αvβ3 antibody could efficiently block suppression of apoptosis. Phorbol ester also induced increased expression of αvβ3 on MCF-7-PKC-α cells by up-regulating expression of a second species of β3 mRNA (Carey et al., 1999; Noti, 2000). Ibrahim et al. (2000) also found that Eta-1/Op is expressed in breast cancer bone metastases, an activity that is related to increased bone resorptive activity by osteoclasts.

Singhal et al. (1997) demonstrated a statistically significant elevation in plasma Eta-1/Op in the majority (approximately 70 percent) of a large series of patients with metastatic breast cancer when compared (ninety-fifth percentile) to healthy women or patients who had completed adjuvant treatment for early-stage breast cancer. Furthermore, higher Eta-1/Op levels in patients with metastatic breast cancer may be associated with an increased number of involved sites and decreased survival. Plasma Eta-1/Op levels were correlated with other biochemical markers related to the extent of disease, such as serum alkaline phosphatase, aspartate succinate aminotransaminase, and albumin (Singhal et al., 1997).

Concluding Remarks

Chronic fatigue syndrome (CFS) is a malady of unknown etiology. Several lines of research indicate that at least some cases of CFS, in particular those with evidence of immunological activation and an acute onset, may have an infectious etiology. A set of genetic factors determines whether an individual infected by a microbe will overcome the infection or go on to succumb to or develop a chronic infection. This book has focused on one such resistance factor, Eta-1/Op, that by itself confers natural resistance to *Rickettsia tsutsugamushi* and is also associated with resistance to other bacteria and viruses. Expression of Eta-1/Op is part of the genetic program of cellular immunity, a component of the immune system whose function is deficient in many CFS patients. Whether CFS patients suffer Eta-1/Op deficiency remains to be determined, as does the role of this potential deficiency on CFS symptomatology.

Therapies targeted at restoring a healthy cellular immunity may help in the treatment of CFS. In this context, Eta-1/Op could also be used as a therapeutic agent, a simile to the use of interferon products. However, one should bear in mind, as is the case with all immunotherapeutic agents used so far, that cytokines are in general pleiotropic, i.e., they are produced and act on many tissues and organs, and therefore their therapeutic use requires appropriate dosing and may lead to undesired side effects. In this respect, Eta-1/Op is expressed in several tissues in which it mediates both shared and tissue-specific functions, including resistance to bacterial and viral infections, and expression of the Eta-1/Op gene by cells of the immune system also affects the function of nonimmunological tissues. In addition, expression of Eta-1/Op by other tissues affects immunological function. Common functions of Eta-1/Op include cell-cell communication, cellular motility, and regulation of phosphate and calcium metabolism.

Generation of different tissue-specific forms of Eta-1/Op may affect the function of this protein in different body compartments and in different pathologies, as exemplified in this book in the section on neoplasia. Different isoforms of Eta-1/Op may reflect alternative splicing of a single transcript (e.g., inclusion or exclusion of exon 4 resulting in similar, but functionally distinct, proteins) and/or posttranslational modifications (e.g., phosphorylation, acetylation, sulfation, or glycosylation). Transgenic mice bearing DNA constructs that abolish or elevate expression of Eta-1/Op have provided additional insight into this protein's function and its benefits as a therapeutic agent. Determination of the appropriate isoforms for particular therapeutic applications is also of paramount importance.

The characterization of gene products, such as Eta-1/Op, promises to be an important paradigm in this postgenomics and antiviral medicine era. Nature provides us with the best paradigms for the discovery of novel therapeutic agents and for understanding the differential survival of individuals to infectious agents or the differential evolution of disease.

References

Aarden EM, Nijweide PJ, van der Plas A, Alblas MJ, Mackie EJ, Horton MA, Helfrich MH: Adhesive properties of isolated chick osteocytes in vitro. *Bone,* 18(4):305-313, 1996.

Aarden EM, Wassenaar AM, Alblas MJ, Nijweide PJ: Immunocytochemical demonstration of extracellular matrix proteins in isolated osteocytes. *Histochemistry and Cellular Biology,* 106(5):495-501, 1996.

Abbate M, Zoja C, Corna D, Capitanio M, Bertani T, Remuzzi G: In progressive nephropathies, overload of tubular cells with filtered proteins translates glomerular permeability dysfunction into cellular signals of interstitial inflammation. *Journal of the American Society of Nephrology,* 9(7):1213-1224, 1998.

Ablashi DV, Josephs SF, Buchbinder A: Human B-lymphotropic virus (human herpesvirus-6). *Journal of Virological Methods (Netherlands),* 21(1-4):49-59, 1988.

Adler B, Ashkar, S, Cantor H, Weber GF: Costimulation by extracellular matrix proteins determines the response to TCR ligation. *Cellular Immunology,* 210(1): 30-40, 2001.

Aeschlimann D, Mosher D, Paulsson M: Tissue transglutaminase and factor XIII in cartilage and bone remodeling. *Seminars in Thrombosis and Hemostasis,* 22(5):437-443, 1996.

Agnihotri R, Crawford HC, Haro H, Matrisian LM, Havrda MC, Liaw L: Osteopontin, a novel substrate for matrix metalloproteinase-3 (stromelysin-1) and matrix metalloproteinase-7 (matrilysin). *Journal of Biological Chemistry,* 276(30): 28261-28267, 2001.

Ahmed S, O'Neill KD, Hood AF, Evan AP, Moe SM: Calciphylaxis is associated with hyperphosphatemia and increased osteopontin expression by vascular smooth muscle cells. *American Journal of Kidney Diseases,* 37(6):1267-1276, 2001.

Ahrens M, Ankenbauer T, Schroder D, Hollnagel A, Mayer H, Gross G: Expression of human bone morphogenetic proteins-2 or -4 in murine mesenchymal progenitor C3H10T1/2 cells induces differentiation into distinct mesenchymal cell lineages. *DNA and Cellular Biology,* 12(10):871-880, 1993.

Airenne S, Surcel HM, Alakarppa H, Laitinen K, Paavonen J, Saikku P, Laurila A: *Chlamydia pneumoniae* infection in human monocytes. *Infection and Immunity,* 67(3):1445-1449, 1999.

Akazawa H, Komuro I, Sugitani Y, Yazaki Y, Nagai R, Noda T: Targeted disruption of the homeobox transcription factor Bapx1 results in lethal skeletal dysplasia with asplenia and gastroduodenal malformation. *Genes and Cells,* 5(6):499-513, 2000.

Alberius P, Gordh M: Failure of onlay bone grafts to integrate over the calvarial suture: Observations in adult isogeneic rats. *Journal of Craniomaxillofacial Surgery,* 24(4):251-255, 1996.

Alberius P, Gordh M: Osteopontin and bone sialoprotein distribution at the bone graft recipient site. *Archives of Otolaryngology and Head Neck Surgery,* 124(12):1382-1386, 1998.

Alberius P, Gordh M, Lindberg L, Johnell O: Effect of cortical perforations of both graft and host bed on onlay incorporation to the rat skull. *European Journal of Oral Science,* 104(5-6):554-561, 1996a.

Alberius P, Gordh M, Lindberg L, Johnell O: Influence of surrounding soft tissues on onlay bone graft incorporation. *Oral Surgery, Oral Medicine, Oral Pathology, Oral Radiology and Endodontics,* 82(1):22-33, 1996b.

Alberius P, Johnell O: Immunohistochemical assessment of cranial suture development in rats. *Journal of Anatomy,* 173:61-68, 1990.

Alberius P, Johnell O: Repair of intra-membranous bone fractures and defects in rats. Immunolocalization of bone and cartilage proteins and proteoglycans. *Journal of Craniomaxillofacial Surgery,* 19(1):15-20, 1991.

Amar S, Chung KM, Nam SH, Karatzas S, Myokai F, Van Dyke TE: Markers of bone and cementum formation accumulate in tissues regenerated in periodontal defects treated with expanded polytetrafluoroethylene membranes. *Journal of Periodontal Research,* 32(1 Pt 2):148-158, 1997.

Amizuka N, Yamada M, Watanabe JI, Hoshi K, Fukushi M, Oda K, Ikehara Y, Ozawa H: Morphological examination of bone synthesis via direct administration of basic fibroblast growth factor into rat bone marrow. *Microscopy Research and Technology,* 41(4):313-322, 1998.

Anderson PG, Boerth NJ, Liu M, McNamara DB, Cornwell TL, Lincoln TM: Cyclic GMP-dependent protein kinase expression in coronary arterial smooth muscle in response to balloon catheter injury. *Arteriosclerosis and Thrombosis Vascular Biology,* 20(10):2192-2197, 2000.

Andersson G, Johansson EK: Adhesion of human myelomonocytic (HL-60) cells induced by 1,25-dihydroxyvitamin D3 and phorbol myristate acetate is dependent on osteopontin synthesis and the alpha v beta 3 integrin. *Connective Tissue Research,* 35(1-4):163-171, 1996.

Anselme K, Bigerelle M, Noel B, Dufresne E, Judas D, Iost A, Hardouin P: Qualitative and quantitative study of human osteoblast adhesion on materials with various surface roughnesses. *Journal of Biomedical Materials Research,* 49(2):155-166, 2000.

Aplin HM, Hirst KL, Crosby AH, Dixon MJ: Mapping of the human dentin matrix acidic phosphoprotein gene (DMP1) to the dentinogenesis imperfecta type II critical region at chromosome 4q21. *Genomics,* 30(2):347-349, 1995.

Arai M, Inoue H, Tsuboi T, Togari A: Involvement of vitamin D in lead-induced cutaneous calcification in rodents. *Journal of Toxicological Sciences,* 23(2):121-128, 1998.

Arai N, Ohya K, Kasugai S, Shimokawa H, Ohida S, Ogura H, Amagasa T: Expression of bone sialoprotein mRNA during bone formation and resorption induced by colchicine in rat tibial bone marrow cavity. *Journal of Bone Mineral Research,* 10(8):1209-1217, 1995.

Arai N, Ohya K, Ogura H: Osteopontin mRNA expression during bone resorption: An in situ hybridization study of induced ectopic bone in the rat. *Bone Minerals,* 22(2):129-145, 1993.

Arase H, Arase-Fukushi N, Good RA, Onoe K: Lymphokine-activated killer cell activity of $CD^{4-}CD^{8-}$ TCR alpha beta+ thymocytes. *Journal of Immunology,* 151(2):546-555, 1993.

Arbelle JE, Chen H, Gaead MA, Allegretto EA, Pike JW, Adams JS: Inhibition of vitamin D receptor-retinoid X receptor-vitamin D response element complex formation by nuclear extracts of vitamin D-resistant New World primate cells. *Endocrinology,* 137(2):786-789, 1996.

Arihiro K, Kaneko M, Fujii S, Inai K, Yokosaki Y: Significance of alpha 9 beta 1 and alpha v beta 6 integrin expression in breast carcinoma. *Breast Cancer,* 7(1):19-26, 2000.

Arzate H, Alvarez-Perez MA, Aguilar-Mendoza ME, Alvarez-Fregoso O: Human cementum tumor cells have different features from human osteoblastic cells in vitro. *Journal of Periodontal Research,* 33(5):249-258, 1998.

Arzate H, Portilla Robertson J, Aguilar Mendoza ME: Recombination of epithelial root sheath and dental papilla cells in vitro. *Archives of Medical Research,* 27(4):573-577, 1996.

Ashizawa N, Graf K, Do YS, Nunohiro T, Giachelli CM, Meehan WP, Tuan TL, Hsueh WA: Osteopontin is produced by rat cardiac fibroblasts and mediates A(II)-induced DNA synthesis and collagen gel contraction. *Journal of Clinical Investigation,* 98(10):2218-2227, 1996.

Ashkar S, Glimcher MJ, Saavedra RA: Mouse osteopontin expressed in *E. coli* exhibits autophosphorylating activity of tyrosine residues. *Biochemical and Biophysical Research Communications,* 194(1):274-279, 1993.

Ashkar S, Schaffer JL, Salih E, Gerstenfeld LC, Glimcher MJ: Phosphorylation of osteopontin by Golgi kinases. *Annals of the New York Academy of Sciences,* 760:296-298, 1995.

Ashkar S, Teplow DB, Glimcher MJ, Saavedra RA: In vitro phosphorylation of mouse osteopontin expressed in *E. coli. Biochemical and Biophysical Research Communications,* 191(1):126-133, 1993.

Ashkar S, Weber GF, Panoutsakopoulou V, Sanchirico ME, Jansson M, Zawaideh S, Rittling SR, Denhardt DT, Glimcher MJ, Cantor H: Eta-1 (osteopontin): An early component of type-1 (cell-mediated) immunity. *Science,* 287(5454):860-864, 2000.

Asou Y, Rittling SR, Yoshitake H, Tsuji K, Shinomiya K, Nifuji A, Denhardt DT, Noda M: Osteopontin facilitates angiogenesis, accumulation of osteoclasts, and resorption in ectopic bone. *Endocrinology,* 142(3):1325-1332, 2001.

Atkins K, Berry JE, Zhang WZ, Harris JF, Chambers AF, Simpson RU, Somerman MJ: Coordinate expression of OPN and associated receptors during monocyte/macrophage differentiation of HL-60 cells. *Journal of Cellular Physiology,* 175(2):229-237, 1998.

Atkins KB, Simpson RU, Somerman MJ: Stimulation of osteopontin mRNA expression in HL-60 cells is independent of differentiation. *Archives of Biochemistry and Biophysics,* 343(2):157-163, 1997.

Atmani F, Glenton PA, Khan SR: Identification of proteins extracted from calcium oxalate and calcium phosphate crystals induced in the urine of healthy and stone forming subjects. *Urology Research,* 26(3):201-207, 1998.

Atmani F, Glenton PA, Khan SR: Role of inter-alpha-inhibitor and its related proteins in experimentally induced calcium oxalate urolithiasis. Localization of proteins and expression of bikunin gene in the rat kidney. *Urology Research,* 27(1):63-67, 1999.

Atmani F, Opalko FJ, Khan SR: Association of urinary macromolecules with calcium oxalate crystals induced in vitro in normal human and rat urine. *Urology Research,* 24(1):45-50, 1996.

Attawia MA, Herbert KM, Uhrich KE, Langer R, Laurencin CT: Proliferation, morphology, and protein expression by osteoblasts cultured on poly(anhydride-coimides). *Journal of Biomedical Materials Research,* 48(3):322-327, 1999.

Attur MG, Dave MN, Clancy RM, Patel IR, Abramson SB, Amin AR: Functional genomic analysis in arthritis-affected cartilage: Yin-yang regulation of inflammatory mediators by alpha 5 beta 1 and alpha v beta 3 integrins. *Journal of Immunology,* 164(5):2684-2691, 2000.

Attur MG, Dave MN, Stuchin S, Kowalski AJ, Steiner G, Abramson SB, Denhardt DT, Amin AR. Osteopontin: An intrinsic inhibitor of inflammation in cartilage. *Arthritis and Rheumatism,* 44(3):578-584, 2001.

Aubin JE: Osteoprogenitor cell frequency in rat bone marrow stromal populations: Role for heterotypic cell-cell interactions in osteoblast differentiation. *Journal of Cellular Biochemistry,* 72(3):396-410, 1999.

Aubin JE, Liu F, Malaval L, Gupta AK: Osteoblast and chondroblast differentiation. *Bone,* 17(Suppl 2):77S-83S, 1995.

Ayres JG, Flint N, Smith EG, Tunnicliffe WS, Fletcher TJ, Hammond K, Ward D, Marmion BP: Post-infection fatigue syndrome following Q fever. *Quarterly Journal of Medicine,* 91(2):105-123, 1998.

Ayukawa Y, Takeshita F, Inoue T, Yoshinari M, Shimono M, Suetsugu T, Tanaka T: An immunoelectron microscopic localization of noncollagenous bone proteins (osteocalcin and osteopontin) at the bone-titanium interface of rat tibiae. *Journal of Biomedical Materials Research,* 41(1):111-119, 1998.

Baccarani-Contri M, Taparelli F, Pasquali-Ronchetti I: Osteopontin is a constitutive component of normal elastic fibers in human skin and aorta. *Matrix Biology,* 14(7):553-560, 1995.

Bai S, Shi X, Yang X, Cao X: Smad6 as a transcriptional corepressor. *Journal of Biological Chemistry,* 275(12):8267-8270, 2000.

Baik MG, Lee MJ, Choi YJ: Gene expression during involution of mammary gland (review). *International Journal of Molecular Medicine,* 2(1):39-44, 1998.

Barak-Shalom T, Schickler M, Knopov V, Shapira R, Hurwitz S, Pines M: Synthesis and phosphorylation of osteopontin by avian epiphyseal growth-plate chondrocytes as affected by differentiation. *Comparative Biochemistry, Physiology, Pharmacology, Toxicology and Endocrinology,* 111(1):49-59, 1995.

BarKana II, Narayanan AS, Grosskop A, Savion N, Pitaru S: Cementum attachment protein enriches putative cementoblastic populations on root surfaces in vitro. *Journal of Dental Research,* 79(7):1482-1488, 2000.

Baron JH, Moiseeva EP, de Bono DP, Abrams KR, Gershlick AH: Inhibition of vascular smooth muscle cell adhesion and migration by c7E3 Fab (abciximab): A possible mechanism for influencing restenosis. *Cardiovascular Research,* 48(3):464-472, 2000.

Barone LM, Aronow MA, Tassinari MS, Conlon D, Canalis E, Stein GS, Lian JB: Differential effects of warfarin on mRNA levels of developmentally regulated vitamin K dependent proteins, osteocalcin, and matrix GLA protein in vitro. *Journal of Cellular Physiology,* 160(2):255-264, 1994.

Barone LM, Owen TA, Tassinari MS, Bortell R, Stein GS, Lian JB: Developmental expression and hormonal regulation of the rat matrix Gla protein (MGP) gene in chondrogenesis and osteogenesis. *Journal of Cellular Biochemistry,* 46(4):351-365, 1991.

Barone LM, Tassinari MS, Bortell R, Owen TA, Zerogian J, Gagne K, Stein GS, Lian JB: Inhibition of induced endochondral bone development in caffeine-treated rats. *Journal of Cellular Biochemistry,* 52(2):171-182, 1993.

Barraclough R, Chen HJ, Davies BR, Davies MP, Ke Y, Lloyd BH, Oates A, Rudland PS: Use of DNA transfer in the induction of metastasis in experimental mammary systems. *Biochemistry Society Symposia,* 63:273-294, 1998.

Barros SS, Gimeno EJ: Cell differentiation and bone protein synthesis in the lungs of sheep with spontaneous calcinosis. *Journal of Comparative Pathology,* 123(4): 270-277, 2000.

Barry ST, Ludbrook SB, Murrison E, Horgan CM: Analysis of the alpha4beta1 integrin-osteopontin interaction. *Experimental Cell Research,* 258(2):342-351, 2000a.

Barry ST, Ludbrook SB, Murrison E, Horgan CM: A regulated interaction between alpha5beta1 integrin and osteopontin. *Biochemical and Biophysical Research Communications,* 267(3):764-769, 2000b.

Baud L: [Tubulointerstitial lesions in progressive renal diseases: Potential role of osteopontin]. *Nephrologie,* 17(2):137-138, 1996.

Bautista DS, Denstedt J, Chambers AF, Harris JF: Low-molecular-weight variants of osteopontin generated by serine proteinases in urine of patients with kidney stones. *Journal of Cellular Biochemistry,* 61(3):402-409, 1996.

Bautista DS, Saad Z, Chambers AF, Tonkin KS, O'Malley FP, Singhal H, Tokmakejian S, Bramwell V, Harris JF: Quantification of osteopontin in human plasma with an ELISA: Basal levels in pre- and postmenopausal women. *Clinical Biochemistry,* 29(3):231-239, 1996.

Bautista DS, Xuan JW, Hota C, Chambers AF, Harris JF: Inhibition of Arg-Gly-Asp (RGD)-mediated cell adhesion to osteopontin by a monoclonal antibody against osteopontin. *Journal of Biological Chemistry,* 269(37):23280-23285, 1994.

Bautista DS, Xuan JW, Hota C, Chambers AF, Harris JF: A monoclonal antibody against osteopontin inhibits RGD-mediated cell adhesion to osteopontin. *Annals of the New York Academy of Sciences,* 760:309-311, 1995.

Bayless KJ, Davis GE: Identification of dual alpha4beta1 integrin binding sites within a 38 amino acid domain in the N-terminal thrombin fragment of human osteopontin. *Journal of Biological Chemistry,* 276(16):13483-13489, 2001.

Bayless KJ, Davis GE, Meininger GA: Isolation and biological properties of osteopontin from bovine milk. *Protein Expression and Purification,* 9(3):309-314, 1997.

Bayless KJ, Meininger GA, Scholtz JM, Davis GE: Osteopontin is a ligand for the alpha4beta1 integrin. *Journal of Cell Sciences,* 111(Pt 9):1165-1174, 1998.

Bazan JF: Haemopoietic receptors and helical cytokines. *Immunology Today,* 11(10): 350-354, 1990.

Beck GR Jr, Sullivan EC, Moran E, Zerler B: Relationship between alkaline phosphatase levels, osteopontin expression, and mineralization in differentiating MC3T3-E1 osteoblasts. *Journal of Cellular Biochemistry,* 68(2):269-280, 1998.

Beck GR Jr, Zerler B, Moran E: Phosphate is a specific signal for induction of osteopontin gene expression. *Proceedings of the National Academy of Sciences of the United States of America,* 97(15):8352-8357, 2000.

Beckman EM, Porcell SA, Morita CT, Behar SM, Furlong ST, Brener MB: Recognition of a lipid antigen by CD1-restricted αβ+ T cells. *Nature,* 372:691-694, 1994.

Beertsen W, van den Bos T, Niehof A, Everts V: Formation of reparative acellular extrinsic fiber cementum in relation to implant materials installed in rat periodontium. *European Journal of Oral Science,* 106(Suppl 1):368-375, 1998.

Behrend EI, Chambers AF, Wilson SM, Denhardt DT: Comparative analysis of two alternative first exons reported for the mouse osteopontin gene. *Journal of Biological Chemistry,* 268(15):11172-11175, 1993.

Behrend EI, Craig AM, Wilson SM, Denhardt DT, Chambers AF: Reduced malignancy of ras-transformed NIH 3T3 cells expressing antisense osteopontin RNA. *Cancer Research,* 54(3):832-837, 1994.

Behrend EI, Craig AM, Wilson SM, Denhardt DT, Chambers AF: Expression of antisense osteopontin RNA in metastatic mouse fibroblasts is associated with reduced malignancy. *Annals of the New York Academy of Sciences,* 760:299-301, 1995.

Bellahcene A, Castronovo V: Increased expression of osteonectin and osteopontin, two bone matrix proteins, in human breast cancer. *American Journal of Pathology,* 146(1):95-100, 1995.

Bellahcene A, Castronovo V: Expression of bone matrix proteins in human breast cancer: Potential roles in microcalcification formation and in the genesis of bone metastases. *Bulletin of Cancer,* 84(1):17-24, 1997.

Bellows CG, Reimers SM, Heersche JN: Expression of mRNAs for type-I collagen, bone sialoprotein, osteocalcin, and osteopontin at different stages of osteoblastic differentiation and their regulation by 1,25 dihydroxyvitamin D3. *Cell and Tissue Research,* 297(2):249-259, 1999.

Benayahu D, Fried A, Shamay A, Cunningham N, Blumberg S, Wientroub S: Differential effects of retinoic acid and growth factors on osteoblastic markers and

CD10/NEP activity in stromal-derived osteoblasts. *Journal of Cellular Biochemistry,* 56(1):62-73, 1994.

Benayahu D, Gurevitz OA, Shamay A: Bone-related matrix proteins expression in vitro and in vivo by marrow stromal cell line. *Tissue and Cell,* 26(5):661-666, 1994.

Benayahu D, Kompier R, Shamay A, Kadouri A, Zipori D, Wientroub S: Mineralization of marrow-stromal osteoblasts MBA-15 on three-dimensional carriers. *Calcified Tissue International,* 55(2):120-127, 1994.

Ben-Bassat S, Genina O, Lavelin I, Leach RM, Pines M: Parathyroid receptor gene expression by epiphyseal growth plates in rickets and tibial dyschondroplasia. *Molecular and Cellular Endocrinology,* 149(1-2):185-195, 1999.

Bendeck MP, Irvin C, Reidy M, Smith L, Mulholland D, Horton M, Giachelli CM: Smooth muscle cell matrix metalloproteinase production is stimulated via alpha(v)beta(3) integrin. *Arteriosclerosis and Thrombosis Vascular Biology,* 20(6): 1467-1472, 2000.

Bendelac A, Olivier L, Quimby ME, Yewdell JW, Bennink JR, Brutkiewicz RR: CD1 recognition by mouse NK1+ T lymphocytes. *Science,* 268:863-865, 1995.

Benigni A, Remuzzi G: Glomerular protein trafficking and progression of renal disease to terminal uremia. *Seminars in Nephrology,* 16(3):151-159, 1996.

Beninati S, Senger DR, Cordella-Miele E, Mukherjee AB, Chackalaparampil I, Shanmugam V, Singh K, Mukherjee BB: Osteopontin: Its transglutaminase-catalyzed posttranslational modifications and cross-linking to fibronectin. *Journal of Biochemistry (Tokyo),* 115(4):675-682, 1994.

Bennett BK, Hickie IB, Vollmer-Conna US, Quigley B, Brennan CM, Wakefield D, Douglas MP, Hansen GR, Tahmindjis AJ, Lloyd AR: The relationship between fatigue, psychological and immunological variables in acute infectious illness. *Australian and New Zealand Journal of Psychiatry,* 32(2):180-186, 1998.

Bennett JS, Catella-Lawson F, Rut AR, Vilaire G, Qi W, Kapoor SC, Murphy S, FitzGerald GA: Effect of the Pl(A2) alloantigen on the function of beta(3)-integrins in platelets. *Blood,* 97(10):3093-3099, 2001.

Bennett JS, Chan C, Vilaire G, Mousa SA, DeGrado WF: Agonist-activated alphavbeta3 on platelets and lymphocytes binds to the matrix protein osteopontin. *Journal of Biological Chemistry,* 272(13):8137-8140, 1997.

Bennett MR, Lindner V, DeBlois D, Reidy MA, Schwartz SM: Effect of phosphorothioated oligonucleotides on neointima formation in the rat carotid artery. Dissecting the mechanism of action. *Arteriosclerosis and Thrombosis Vascular Biology,* 17(11):2326-2332, 1997.

Bennett WM: Insights into chronic cyclosporine nephrotoxicity. *International Journal of Clinical Pharmacology and Therapy,* 34(11):515-519, 1996.

Ber R, Kubota T, Sodek J, Aubin JE: Effects of transforming growth factor-beta on normal clonal bone cell populations. *Biochemical and Cellular Biology,* 69 (2-3):132-140, 1991.

Berdal A: [Vitamin D: Biosynthesis, metabolism and mechanism of action at the cellular level]. *Jiornale di Biologia Buccale,* 20(2):71-83, 1992.

Beresford JN, Joyner CJ, Devlin C, Triffitt JT: The effects of dexamethasone and 1,25-dihydroxyvitamin D3 on osteogenic differentiation of human marrow stromal cells in vitro. *Archives of Oral Biology*, 39(11):941-947, 1994.

Berghofer-Hochheimer Y, Zurek C, Langer G, Munder T: Expression of the vitamin D and the retinoid X receptors in *Saccharomyces cerevisiae:* Alternative in vivo models for ligand-induced transactivation. *Journal of Cellular Biochemistry*, 66(2):184-196, 1997.

Bernit E, Pouget J, Janbon F, Dutronc H, Martinez P, Brouqui P, Raoult D: Neurological involvement in acute Q fever. *Archives of Internal Medicine*, 162:693-700, 2002.

Berry JE, Somerman MJ, Khalkhali-Ellis Z, Osdoby P, Simpson RU: HL-60 cell differentiation and osteopontin expression. *Annals of the New York Academy of Sciences*, 760:302-304, 1995.

Bhalerao J, Bogers J, Van Marck E, Merregaert J: Establishment and characterization of two clonal cell lines derived from murine mandibular condyles. *Tissue and Cell*, 27(4):369-382, 1995.

Bidder M, Latifi T, Towler DA: Reciprocal temporospatial patterns of Msx2 and Osteocalcin gene expression during murine odontogenesis. *Journal of Bone Mineral Research*, 13(4):609-619, 1998.

Binette F, McQuaid DP, Haudenschild DR, Yaeger PC, McPherson JM, Tubo R: Expression of a stable articular cartilage phenotype without evidence of hypertrophy by adult human articular chondrocytes in vitro. *Journal of Orthopedic Research*, 16(2):207-216, 1998.

Bini A, Mann KG, Kudryk BJ, Schoen FJ: Noncollagenous bone matrix proteins, calcification, and thrombosis in carotid artery atherosclerosis. *Arteriosclerosis and Thrombosis Vascular Biology*, 19(8):1852-1861, 1999.

Binkert C, Demetriou M, Sukhu B, Szweras M, Tenenbaum HC, Dennis JW: Regulation of osteogenesis by fetuin. *Journal of Biological Chemistry*, 274(40): 28514-28520, 1999.

Blaese RM, Grayson J, Steinberg AD: Elevated immunoglobulin secreting cells in the blood of patients with active SLE: Correlation of laboratory and clinical assessment of disease activity. *American Journal of Medicine*, 69:345, 1980.

Bliziotes M, Murtagh J, Wiren K: Beta-adrenergic receptor kinage-like activity and beta-arrestin are expressed in osteoblastic cells. *Journal of Bone Mineral Research*, 11(6):820-826, 1996.

Bobe J, Goetz FW: A novel osteopontin-like protein is expressed in the trout ovary during ovulation. *FEBS Letters*, 489(2-3):119-124, 2001.

Bock GR, Whelan J, eds., *Chronic Fatigue Syndrome*. Chichester: John Wiley and Sons, 1993, pp. 280-297.

Bonin LR, Madden K, Shera K, Ihle J, Matthews C, Aziz S, Perez-Reyes N, McDougall JK, Conroy SC: Generation and characterization of human smooth muscle cell lines derived from atherosclerotic plaque. *Arteriosclerosis and Thrombosis Vascular Biology*, 19(3):575-587, 1999.

Bonnelye E, Merdad L, Kung V, Aubin JE: The orphan nuclear estrogen receptor-related receptor alpha (ERRalpha) is expressed throughout osteoblast differentiation and regulates bone formation in vitro. *Journal of Cell Biology,* 153(5):971-984, 2001.

Bonnelye E, Vanacker JM, Dittmar T, Begue A, Desbiens X, Denhardt DT, Aubin JE, Laudet V, Fournier B: The ERR-1 orphan receptor is a transcriptional activator expressed during bone development. *Molecular Endocrinology,* 11(7):905-916, 1997.

Bonvini JM, Schatzmann U, Beck-Schimmer B, Sun LK, Rittling SR, Denhardt DT, Le Hir M, Wuthrich RP: Lack of in vivo function of osteopontin in experimental anti-GBM nephritis. *Journal of the American Society of Nephrology,* 11(9):1647-1655, 2000.

Boot RG, van Achterberg TA, van Aken BE, Renkema GH, Jacobs MJ, Aerts JM, de Vries CJ: Strong induction of members of the chitinase family of proteins in atherosclerosis: Chitotriosidase and human cartilage gp-39 expressed in lesion macrophages. *Arteriosclerosis and Thrombosis Vascular Biology,* 19(3):687-694, 1999.

Boskey AL: Osteopontin and related phosphorylated sialoproteins: Effects on mineralization. *Annals of the New York Academy of Sciences,* 760:249-256, 1995.

Boskey AL, Maresca M, Ullrich W, Doty SB, Butler WT, Prince CW: Osteopontin-hydroxyapatite interactions in vitro: Inhibition of hydroxyapatite formation and growth in a gelatin-gel. *Bone Minerals,* 22(2):147-159, 1993.

Boskey A, Spevak L, Tan M, Doty SB, Butler WT: Dentin sialoprotein (DSP) has limited effects on in vitro apatite formation and growth. *Calcified Tissue International,* 67(6):472-478, 2000.

Bosshardt DD, Nanci A: Immunodetection of enamel- and cementum-related (bone) proteins at the enamel-free area and cervical portion of the tooth in rat molars. *Journal of Bone Mineral Research,* 12(3):367-379, 1997.

Bosshardt DD, Nanci A: Immunolocalization of epithelial and mesenchymal matrix constituents in association with inner enamel epithelial cells. *Journal of Histochemistry and Cytochemistry,* 46(2):135-142, 1998.

Bosshardt DD, Zalzal S, McKee MD, Nanci A: Developmental appearance and distribution of bone sialoprotein and osteopontin in human and rat cementum. *Anatomy Records,* 250(1):13-33, 1998.

Botquin V, Hess H, Fuhrmann G, Anastassiadis C, Gross MK, Vriend G, Scholer HR: New POU dimer configuration mediates antagonistic control of an osteopontin preimplantation enhancer by Oct-4 and Sox-2. *Genes and Development,* 12(13): 2073-2090, 1998.

Bottero P: Role of Pickettsiae and Chlamydiae in the psychopathology of chronic fatigue syndrome (CFS) patients: A diagnostic and therapeutic report. *Journal of Chronic Fatigue Syndrome,* 6(3/4):147-161, 2000.

Bowers MR, Fisher LW, Termine JD, Somerman MJ: Connective tissue-associated proteins in crevicular fluid: Potential markers for periodontal diseases. *Journal of Periodontology,* 60(8):448-451, 1989.

Breen EC, Ignotz RA, McCabe L, Stein JL, Stein GS, Lian JB: TGF beta alters growth and differentiation related gene expression in proliferating osteoblasts in vitro, preventing development of the mature bone phenotype. *Journal of Cell Physiology,* 160(2):323-335, 1994.

Broess M, Riva A, Gerstenfeld LC: Inhibitory effects of 1,25(OH)2 vitamin D3 on collagen type I, osteopontin, and osteocalcin gene expression in chicken osteoblasts. *Journal of Cellular Biochemistry,* 57(3):440-451, 1995.

Bronckers AL, Farach-Carson MC, Van Waveren E, Butler WT: Immunolocalization of osteopontin, osteocalcin, and dentin sialoprotein during dental root formation and early cementogenesis in the rat. *Journal of Bone Mineral Research,* 9(6):833-841, 1994.

Bronckers AL, Lyaruu DM, Woltgens JH: Immunohistochemistry of extracellular matrix proteins during various stages of dentinogenesis. *Connective Tissue Research,* 22(1-4):65-70, 1989.

Brown LF, Berse B, Van de Water L, Papadopoulos-Sergiou A, Perruzzi CA, Manseau EJ, Dvorak HF, Senger DR: Expression and distribution of osteopontin in human tissues: Widespread association with luminal epithelial surfaces. *Molecular Biology and Cells,* 3(10):1169-1180, 1992.

Brown LF, Papadopoulos-Sergiou A, Berse B, Manseau EJ, Tognazzi K, Perruzzi CA, Dvorak HF, Senger DR: Osteopontin expression and distribution in human carcinomas. *American Journal of Pathology,* 145(3):610-623, 1994.

Brzeska H, Lynch TJ, Martin B, Korn ED: The localization and sequence of the phosphorylation sites of *Acanthamoeba* myosin I: An improved method for locating the phosphorylated amino acids. *Journal of Biological Chemistry,* 264:19340, 1989.

Buchwald D, Cheney PR, Peterson DL, Henry B, Wormsley SB, Geiger A, Ablashi DV, Salahuddin SZ, Saxinger C, Biddle R, et al.: A chronic illness characterized by fatigue, neurologic and immunologic disorders, and active human herpes virus type 6 infection. *Annals of Internal Medicine,* 116(2):103-113, 1992.

Buchwald D, Komaroff A: Review of laboratory finding for patients with chronic fatigue syndrome. *Review of Infectious Diseases,* 13(Suppl 1):S12-S18, 1991.

Buchwald D, Sullivan J, Komaroff A: Frequency of "chronic active Epstein-Barr virus infection" in a general medical practice. *Journal of the American Medical Association,* 257(17):2303-2307, 1987.

Budman DR, Merchant EB, Steinberg AD, Doft B, Gershwin ME, Lizzio E, Reeves JP: Increased spontaneous activity of antibody-forming cells in the peripheral blood of patients with active SLE. *Arthritis and Rheumatism,* 20(3):829-833, 1977.

Butler WT: The nature and significance of osteopontin. *Connective Tissue Research,* 23(2-3):123-136, 1989.

Butler WT: Sialoproteins of bone and dentin. *Jiornale de Biologia Buccale,* 19(1): 83-89, 1991.

Butler WT: Structural and functional domains of osteopontin. *Annals of the New York Academy of Sciences,* 760:6-11, 1995.

Butler WT, Bhown M, Brunn JC, D'Souza RN, Farach-Carson MC, Happonen RP, Schrohenloher RE, Seyer JM, Somerman MJ, Foster RA, et al.: Isolation, characterization and immunolocalization of a 53-kDal dentin sialoprotein (DSP). *Matrix,* 12(5):343-351, 1992.

Butler WT, Ritchie H: The nature and functional significance of dentin extracellular matrix proteins. *International Journal of Developmental Biology,* 39(1):169-179, 1995.

Butt HL, Dunstan RH, McGregor NR, Roberts TK, Zerbes M, Klineberg IJ: An association of membrane damaging toxins form coagulase-negative staphylococcus and chronic orofacial muscle pain. *Journal of Medical Microbiology,* 47(7):577-584, 1998.

Byers RJ, Brown J, Brandwood C, Wood P, Staley W, Hainey L, Freemont AJ, Hoyland JA: Osteoblastic differentiation and mRNA analysis of STRO-1-positive human bone marrow stromal cells using primary in vitro culture and poly (A) PCR. *Journal of Pathology,* 187(3):374-381, 1999.

Caceres-Rios H, Rodriguez-Tafur J, Bravo-Puccio F, Maguiña-Vargas C, Sanguineti Diaz C, Carrillo Ramos D, Patarca R: Verruga peruana: An infectious endemic angiomatosis. *Critical Reviews in Oncogenesis,* 6(1):47-56, 1995.

Cachau RE, Serpersu EH, Mildvan AS, August JT, Amzel LM: Recognition in cell adhesion. A comparative study of the conformations of RGD-containing peptides by Monte Carlo and NMR methods. *Journal of Molecular Recognition,* 2(4):179-186, 1989.

Caltabiano S, Hum WT, Attwell GJ, Gralnick DN, Budman LJ, Cannistraci AM, Bex FJ: The integrin specificity of human recombinant osteopontin. *Biochemical Pharmacology,* 58(10):1567-1578, 1999.

Camussi G, Montrucchio G, Lupia E, De Martino A, Perona L, Arese M, Vercellone A, Toniolo A, Bussolino F: Platelet-activating factor directly stimulates in vitro migration of endothelial cells and promotes in vivo angiogenesis by a heparin-dependent mechanism. *Journal of Immunology,* 154:6492-6501, 1995.

Cancel AM, Chapman DA, Killian GJ: Osteopontin is the 55-kilodalton fertility-associated protein in Holstein bull seminal plasma. *Biology and Reproduction,* 57(6):1293-1301, 1997.

Cancel AM, Chapman DA, Killian GJ: Osteopontin localization in the Holstein bull reproductive tract. *Biology and Reproduction,* 60(2):454-460, 1999.

Candeliere GA, Liu F, Aubin JE: Individual osteoblasts in the developing calvaria express different gene repertoires. *Bone,* 28(4):351-361, 2001.

Cantor H: The role of Eta-1/osteopontin in the pathogenesis of immunological disorders. *Annals of the New York Academy of Sciences,* 760:143-150, 1995.

Cantor H: T-cell receptor crossreactivity and autoimmune disease. *Advances in Immunology,* 75:209-233, 2000.

Canver CC, Gregory RD, Cooler SD, Voytovich MC: Association of osteopontin with calcification in human mitral valves. *Journal of Cardiovascular Surgery (Torino),* 41(2):171-174, 2000.

Cao Z, Kelly DJ, Cox A, Casley D, Forbes JM, Martinello P, Dean R, Gilbert RE, Cooper ME: Angiotensin type 2 receptor is expressed in the adult rat kidney and promotes cellular proliferation and apoptosis. *Kidney International,* 58(6):2437-2451, 2000.

Cappadona C, Redmond EM, Theodorakis NG, McKillop IH, Hendrickson R, Chhabra A, Sitzmann JV, Cahill PA: Phenotype dictates the growth response of vascular smooth muscle cells to pulse pressure in vitro. *Experimental Cell Research,* 250(1):174-186, 1999.

Carey I, Williams CL, Ways DK, Noti JD: Overexpression of protein kinase C-alpha in MCF-7 breast cancer cells results in differential regulation and expression of alphavbeta3 and alphavbeta5. *International Journal of Oncology,* 15(1):127-136, 1999.

Carlberg C, Mathiasen IS, Saurat JH, Binderup L: The 1,25-dihydroxyvitamin D3 (VD) analogues MC903, EB1089 and KH1060 activate the VD receptor: Homodimers show higher ligand sensitivity than heterodimers with retinoid X receptors. *Journal of Steroid Biochemistry and Molecular Biology,* 51(3-4):137-142, 1994.

Carlson CS, Tulli HM, Jayo MJ, Loeser RF, Tracy RP, Mann KG, Adams MR: Immunolocalization of noncollagenous bone matrix proteins in lumbar vertebrae from intact and surgically menopausal cynomolgus monkeys. *Journal of Bone Mineral Research,* 8(1):71-81, 1993.

Carlson I, Tognazzi K, Manseau EJ, Dvorak HF, Brown LF: Osteopontin is strongly expressed by histiocytes in granulomas of diverse etiology. *Laboratory Investigation,* 77(1):103-108, 1997.

Carron CP, Meyer DM, Engleman VW, Rico JG, Ruminski PG, Ornberg RL, Westlin WF, Nickols GA: Peptidomimetic antagonists of alphavbeta3 inhibit bone resorption by inhibiting osteoclast bone resorptive activity, not osteoclast adhesion to bone. *Journal of Endocrinology,* 165(3):587-598, 2000.

Carter DH, Scully AJ, Davies RM, Aaron JE: Evidence for phosphoprotein microspheres in bone. *Histochemistry Journal,* 30(9):677-686, 1998.

Carvalho RS, Schaffer JL, Gerstenfeld LC: Osteoblasts induce osteopontin expression in response to attachment on fibronectin: Demonstration of a common role for integrin receptors in the signal transduction processes of cell attachment and mechanical stimulation. *Journal of Cellular Biochemistry,* 70(3):376-390, 1998.

Cassell GH: Infectious causes of chronic inflammatory diseases and cancer. *Emerging Infectious Diseases,* 4(3):475-487, 1998.

Casson AG, Wilson SM, McCart JA, O'Malley FP, Ozcelik H, Tsao MS, Chambers AF: ras mutation and expression of the ras-regulated genes osteopontin and cathepsin L in human esophageal cancer. *International Journal of Cancer,* 72(5):739-745, 1997.

Castagnola P, Bet P, Quarto R, Gennari M, Cancedda R: cDNA cloning and gene expression of chicken osteopontin. Expression of osteopontin mRNA in chondrocytes is enhanced by trypsin treatment of cells. *Journal of Biological Chemistry,* 266(15):9944-9949, 1991.

Castronovo V, Bellahcene A: Evidence that breast cancer associated microcalcifications are mineralized malignant cells. *International Journal of Oncology,* 12(2):305-308, 1998.

Celic S, Katayama Y, Chilco PJ, Martin TJ, Findlay DM: Type I collagen influence on gene expression in UMR106-06 osteoblast-like cells is inhibited by genistein. *Journal of Endocrinology,* 158(3):377-388, 1998.

Cha JH, Ahn YH, Lim SW, Kim YH, Han KH, Jung JY, Kim J: Decreased osteopontin expression in the rat kidney on a sodium deficient diet. *Yonsei Medical Journal,* 41(1):128-135, 2000.

Chackalaparampil I, Peri A, Nemir M, Mckee MD, Lin PH, Mukherjee BB, Mukherjee AB: Cells in vivo and in vitro from osteopetrotic mice homozygous for c-src disruption show suppression of synthesis of osteopontin, a multifunctional extracellular matrix protein. *Oncogene,* 12(7):1457-1467, 1996.

Chambers AF: Regulation and function of osteopontin in ras-transformed cells. *Annals of the New York Academy of Sciences,* 760:101-108, 1995.

Chambers AF, Behrend EI, Wilson SM, Denhardt DT: Induction of expression of osteopontin (OPN; secreted phosphoprotein) in metastatic, ras-transformed NIH 3T3 cells. *Anticancer Research,* 12(1):43-47, 1992.

Chambers AF, Hota C, Prince CW: Adhesion of metastatic, ras-transformed NIH 3T3 cells to osteopontin, fibronectin, and laminin. *Cancer Research,* 53(3):701-706, 1993.

Chambers AF, Tuck AB: ras-responsive genes and tumor metastasis. *Critical Reviews in Oncogenesis,* 4(2):95-114, 1993.

Chambers AF, Wilson SM, Kerkvliet N, O'Malley FP, Harris JF, Casson AG: Osteopontin expression in lung cancer. *Lung Cancer,* 15(3):311-323, 1996.

Chan JC, Scanlon M, Denhardt DT, Singh K, Mukherjee BB, Farach-Carson MC, Butler WT: Immunochemical comparison of transformation-associated protein and secreted phosphoprotein. *International Journal of Cancer,* 46(5):864-870, 1990.

Chang PL, Chambers AF: Transforming JB6 cells exhibit enhanced integrin-mediated adhesion to osteopontin. *Journal of Cellular Biochemistry,* 78(1):8-23, 2000.

Chang PL, Lee TF, Garretson K, Prince CW: Calcitriol enhancement of TPA-induced tumorigenic transformation is mediated through vitamin D receptor-dependent and -independent pathways. *Clinical and Experimental Metastasis,* 15(6):580-592, 1997.

Chang PL, Prince CW: 1 alpha,25-dihydroxyvitamin D3 stimulates synthesis and secretion of nonphosphorylated osteopontin (secreted phosphoprotein 1) in mouse JB6 epidermal cells. *Cancer Research,* 51(8):2144-2150, 1991.

Chang PL, Prince CW: 1 alpha,25-dihydroxyvitamin D3 enhances 12-O-tetradecanoylphorbol-13-acetate-induced tumorigenic transformation and osteopontin expression in mouse JB6 epidermal cells. *Cancer Research,* 53(Suppl 10):2217-2220, 1993.

Chang PL, Ridall AL, Prince CW: Calcitriol regulation of osteopontin expression in mouse epidermal cells. *Endocrinology,* 135(3):863-869, 1994.

Chang PL, Yang WC, Prince CW: Effects of okadaic acid on calcitriol- and phorbol ester-induced expression and phosphorylation of osteopontin in mouse JB6 epidermal cells. *Annals of the New York Academy of Sciences,* 760:24-34, 1995.

Chatterjee M: Vitamin D and genomic stability. *Mutation Research,* 475(1-2): 69-87, 2001.

Cheifetz S, Li IW, McCulloch CA, Sampath K, Sodek J: Influence of osteogenic protein-1 (OP-1;BMP-7) and transforming growth factor-beta 1 on bone formation in vitro. *Connective Tissue Research,* 35(1-4):71-78, 1996.

Chellaiah MA, Fitzgerald C, Alvarez U, Hruska K: c-Src is required for stimulation of gelsolin-associated phosphatidylinositol 3-kinase. *Journal of Biological Chemistry,* 273(19):11908-11916, 1998.

Chellaiah MA, Fitzgerald C, Filardo EJ, Cheresh DA, Hruska KA: Osteopontin activation of c-src in human melanoma cells requires the cytoplasmic domain of the integrin alpha v-subunit. *Endocrinology,* 137(6):2432-2440, 1996.

Chellaiah MA, Hruska K: Osteopontin stimulates gelsolin-associated phosphoinositide levels and phosphatidylinositol triphosphate-hydroxyl kinase. *Molecular Biology and Cell,* 7(5):743-753, 1996.

Chellaiah MA, Kizer N, Silva M, Alvarez U, Kwiatkowski D, Hruska KA: Gelsolin deficiency blocks podosome assembly and produces increased bone mass and strength. *Journal of Cell Biology,* 148(4):665-678, 2000.

Chellaiah MA, Soga N, Swanson S, McAllister S, Alvarez U, Wang D, Dowdy SF, Hruska KA: Rho-A is critical for osteoclast podosome organization, motility, and bone resorption. *Journal of Biological Chemistry,* 275(16):11993-12002, 2000.

Chen D, Harris MA, Rossini G, Dunstan CR, Dallas SL, Feng JQ, Mundy GR, Harris SE: Bone morphogenetic protein 2 (BMP-2) enhances BMP-3, BMP-4, and bone cell differentiation marker gene expression during the induction of mineralized bone matrix formation in cultures of fetal rat calvarial osteoblasts. *Calcified Tissue International,* 60(3):283-290, 1997.

Chen H, Ke Y, Oates AJ, Barraclough R, Rudland PS: Isolation of and effector for metastasis-inducing DNAs from a human metastatic carcinoma cell line. *Oncogene,* 14(13):1581-1588, 1997.

Chen JJ, Jin H, Ranly DM, Sodek J, Boyan BD: Altered expression of bone sialoproteins in vitamin D-deficient rBSP2.7Luc transgenic mice. *Journal of Bone Mineral Research,* 14(2):221-229, 1999.

Chen J, McCulloch CA, Sodek J: Bone sialoprotein in developing porcine dental tissues: Cellular expression and comparison of tissue localization with osteopontin and osteonectin. *Archives of Oral Biology,* 38(3):241-249, 1993.

Chen J, McKee MD, Nanci A, Sodek J: Bone sialoprotein mRNA expression and ultrastructural localization in fetal porcine calvarial bone: Comparisons with osteopontin. *Histochemistry Journal,* 26(1):67-78, 1994.

Chen J, Shapiro HS, Sodek J: Development expression of bone sialoprotein mRNA in rat mineralized connective tissues. *Journal of Bone Mineral Research,* 7(8):987-997, 1992.

Chen J, Singh K, Mukherjee BB, Sodek J: Developmental expression of osteopontin (OPN) mRNA in rat tissues: Evidence for a role for OPN in bone formation and resorption. *Matrix,* 13(2):113-123, 1993.

Chen J, Thomas HF, Sodek J: Regulation of bone sialoprotein and osteopontin mRNA expression by dexamethasone and 1,25-dihydroxyvitamin D3 in rat bone organ cultures. *Connective Tissue Research,* 34(1):41-51, 1996.

Chen J, Zhang Q, McCulloch CA, Sodek J: Immunohistochemical localization of bone sialoprotein in foetal porcine bone tissues: Comparisons with secreted phosphoprotein 1 (SPP-1, osteopontin) and SPARC (osteonectin). *Histochemistry Journal,* 23(6):281-289, 1991.

Chen L, Adar R, Yang X, Monsonego EO, Li C, Hauschka PV, Yayon A, Deng CX: Gly369Cys mutation in mouse FGFR3 causes achondroplasia by affecting both chondrogenesis and osteogenesis. *Journal of Clinical Investigation,* 104(11): 1517-1525, 1999.

Chen Y, Bal BS, Gorski JP: Calcium and collagen binding properties of osteopontin, bone sialoprotein, and bone acidic glycoprotein-75 from bone. *Journal of Biological Chemistry,* 267(34):24871-24878, 1992.

Cheng SL, Lai CF, Blystone SD, Avioli LV: Bone mineralization and osteoblast differentiation are negatively modulated by integrin alpha(v)beta3. *Journal of Bone Mineral Research,* 16(2):277-288, 2001.

Cheng SL, Lai CF, Fausto A, Chellaiah M, Feng X, McHugh KP, Teitelbaum SL, Civitelli R, Hruska KA, Ross FP, et al.: Regulation of alphaVbeta3 and alphaVbeta5 integrins by dexamethasone in normal human osteoblastic cells. *Journal of Cellular Biochemistry,* 77(2):265-276, 2000.

Cheng SL, Lou J, Wright NM, Lai CF, Avioli LV, Riew KD: In vitro and in vivo induction of bone formation using a recombinant adenoviral vector carrying the human BMP-2 gene. *Calcified Tissue International,* 68(2):87-94, 2001.

Cheng SL, Shin CS, Towler DA, Civitelli R: A dominant negative cadherin inhibits osteoblast differentiation. *Journal of Bone Mineral Research,* 15(12):2362-2370, 2000.

Cheng SL, Zhang SF, Avioli LV: Expression of bone matrix proteins during dexamethasone-induced mineralization of human bone marrow stromal cells. *Journal of Cellular Biochemistry,* 61(2):182-193, 1996.

Cheng SL, Zhang SF, Nelson TL, Warlow PM, Civitelli R: Stimulation of human osteoblast differentiation and function by ipriflavone and its metabolites. *Calcified Tissue International,* 55(5):356-362, 1994.

Chenoufi HL, Diamant M, Rieneck K, Lund B, Stein GS, Lian JB: Increased mRNA expression and protein secretion of interleukin-6 in primary human osteoblasts differentiated in vitro from rheumatoid and osteoarthritic bone. *Journal of Cellular Biochemistry,* 81(4):666-678, 2001.

Chenu C, Colucci S, Grano M, Zigrino P, Barattolo R, Zambonin G, Baldini N, Vergnaud P, Delmas PD, Zallone AZ: Osteocalcin induces chemotaxis, secretion of matrix proteins, and calcium-mediated intracellular signaling in human osteoclast-like cells. *Journal of Cell Biology,* 127(4):1149-1158, 1994.

Chenu C, Delmas PD: Platelets contribute to circulating levels of bone sialoprotein in human. *Journal of Bone Mineral Research,* 7(1):47-54, 1992.

Chia JKS, Chia LY: Chronic *Chlamydia pneumoniae* infection: A treatable cause of chronic fatigue syndrome. *Clinical Infectious Disease,* 29(2):452-453, 1999.

Chiba S, Rashid MM, Okamoto H, Shiraiwa H, Kon S, Maeda M, Murakami M, Inobe M, Kitabatake A, Chambers AF, Uede T: The role of osteopontin in the development of granulomatous lesions in lung. *Microbiology and Immunology,* 44(4):319-332, 2000.

Chien HH, Lin WL, Cho MI: Expression of TGF-beta isoforms and their receptors during mineralized nodule formation by rat periodontal ligament cells in vitro. *Journal of Periodontal Research,* 34(6):301-309, 1999a.

Chien HH, Lin WL, Cho MI: Interleukin-1beta-induced release of matrix proteins into culture media causes inhibition of mineralization of nodules formed by periodontal ligament cells in vitro. *Calcified Tissue International,* 64(5):402-413, 1999b.

Chimal-Monroy J, Bravo-Ruiz T, Furuzawa-Carballeda GJ, Lira JM, de la Cruz JC, Almazan A, Krotzsch-Gomez FE, Arrellin G, Diaz de Leon L: Collagen-PVP accelerates new bone formation of experimentally induced bone defects in rat skull and promotes the expression of osteopontin and SPARC during bone repair of rat femora fractures. *Annals of the New York Academy of Sciences,* 857:232-236, 1998.

Choi S, Kobayashi M, Wang J, Habelhah H, Okada F, Hamada J, Moriuchi T, Totsuka Y, Hosokawa M: Activated leukocyte cell adhesion molecule (ALCAM) and annexin II are involved in the metastatic progression of tumor cells after chemotherapy with Adriamycin. *Clinical and Experimental Metastasis,* 18(1): 45-50, 2000.

Choong PF, Martin TJ, Ng KW: Effects of ascorbic acid, calcitriol, and retinoic acid on the differentiation of preosteoblasts. *Journal of Orthopedic Research,* 11(5): 638-647, 1993.

Choppa PC, Vojdani A, Tagle C, Andrin R, Magtoto L: Multiplex PCR for the detection of *Mycoplasma fermentans, M. hominis,* and *M. penetrans* in cell cultures and blood samples of patients with chronic fatigue syndrome. *Molecular and Cellular Probes,* 12(5):301-308, 1998.

Chou PY, Fasman GD: Prediction of the secondary structure of proteins from their amino acid sequences. *Advances in Enzymology,* 47:45-148, 1978.

Chou SY, Hannah SS, Lowe KE, Norman AW, Henry HL: Tissue-specific regulation by vitamin D status of nuclear and mitochondrial gene expression in kidney and intestine. *Endocrinology,* 136(12):5520-5526, 1995.

Churchill WH Jr, Piessens WF, Sulis CA, David JR: Macrophages activated as suspension cultures with lymphocyte mediators devoid of antigen become cytotoxic for tumor cells. *Journal of Immunology,* 115(3):781-786, 1975.

Clauss IM, Gravallese EM, Darling JM, Shapiro F, Glimcher MJ, Glimcher LH: In situ hybridization studies suggest a role for the basic region-leucine zipper protein hXBP-1 in exocrine gland and skeletal development during mouse embryogenesis. *Developmental Dynamics,* 197(2):146-156, 1993.

Cockerell C, Tierno P, Friedman-Kien A, Kim KS: Clinical, histologic, microbiologic, and biochemical characterization of the causative agent of bacillary (epithelioid) angiomatosis: A rickettsial illness with features of bartonellosis. *Journal of Investigative Dermatology,* 97:812-817, 1991.

Coller BS: Potential non-glycoprotein IIb/IIIa effects of abciximab. *American Heart Journal,* 138(1 Pt 2):S1-S5, 1999.

Colnot S, Lambert M, Blin C, Thomasset M, Perret C: Identification of DNA sequences that bind retinoid X receptor-1,25(OH)2D3-receptor heterodimers with high affinity. *Molecular and Cellular Endocrinology,* 113(1):89-98, 1995.

Cometta-Morini C, Maguire PA, Loew GH: Molecular determinants of mu receptor recognition for the fentanyl class of compounds. *Molecular Pharmacology,* 41(1):185-196, 1992.

Connor JR, Dodds RA, James IE, Gowen M: Human osteoclast and giant cell differentiation: The apparent switch from nonspecific esterase to tartrate resistant acid phosphatase activity coincides with the in situ expression of osteopontin mRNA. *Journal of Histochemistry and Cytochemistry,* 43(12):1193-1201, 1995.

Constant P, Davodeau F, Peyrat MA, Poquet Y, Puzo G, Bonneville M, Fournie JJ: Stimulation of human γδ T cells by nonpeptidic mycobacterial ligands. *Science*, 264:267-270, 1995.

Contri MB, Boraldi F, Taparelli F, De Paepe A, Ronchetti IP: Matrix proteins with high affinity for calcium ions are associated with mineralization within the elastic fibers of pseudoxanthoma elasticum dermis. *American Journal of Pathology*, 148(2):569-577, 1996.

Cooper LF, Yliheikkila PK, Felton DA, Whitson SW: Spatiotemporal assessment of fetal bovine osteoblast culture differentiation indicates a role for BSP in promoting differentiation. *Journal of Bone Mineral Research*, 13(4):620-632, 1998.

Corjay MH, Diamond SM, Schlingmann KL, Gibbs SK, Stoltenborg JK, Racanelli AL: Alphavbeta3, alphavbeta5, and osteopontin are coordinately upregulated at early time points in a rabbit model of neointima formation. *Journal of Cellular Biochemistry*, 75(3):492-504, 1999.

Cosman D, Cerretti DP, Larsen A, Park L, March C, Dower S, Gillis S, Urdal D: Cloning, sequencing and expression of human interleukin-2 receptor. *Nature*, 312(5996):768-771, 1984.

Couser WG, Johnson RJ: Mechanisms of progressive renal disease in glomerulonephritis. *American Journal of Kidney Diseases*, 23(2):193-198, 1994.

Cowan KN, Jones PL, Rabinovitch M: Elastase and matrix metalloproteinase inhibitors induce regression, and tenascin-C antisense prevents progression, of vascular disease. *Journal of Clinical Investigation*, 105(1):21-34, 2000.

Cowles EA, DeRome ME, Pastizzo G, Brailey LL, Gronowicz GA: Mineralization and the expression of matrix proteins during in vivo bone development. *Calcified Tissue International*, 62(1):74-82, 1998.

Craig AM, Bowden GT, Chambers AF, Spearman MA, Greenberg AH, Wright JA, McLeod M, Denhardt DT: Secreted phosphoprotein mRNA is induced during multi-stage carcinogenesis in mouse skin and correlates with the metastatic potential of murine fibroblasts. *International Journal of Cancer*, 46(1):133-137, 1990.

Craig AM, Denhardt DT: The murine gene encoding secreted phosphoprotein 1 (osteopontin): Promoter structure, activity, and induction in vivo by estrogen and progesterone. *Gene*, 100:163-171, 1991.

Craig AM, Nemir M, Mukherjee BB, Chambers AF, Denhardt DT: Identification of the major phosphoprotein secreted by many rodent cell lines as 2ar/osteopontin: Enhanced expression in H-ras-transformed 3T3 cells. *Biochemical and Biophysical Research Communications*, 157(1):166-173, 1988.

Craig AM, Smith JH, Denhardt DT: Osteopontin, a transformation-associated cell adhesion phosphoprotein, is induced by 12-O-tetradecanoylphorbol 13-acetate in mouse epidermis. *Journal of Biological Chemistry*, 264(16):9682-9689, 1989.

Craig TA, Benson LM, Naylor S, Kumar R: Modulation effects of zinc on the formation of vitamin D receptor and retinoid X receptor alpha-DNA transcription complexes: Analysis by microelectrospray mass spectrometry. *Rapid Communications in Mass Spectrometry*, 15(12):1011-1016, 2001.

Craig TA, Benson LM, Tomlinson AJ, Veenstra TD, Naylor S, Kumar R: Analysis of transcription complexes and effects of ligands by microelectrospray ionization mass spectrometry. *Nature Biotechnology,* 17(12):1214-1218, 1999.

Crawford HC, Matrisian LM, Liaw L: Distinct roles of osteopontin in host defense activity and tumor survival during squamous cell carcinoma progression in vivo. *Cancer Research,* 58(22):5206-5215, 1998.

Crivello JF, Delvin E: Isolation and characterization of a cDNA for osteopontin-k: A kidney cell adhesion molecule with high homology to osteopontins. *Journal of Bone Mineral Research,* 7(6):693-699, 1992.

Crocker PR, Kelm S, Dubois C, Martin B, McWilliams AS, Shotton DM, Paulson JC, Gordon S: Purification and properties of sialoadhesin, a sialic acid-binding receptor of murine tissue macrophages. *EMBO Journal,* 10(7):1661-1669, 1991.

Crosby AH, Edwards SJ, Murray JC, Dixon MJ: Genomic organization of the human osteopontin gene: Exclusion of the locus from a causative role in the pathogenesis of dentinogenesis imperfecta type II. *Genomics,* 27(1):155-160, 1995.

Crosby AH, Lyu MS, Lin K, McBride OW, Kerr JM, Aplin HM, Fisher LW, Young MF, Kozak CA, Dixon MJ: Mapping of the human and mouse bone sialoprotein and osteopontin loci. *Mammalian Genome,* 7(2):149-151, 1996.

Culbert AA, Wallis GA, Kadler KE: Tracing the pathway between mutation and phenotype in osteogenesis imperfecta: Isolation of mineralization-specific genes. *American Journal of Medical Genetics,* 63(1):167-174, 1996.

Cummings TJ, Hulette CM, Bigner SH, Riggins GJ, McLendon RE: Ham56-immunoreactive macrophages in untreated infiltrating gliomas. *Archives of Pathology and Laboratory Medicine,* 125(5):637-641, 2001.

Daculsi G, Pilet P, Cottrel M, Guicheux G: Role of fibronectin during biological apatite crystal nucleation: Ultrastructural characterization. *Journal of Biomedical Materials Research,* 47(2):228-233, 1999.

Daiter E, Omigbodun A, Wang S, Walinsky D, Strauss JF 3rd, Hoyer JR, Coutifaris C: Cell differentiation and endogenous cyclic adenosine 3',5'-monophosphate regulate osteopontin expression in human trophoblasts. *Endocrinology,* 137(5):1785-1790, 1996.

Dallo SF, Lazzell AL, Chavoya A, Reddy SP, Baseman JB: Biofunctional domains of the *Mycoplasma pneumoniae* P30 adhesin. *Infection and Immunity,* 64(7):2595-2601, 1996.

Damjanovski S, Karp X, Funk S, Sage EH, Ringuette MJ: Ectopic expression of SPARC in Xenopus embryos interferes with tissue morphogenesis: Identification of a bioactive sequence in the C-terminal EF hand. *Journal of Histochemistry and Cytochemistry,* 45(5):643-655, 1997.

Dano K, Andreasen PA, Gronhald-Hansen J, Kristensen P, Nielsen LS, Skriver L: Plasminogen activators, tissue degradation, and cancer. *Advances in Cancer Research,* 44:139-266, 1985.

D'Aoust P, McCulloch CA, Tenenbaum HC, Lekic PC: Etidronate (HEBP) promotes osteoblast differentiation and wound closure in rat calvaria. *Cell and Tissue Research,* 302(3):353-363, 2000.

Darwish H, DeLuca HF: Vitamin D-regulated gene expression. *Critical Reviews in Eukaryotic Gene Expression,* 3(2):89-116, 1993.

Darwish HM, DeLuca HF: Analysis of binding of the 1,25-dihydroxyvitamin D3 receptor to positive and negative vitamin D response elements. *Archives of Biochemistry and Biophysics,* 334(2):223-234, 1996.

Davey RA, Hahn CN, May BK, Morris HA: Osteoblast gene expression in rat long bones: Effects of ovariectomy and dihydrotestosterone on mRNA levels. *Calcified Tissue International,* 67(1):75-79, 2000.

Davies JE: In vitro modeling of the bone/implant interface. *Anatomy Records,* 245(2):426-445, 1996.

Davis RL, Lopez CA, Mou K: Expression of osteopontin in the inner ear. *Annals of the New York Academy of Sciences,* 760:279-295, 1995.

De Bri E, Reinholt FP, Heinegard D, Mengarelli-Widholm S, Norgard M, Svensson O: Bone sialoprotein and osteopontin distribution at the osteocartilaginous interface. *Clinical Orthopedics,* 330:251-260, 1996.

De Bruijn WC, de Water R, Boeve ER, van Run PR, Vermaire PJ, van Miert PP, Romijn JC, Verkoelen CF, Cao LC, Schroder FH: Lectin-cytochemistry of experimental rat nephrolithiasis. *Scanning Microscopy,* 10(2):557-576, 1996.

De Bruijn WC, de Water R, van Run PR, Boeve ER, Kok DJ, Cao LC, Romijn HC, Verkoelen CF, Schroder FH: Ultrastructural osteopontin localization in papillary stones induced in rats. *European Urology,* 32(3):360-367, 1997.

De Freitas E, Hilliard B, Cheney PR, Bell DS, Kiggundu E, Sankey D, Wroblewska Z, Palladino M, Woodward JP, Koprowski H: Retroviral sequences related to human T-lymphotropic virus type II in patients with chronic fatigue immune dysfunction syndrome. *Proceedings of the National Academy of Sciences of the United States of America,* 88(7):2922-2926, 1991.

De Meirleir K: Pulmonary function testing in chronic fatigue syndrome (CFS). *Chest,* 116:331S, 1999.

DeBlois D, Lombardi DM, Su EJ, Clowes AW, Schwartz SM, Giachelli CM: Angiotensin II induction of osteopontin expression and DNA replication in rat arteries. *Hypertension,* 28(6):1055-1063, 1996.

DeLuca HF: New concepts of vitamin D functions. *Annals of the New York Academy of Sciences,* 669:59-68; discussion 68-69, 1992.

Demer LL: A skeleton in the atherosclerosis closet. *Circulation,* 92(8):2029-2032, 1995.

Demer LL, Tintut Y: Osteopontin. Between a rock and a hard plaque. *Circulation Research,* 84(2):250-252, 1999.

Denda S: [The role of integrin alpha 8 beta 1 in kidney morphogenesis]. *Tanpakushitsu Kakusan Koso,* 44(2):136-142, 1999.

Denda S, Reichardt LF, Muller U: Identification of osteopontin as a novel ligand for the integrin alpha8 beta1 and potential roles for this integrin-ligand interaction in kidney morphogenesis. *Molecular Biology and Cell,* 9(6):1425-1435, 1998.

Denhardt DT, Chambers AF: Overcoming obstacles to metastasis—defenses against host defenses: Osteopontin (OPN) as a shield against attack by cytotoxic host cells. *Journal of Cellular Biochemistry,* 56(1):48-51, 1994.

Denhardt DT, Giachelli CM, Rittling SR: Role of osteopontin in cellular signaling and toxicant injury. *Annual Reviews of Pharmacology and Toxicology,* 41:723-749, 2001.

Denhardt DT, Guo X: Osteopontin: A protein with diverse functions. *FASEB Journal,* 7(15):1475-1482, 1993.

Denhardt DT, Lopez CA, Rollo EE, Hwang SM, An XR, Walther SE: Osteopontin-induced modifications of cellular functions. *Annals of the New York Academy of Sciences,* 760:127-142, 1995.

Denhardt DT, Noda M: Osteopontin expression and function: Role in bone remodeling. *Journal of Cellular Biochemistry Supplement,* 30-31:92-102, 1998.

Denhardt DT, Noda M: Enhancement of osteoclastic bone resorption and suppression of osteoblastic bone formation in response to reduced mechanical stress do not occur in the absence of osteopontin. *Journal of Experimental Medicine,* 193(3):399-404, 2001.

Denhardt DT, Noda M, O'Regan AW, Pavlin D, Berman JS: Osteopontin as a means to cope with environmental insults: Regulation of inflammation, tissue remodeling, and cell survival. *Journal of Clinical Investigation,* 107(9):1055-1061, 2001.

Derkx P, Nigg AL, Bosman FT, Birkenhager-Frenkel DH, Houtsmuller AB, Pols HA, van Leeuwen JP: Immunolocalization and quantification of noncollagenous bone matrix proteins in methylmethacrylate-embedded adult human bone in combination with histomorphometry. *Bone,* 22(4):367-373, 1998.

D'Errico JA, Berry JE, Ouyang H, Strayhorn CL, Windle JJ, Somerman MJ: Employing a transgenic animal model to obtain cementoblasts in vitro. *Journal of Periodontology,* 71(1):63-72, 2000.

D'Errico JA, MacNeil RL, Takata T, Berry J, Strayhorn C, Somerman MJ: Expression of bone associated markers by tooth root lining cells, in situ and in vitro. *Bone,* 20(2):117-126, 1997.

D'Errico JA, Ouyang H, Berry JE, MacNeil RL, Strayhorn C, Imperiale MJ, Harris NL, Goldberg H, Somerman MJ: Immortalized cementoblasts and periodontal ligament cells in culture. *Bone,* 25(1):39-47, 1999.

D'Errico JA, Sauk JJ, Prince CW, Somerman MJ: Osteopontin adhesion receptors on gingival fibroblasts. *Journal of Periodontal Research,* 30(1):34-41, 1995.

Desai RK, van Wijnen AJ, Stein JL, Stein GS, Lian JB: Control of 1,25-dihydroxyvitamin D3 receptor-mediated enhancement of osteocalcin gene transcription: Effects of perturbing phosphorylation pathways by okadaic acid and staurosporine. *Endocrinology,* 136(12):5685-5693, 1995.

Dever TE, Glynias MJ, Merrick WC: GTP-binding domain: Three consensus sequence elements with distinct spacing. *Proceedings of the National Academy of Sciences of the United States of America,* 84(7):1814-1817, 1987.

Devoll RE, Li W, Woods KV, Pinero GJ, Butler WT, Farach-Carson MC, Happonen RP: Osteopontin (OPN) distribution in premalignant and malignant lesions of oral epithelium and expression in cell lines derived from squamous cell carcinoma of the oral cavity. *Journal of Oral Pathology and Medicine,* 28(3):97-101, 1999.

Devoll RE, Pinero GJ, Appelbaum ER, Dul E, Troncoso P, Butler WT, Farach-Carson MC: Improved immunohistochemical staining of osteopontin (OPN) in paraffin-embedded archival bone specimens following antigen retrieval: Anti-human OPN antibody recognizes multiple molecular forms. *Calcified Tissue International,* 60(4):380-386, 1997.

Dey NB, Boerth NJ, Murphy-Ullrich JE, Chang PL, Prince CW, Lincoln TM: Cyclic GMP-dependent protein kinase inhibits osteopontin and thrombospondin production in rat aortic smooth muscle cells. *Circulation Research,* 82(2):139-146, 1998.

Dhanireddy R, Senger D, Mukherjee BB, Mukherjee AB: Osteopontin in human milk from mothers of premature infants. *Acta Paediatrica,* 82(10):821-822, 1993.

Diamond JR, Kees-Folts D, Ricardo SD, Pruznak A, Eufemio M: Early and persistent up-regulated expression of renal cortical osteopontin in experimental hydronephrosis. *American Journal of Pathology,* 146(6):1455-1466, 1995.

Diamond JR, Kreisberg R, Evans R, Nguyen TA, Ricardo SD: Regulation of proximal tubular osteopontin in experimental hydronephrosis in the rat. *Kidney International,* 54(5):1501-1509, 1998.

Diamond JR, Ricardo SD, Klahr S: Mechanisms of interstitial fibrosis in obstructive nephropathy. *Seminars in Nephrology,* 18(6):594-602, 1998.

Dieudonne SC, Xu T, Chou JY, Kuznetsov SA, Satomura K, Mankani M, Fedarko NS, Smith EP, Robey PG, Young MF: Immortalization and characterization of bone marrow stromal fibroblasts from a patient with a loss of function mutation in the estrogen receptor-alpha gene. *Journal of Bone Mineral Research,* 13(4):598-608, 1998.

Dilworth FJ, Williams GR, Kissmeyer AM, Nielsen JL, Binderup E, Calverley MJ, Makin HL, Jones G: The vitamin D analog, KH1060, is rapidly degraded both in vivo and in vitro via several pathways: Principal metabolites generated retain significant biological activity. *Endocrinology,* 138(12):5485-5496, 1997.

Dodds RA, Connor JR, James IE, Rykaczewski EL, Appelbaum E, Dul E, Gowen M: Human osteoclasts, not osteoblasts, deposit osteopontin onto resorption surfaces: An in vitro and ex vivo study of remodeling bone. *Journal of Bone Minerals Research,* 10(11):1666-1680, 1995.

Doherty MJ, Ashton BA, Walsh S, Beresford JN, Grant ME, Canfield AE: Vascular pericytes express osteogenic potential in vitro and in vivo. *Journal of Bone Minerals Research,* 13(5):828-838, 1998.

Donahue HJ, Zhou Z, Li Z, McCauley LK: Age-related decreases in stimulatory G protein-coupled adenylate cyclase activity in osteoblastic cells. *American Journal of Physiology,* 273(4 Pt 1):E776-E781, 1997.

Dorheim MA, Sullivan M, Dandapani V, Wu X, Hudson J, Segarini PR, Rosen DM, Aulthouse AL, Gimble JM: Osteoblastic gene expression during adipogenesis in hematopoietic supporting murine bone marrow stromal cells. *Journal of Cellular Physiology,* 154(2):317-328, 1993.

Duncan EL, Brown MA, Sinsheimer J, Bell J, Carr AJ, Wordsworth BP, Wass JA: Suggestive linkage of the parathyroid receptor type 1 to osteoporosis. *Journal of Bone Minerals Research,* 14(12):1993-1999, 1999.

Duong LT, Lakkakorpi PT, Nakamura I, Machwate M, Nagy RM, Rodan GA: PYK2 in osteoclasts is an adhesion kinase, localized in the sealing zone, activated by ligation of alpha(v)beta3 integrin, and phosphorylated by src kinase. *Journal of Clinical Investigation,* 102(5):881-892, 1998.

Duong LT, Lakkakorpi P, Nakamura I, Rodan GA: Integrins and signaling in osteoclast function. *Matrix Biology,* 19(2):97-105, 2000.

Duong LT, Rodan GA: Integrin-mediated signaling in the regulation of osteoclast adhesion and activation. *Frontiers in Bioscience,* 3:D757-D768, 1998.

Ecarot-Charrier B, Bouchard F, Delloye C: Bone sialoprotein II synthesized by cultured osteoblasts contains tyrosine sulfate. *Journal of Biological Chemistry,* 264(33):20049-20053, 1989.

Eddy AA: Experimental insights into the tubulointerstitial disease accompanying primary glomerular lesions. *Journal of the American Society of Nephrology,* 5(6):1273-1287, 1994.

Eddy AA: Interstitial inflammation and fibrosis in rats with diet-induced hypercholesterolemia. *Kidney International,* 50(4):1139-1149, 1996.

Eddy AA, Giachelli CM: Renal expression of genes that promote interstitial inflammation and fibrosis in rats with protein-overload proteinuria. *Kidney International,* 47(6):1546-1557, 1995.

Effah Kaufmann EA, Ducheyne P, Shapiro IM: Evaluation of osteoblast response to porous bioactive glass (45S5) substrates by RT-PCR analysis. *Tissue Engineering,* 6(1):19-28, 2000.

Ehrchen J, Heuer H, Sigmund R, Schafer MK, Bauer K: Expression and regulation of osteopontin and connective tissue growth factor transcripts in rat anterior pituitary. *Journal of Endocrinology,* 169(1):87-96, 2001.

Einhorn TA: The cell and molecular biology of fracture healing. *Clinical Orthopedics,* 355:S7-S21, 1998.

Ek-Rylander B, Flores M, Wendel M, Heinegard D, Andersson G: Dephosphorylation of osteopontin and bone sialoprotein by osteoclastic tartrate-resistant acid phosphatase. Modulation of osteoclast adhesion in vitro. *Journal of Biological Chemistry,* 269(21):14853-14856, 1994.

Elgavish A, Prince C, Chang PL, Lloyd K, Lindsey R, Reed R: Osteopontin stimulates a subpopulation of quiescent human prostate epithelial cells with high proliferative potential to divide in vitro. *Prostate,* 35(2):83-94, 1998.

El-Ghannam A, Ducheyne P, Shapiro IM: Porous bioactive glass and hydroxyapatite ceramic affect bone cell function in vitro along different time lines. *Journal of Biomedical Materials Research,* 36(2):167-180, 1997.

Ellegren H, Fredholm M, Edfors-Lilja I, Wintero AK, Andersson L: Conserved synteny between pig chromosome 8 and human chromosome 4 but rearranged and distorted linkage maps. *Genomics,* 17(3):599-603, 1993.

Ellison JA, Barone FC, Feuerstein GZ: Matrix remodeling after stroke. De novo expression of matrix proteins and integrin receptors. *Annals of the New York Academy of Sciences,* 890:204-222, 1999.

Ellison JA, Velier JJ, Spera P, Jonak ZL, Wang X, Barone FC, Feuerstein GZ: Osteopontin and its integrin receptor alpha(v)beta3 are upregulated during formation of the glial scar after focal stroke. *Stroke,* 29(8):1698-1706; discussion 1707, 1998.

El-Tanani MK, Barraclough R, Wilkinson MC, Rudland PS: Regulatory region of metastasis-inducing DNA is the binding site for T cell factor-4. *Oncogene,* 20(14):1793-1797, 2001.

Erard F, Wild MT, Garcia-Sanz JA, Le Gros G: Switch of CD8 T cells to noncytolytic CD8-CD4- that make TH2 cytokines and help B cells. *Science,* 260(5115):1802-1805, 1993.

Evans JF, Yeh JK, Aloia JF: Osteoblast-like cells of the hypophysectomized rat: A model of aberrant osteoblast development. *American Journal of Physiology, Endocrinology and Metabolism,* 278(5):E832-E838, 2000.

Faccio R, Grano M, Colucci S, Zallone AZ, Quaranta V, Pelletier AJ: Activation of alphav beta3 integrin on human osteoclast-like cells stimulates adhesion and migration in response to osteopontin. *Biochemical and Biophysical Research Communications,* 249(2):522-525, 1998.

Fagenholz PJ, Warren SM, Greenwald JA, Bouletreau PJ, Spector JA, Crisera FE, Longaker MT: Osteoblast gene expression is differentially regulated by TGF-beta isoforms. *Journal of Craniofacial Surgery,* 12(2):183-190, 2001.

Fajardo LF, Kwan HH, Kowalski J, Prionas SD, Wilson AC: Dual role of tumor necrosis factor-α in angiogenesis. *American Journal of Pathology,* 140:539-544, 1992.

Farach-Carson MC: Bioactive analogs that simulate subsets of biological activities of 1alpha,25(OH)(2)D(3) in osteoblasts. *Steroids,* 66(3-5):357-361, 2001.

Farach-Carson MC, Abe J, Nishii Y, Khoury R, Wright GC, Norman AW: 22-Oxacalcitriol: Dissection of 1,25(OH)2D3 receptor-mediated and Ca2+ entry-stimulating pathways. *American Journal of Physiology,* 265(5 Pt 2):F705-F711, 1993.

Farach-Carson MC, Ridall AL: Dual 1,25-dihydroxyvitamin D3 signal response pathways in osteoblasts: Cross-talk between genomic and membrane-initiated pathways. *American Journal of Kidney Diseases,* 31(4):729-742, 1998.

Farach-Carson MC, Wright GC, Butler WT: Improved binding of acidic bone matrix proteins to cationized filters during solid phase assays. *Bone Minerals,* 16(1):1-9, 1992.

Farrington C, Roberts IS, Heagerty AM, Canfield AE: The expression of cartilage oligomeric matrix protein, thrombospondin-1, bone sialoprotein and osteopontin in calcified and non-calcified arterial lesions. *Biochemistry Society Transactions,* 26(1):S3, 1998.

Faucheux C, Bareille R, Amedee J: Synthesis of calbindin-D28K during mineralization in human bone marrow stromal cells. *Biochemistry Journal,* 333(Pt 3):817-823, 1998.

Fazleabas AT, Bell SC, Fleming S, Sun J, Lessey BA: Distribution of integrins and the extracellular matrix proteins in the baboon endometrium during the menstrual cycle and early pregnancy. *Biology and Reproduction,* 56(2):348-356, 1997.

Fedarko NS, Fohr B, Robey PG, Young MF, Fisher LW: Factor H binding to bone sialoprotein and osteopontin enables tumor cell evasion of complement-mediated attack. *Journal of Biological Chemistry,* 275(22):16666-16672, 2000.

Feinleib JL, Krauss RS: Dissociation of ras oncogene-induced gene expression and anchorage-independent growth in a series of somatic cell mutants. *Molecular Carcinogenesis,* 16(3):139-148, 1996.

Feng B, Rollo EE, Denhardt DT: Osteopontin (OPN) may facilitate metastasis by protecting cells from macrophage NO-mediated cytotoxicity: Evidence from cell lines down-regulated for OPN expression by a targeted ribozyme. *Clinical and Experimental Metastasis,* 13(6):453-462, 1995.

Feng F, Rittling SR: Mammary tumor development in MMTV-c-myc/MMTV-v-Ha-ras transgenic mice is unaffected by osteopontin deficiency. *Breast Cancer Research and Treatment,* 63(1):71-79, 2000.

Ferrara J, McCuaig K, Hendy GN, Uskokovic M, White JH: Highly potent transcriptional activation by 16-ene derivatives of 1,25-dihydroxyvitamin D3. Lack of modulation by 9-cis-retinoic acid of response to 1,25-dihydroxyvitamin D3 or its derivatives. *Journal of Biological Chemistry,* 269(4):2971-2981, 1994.

Ferraz MP, Knowles JC, Olsen I, Monteiro FJ, Santos JD: Flow cytometry analysis of effects of glass on response of osteosarcoma cells to plasma-sprayed hydroxyapatite/CaO-P(2)O(5) coatings. *Journal of Biomedical Materials Research,* 47(4): 603-611, 1999.

Fet V, Dickinson ME, Hogan BL: Localization of the mouse gene for secreted phosphoprotein 1 (Spp-1) (2ar, osteopontin, bone sialoprotein 1, 44-kDa bone phosphoprotein, tumor-secreted phosphoprotein) to chromosome 5, closely linked to Ric (Rickettsia resistance). *Genomics,* 5(2):375-377, 1989.

Feuerbach D, Loetscher E, Buerki K, Sampath TK, Feyen JH: Establishment and characterization of conditionally immortalized stromal cell lines from a temperature-sensitive T-Ag transgenic mouse. *Journal of Bone Minerals Research,* 12(2):179-190, 1997.

Fierabracci A, Biro PA, Yiangou Y, Mennuni C, Luzzago A, Ludvigsson J, Cortese R, Bottazzo GF: Osteopontin is an autoantigen of the somatostatin cells in human islets: Identification by screening random peptide libraries with sera of patients with insulin-dependent diabetes mellitus. *Vaccine,* 18(3-4):342-354, 1999.

Filippini P, Rainaldi G, Ferrante A, Mecheri B, Gabrielli G, Bombace M, Indovina PL, Santini MT: Modulation of osteosarcoma cell growth and differentiation by silane-modified surfaces. *Journal of Biomedical Materials Research,* 55(3):338-349, 2001.

Fischer JW, Tschope C, Reinecke A, Giachelli CM, Unger T: Upregulation of osteopontin expression in renal cortex of streptozotocin-induced diabetic rats is mediated by bradykinin. *Diabetes,* 47(9):1512-1518, 1998.

Fisher JL, Field CL, Zhou H, Harris TL, Henderson MA, Choong PF: Urokinase plasminogen activator system gene expression is increased in human breast carcinoma and its bone metastases—a comparison of normal breast tissue, noninvasive and invasive carcinoma and osseous metastases. *Breast Cancer Research and Treatment,* 61(1):1-12, 2000.

Fisher JL, Mackie PS, Howard ML, Zhou H, Choong PF: The expression of the urokinase plasminogen activator system in metastatic murine osteosarcoma: An in vivo mouse model. *Clinical Cancer Research,* 7(6):1654-1660, 2001.

Fisher LW: Structure/function of the sialo-glycoproteins and proteoglycans of bone: It is still the early days. In *Chemistry and Biology of Mineralized Tissues,* Slavkin H and Price P, Eds. Excerpta Medica, Amsterdam, pp. 177 ff., 1992.

Fisher LW, Torchia DA, Fohr B, Young MF, Fedarko NS: Flexible structures of SIBLING proteins, bone sialoprotein, and osteopontin. *Biochemical and Biophysical Research Communications,* 280(2):460-465, 2001.

Fitzpatrick LA: Gender-related differences in the development of atherosclerosis: Studies at the cellular level. *Clinical and Experimental Pharmacology and Physiology,* 23(3):267-279, 1996.

Fitzpatrick LA, Severson A, Edwards WD, Ingram RT: Diffuse calcification in human coronary arteries. Association of osteopontin with atherosclerosis. *Journal of Clinical Investigation,* 94(4):1597-1604, 1994.

Floege J, Hackmann B, Kliem V, Kriz W, Alpers CE, Johnson RJ, Kuhn KW, Koch KM, Brunkhorst R: Age-related glomerulosclerosis and interstitial fibrosis in Milan normotensive rats: A podocyte disease. *Kidney International,* 51(1):230-243, 1997.

Flores ME, Heinegard D, Reinholt FP, Andersson G: Bone sialoprotein coated on glass and plastic surfaces is recognized by different beta 3 integrins. *Experimental Cell Research,* 227(1):40-46, 1996.

Flores ME, Norgard M, Heinegard D, Reinholt FP, Andersson G: RGD-directed attachment of isolated rat osteoclasts to osteopontin, bone sialoprotein, and fibronectin. *Experimental Cell Research,* 201(2):526-530, 1992.

Fong YM, Maranao MA, Moldawer LL, Wei H, Calvano SE, Kenney JS, Allison AC, Cerami A, Shires GT, Lowry SF: The acute splanchnic and peripheral tissue metabolic response to endotoxin in humans. *Journal of Clinical Investigation,* 85(6):1896-1904, 1990.

Fragale A, Tartaglia M, Bernardini S, Di Stasi AM, Di Rocco C, Velardi F, Teti A, Battaglia PA, Migliaccio S: Decreased proliferation and altered differentiation in osteoblasts from genetically and clinically distinct craniosynostotic disorders. *American Journal of Pathology,* 154(5):1465-1477, 1999.

Frangogiannis NG, Youker KA, Rossen RD, Gwechenberger M, Lindsey MH, Mendoza LH, Michael LH, Ballantyne CM, Smith CW, Entman ML: Cytokines and the microcirculation in ischemia and reperfusion. *Journal of Molecular and Cellular Cardiology,* 30(12):2567-2576, 1998.

Frank JD, Balena R, Masarachia P, Seedor JG, Cartwright ME: The effects of three different demineralization agents on osteopontin localization in adult rat bone using immunohistochemistry. *Histochemistry,* 99(4):295-301, 1993.

Franzen A, Heinegard D: Isolation and characterization of two sialoproteins present only in bone calcified matrix. *Biochemistry Journal,* 232:715, 1985.

Franzen A, Oldberg A, Solursh M: Possible recruitment of osteoblastic precursor cells from hypertrophic chondrocytes during initial osteogenesis in cartilaginous limbs of young rats. *Matrix,* 9(4):261-265, 1989.

Freedman LP, Arce V, Perez Fernandez R: DNA sequences that act as high affinity targets for the vitamin D3 receptor in the absence of the retinoid X receptor. *Molecular Endocrinology,* 8(3):265-273, 1994.

Freedman LP, Towers TL: DNA binding properties of the vitamin D3 receptor zinc finger region. *Molecular Endocrinology,* 5(12):1815-1826, 1991.

Freyen JHM, Elford P, DiPadova FE, Treschel U: Interleukin 6 is produced by bone and modulated by parathyroid hormone. *Journal of Bone Minerals Research,* 4:633, 1989.

Frick KK, Bushinsky DA: Chronic metabolic acidosis reversibly inhibits extracellular matrix gene expression in mouse osteoblasts. *American Journal of Physiology,* 275(5 Pt 2):F840-F847, 1998.

Frick KK, Bushinsky DA: In vitro metabolic and respiratory acidosis selectively inhibit osteoblastic matrix gene expression. *American Journal of Physiology,* 277(5 Pt 2):F750-F755, 1999.

Fried A, Shamay A, Wientroub S, Benayahu D: Phenotypic expression of marrow cells when grown on various substrata. *Journal of Cellular Biochemistry,* 61(2): 246-254, 1996.

Fromigue O, Marie PJ, Lomri A: Differential effects of transforming growth factor beta2, dexamethasone and 1,25-dihydroxyvitamin D on human bone marrow stromal cells. *Cytokine,* 9(8):613-623, 1997.

Fujisaki S: [A study on development of enzyme immunoassay of human osteopontin: molecular fragility of serum osteopontin]. *Hokkaido Igaku Zasshi,* 75(1): 45-52, 2000.

Fujisawa R, Butler WT, Brunn JC, Zhou HY, Kuboki Y: Differences in composition of cell-attachment sialoproteins between dentin and bone. *Journal of Dentistry Research,* 72(8):1222-1226, 1993.

Fujisawa R, Kuboki Y: [Bone matrix proteins]. *Nippon Rinsho,* 56(6):1425-1429, 1998.

Fujita Y: [Osteopontin mRNA expression in remodeling alveolar bone incident to tooth movement—visualized by in situ hybridization]. *Kokubyo Gakkai Zasshi,* 60(1):183-198, 1993.

Gabinskaya T, Salafia CM, Gulle VE, Holzman IR, Weintraub AS: Gestational age-dependent extravillous cytotrophoblast osteopontin immunolocalization differentiates between normal and preeclamptic pregnancies. *American Journal of Reproductive Immunology,* 40(5):339-346, 1998.

Gadeau AP, Campan M, Millet D, Candresse T, Desgranges C: Osteopontin overexpression is associated with arterial smooth muscle cell proliferation in vitro. *Arteriosclerosis and Thrombosis,* 13(1):120-125, 1993.

Gadeau AP, Chaulet H, Daret D, Kockx M, Daniel-Lamaziere JM, Desgranges C: Time course of osteopontin, osteocalcin, and osteonectin accumulation and calcification after acute vessel wall injury. *Journal of Histochemistry and Cytochemistry,* 49(1):79-86, 2001.

Gang X, Ueki K, Kon S, Maeda M, Naruse T, Nojima Y: Reduced urinary excretion of intact osteopontin in patients with IgA nephropathy. *American Journal of Kidney Diseases,* 37(2):374-349, 2001.

Ganss B, Cheifetz S: Expression of bone sialoprotein and osteopontin in breast cancer bone metastases. *Clinical and Experimental Metastasis,* 18(3):253-260, 2000.

Gardner HA, Berse B, Senger DR: Specific reduction in osteopontin synthesis by antisense RNA inhibits the tumorigenicity of transformed Rat1 fibroblasts. *Oncogene,* 9(8):2321-2326, 1994.

Gerstenfeld LC: Osteopontin in skeletal tissue homeostasis: An emerging picture of the autocrine/paracrine functions of the extracellular matrix. *Journal of Bone Mineral Research,* 14(6):850-855, 1999.

Gerstenfeld LC, Feng M, Gotoh Y, Glimcher MJ: Selective extractability of noncollagenous proteins from chicken bone. *Calcified Tissue International,* 55(3):230-235, 1994.

Gerstenfeld LC, Shapiro FD: Expression of bone-specific genes by hypertrophic chondrocytes: Implication of the complex functions of the hypertrophic chondrocyte during endochondral bone development. *Journal of Cellular Biochemistry,* 62(1):1-9, 1996.

Gerstenfeld LC, Uporova T, Ashkar S, Salih E, Gotoh Y, McKee MD, Nanci A, Glimcher MJ: Regulation of avian osteopontin pre- and posttranscriptional expression in skeletal tissues. *Annals of the New York Academy of Sciences,* 760:67-82, 1995.

Gerstenfeld LC, Uporova T, Schmidt J, Strauss PG, Shih SD, Huang LF, Gundberg C, Mizuno S, Glowacki J: Osteogenic potential of murine osteosarcoma cells: Comparison of bone-specific gene expression in in vitro and in vivo conditions. *Laboratory Investigation,* 74(5):895-906, 1996.

Gerstenfeld LC, Zurakowski D, Schaffer JL, Nichols DP, Toma CD, Broess M, Bruder SP, Caplan AI: Variable hormone responsiveness of osteoblast populations isolated at different stages of embryogenesis and its relationship to the osteogenic lineage. *Endocrinology,* 137(9):3957-3968, 1996.

Ghilzon R, McCulloch CA, Zohar R: Stromal mesenchymal progenitor cells. *Leukemia and Lymphoma,* 32(3-4):211-221, 1999.

Giachelli CM: Ectopic calcification: New concepts in cellular regulation. *Zeitschrift Kardiologie* 3(Suppl 90):31-37, 2001.

Giachelli CM, Bae N, Almeida M, Denhardt DT, Alpers CE, Schwartz SM: Osteopontin is elevated during neointima formation in rat arteries and is a novel component of human atherosclerotic plaques. *Journal of Clinical Investigation,* 92(4):1686-1696, 1993.

Giachelli C, Bae N, Lombardi D, Majesky M, Schwartz S: Molecular cloning and characterization of 2B7, a rat mRNA which distinguishes smooth muscle cell phenotypes in vitro and is identical to osteopontin (secreted phosphoprotein I, 2aR). *Biochemical and Biophysical Research Communications,* 177(2):867-873, 1991.

Giachelli CM, Liaw L, Murry CE, Schwartz SM, Almeida M: Osteopontin expression in cardiovascular diseases. *Annals of the New York Academy of Sciences,* 760:109-126, 1995.

Giachelli CM, Lombardi D, Johnson RJ, Murry CE, Almeida M: Evidence for a role of osteopontin in macrophage infiltration in response to pathological stimuli in vivo. *American Journal of Pathology,* 152(2):353-358, 1998.

Giachelli CM, Pichler R, Lombardi D, Denhardt DT, Alpers CE, Schwartz SM, Johnson RJ: Osteopontin expression in angiotensin II-induced tubulointerstitial nephritis. *Kidney International,* 45(2):515-524, 1994.

Giachelli CM, Steitz S: Osteopontin: A versatile regulator of inflammation and biomineralization. *Matrix Biology,* 19(7):615-622, 2000.

Giannobile WV, Lee CS, Tomala MP, Tejeda KM, Zhu Z: Platelet-derived growth factor (PDGF) gene delivery for application in periodontal tissue engineering. *Journal of Periodontology,* 72(6):815-823, 2001.

Gil JC, Cedillo RL, Mayagoitia BG, Paz MD: Isolation of *Mycoplasma pneumoniae* from asthmatic patients. *Annals of Allergy,* 70(1):23-25, 1993.

Gilbert M, Shaw WJ, Long JR, Nelson K, Drobny GP, Giachelli CM, Stayton PS: Chimeric peptides of statherin and osteopontin that bind hydroxyapatite and mediate cell adhesion. *Journal of Biological Chemistry,* 275(21):16213-16218, 2000.

Gillespie MT, Thomas RJ, Pu ZY, Zhou H, Martin TJ, Findlay DM: Calcitonin receptors, bone sialoprotein and osteopontin are expressed in primary breast cancers. *International Journal of Cancer,* 73(6):812-815, 1997.

Gladson CL: The extracellular matrix of gliomas: Modulation of cell function. *Journal of Neuropathology and Experimental Neurology,* 58(10):1029-1040, 1999.

Gladson CL, Dennis C, Rotolo TC, Kelly DR, Grammer JR: Vitronectin expression in differentiating neuroblastic tumors: Integrin alpha v beta 5 mediates vitronectin-dependent adhesion of retinoic-acid-differentiated neuroblastoma cells. *American Journal of Pathology,* 150(5):1631-1646, 1997.

Glimcher MJ: Composition, structure, and organization of bone and other mineralized tissues and the mechanism of calcification. In *Handbook of Physiology, Section 7: Endocrinology,* Vol. BII, Greep RD and Astwood EB, eds. American Physiological Society, Washington, DC, p. 25, 1976.

Glimcher MJ: Mechanism of calcification: Role of collagen fibrils and collagen-phosphoprotein complexes in vitro and in vivo. *Anatomy Records,* 224(2):139-153, 1989.

Gokhale JA, Glenton PA, Khan SR: Localization of tamm-horsfall protein and osteopontin in a rat nephrolithiasis model. *Nephron,* 73(3):456-461, 1996.

Gold D, Bowden R, Sixbey J, Riggs R, Katon WJ, Ashley R, Obrigewitch RM, Coey L: Chronic fatigue. A prospective clinical and virological study. *Journal of the American Medical Association,* 264(1):48-53, 1990.

Goldberg HA, Hunter GK: The inhibitory activity of osteopontin on hydroxyapatite formation in vitro. *Annals of the New York Academy of Sciences,* 760:305-308, 1995.

Goldberg HA, Warner KJ: The staining of acidic proteins on polyacrylamide gels: Enhanced sensitivity and stability of "Stains-all" staining in combination with silver nitrate. *Analytical Biochemistry,* 251(2):227-233, 1997.

Goldberg HA, Warner KJ, Stillman MJ, Hunter GK: Determination of the hydroxyapatite-nucleating region of bone sialoprotein. *Connective Tissue Research,* 35(1-4):385-392, 1996.

Gong H, Zolzer F, von Recklinghausen G, Rossler J, Breit S, Havers W, Fotsis T, Schweigerer L: Arginine deaminase inhibits cell proliferation by arresting cell cycle and inducing apoptosis. *Biochemical and Biophysical Research Communications,* 261(1):10-14, 1999.

Goodison S, Urquidi V, Tarin D: CD44 cell adhesion molecules. *Molecular Pathology,* 52(4):189-196, 1999.

Goodman GT, Koprowski H: Macrophages as cellular expression of inherited natural resistance. *Proceedings of the National Academy of Sciences of the United States of America,* 48:160-165, 1962.

Goppelt-Struebe M, Wiedemann T, Heusinger-Ribeiro J, Vucadinovic M, Rehm M, Prols F: Cox-2 and osteopontin in cocultured platelets and mesangial cells: Role of glucocorticoids. *Kidney International,* 57(6):2229-2238, 2000.

Goralczyk R, Appold A, Luz A, Riemann S, Strauss PG, Erfle V, Schmidt J: Establishment and characterization of osteoblast-like cell lines from retrovirus (RFB MuLV)-induced osteomas in mice. *Differentiation,* 63(5):253-262, 1998.

Goronzy J, Weyand CM, Fathman CG: Long-term humoral unresponsiveness in vivo, induced by treatment with monoclonal antibody against L3T4. *Journal of Experimental Medicine,* 164(3):911-925, 1986.

Gorski JP: Acidic phosphoproteins from bone matrix: A structural rationalization of their role in biomineralization. *Calcified Tissue International,* 50(5):391-396, 1992.

Gorski JP: Is all bone the same? Distinctive distributions and properties of non-collagenous matrix proteins in lamellar vs. woven bone imply the existence of different underlying osteogenic mechanisms. *Critical Reviews in Oral Biology and Medicine,* 9(2):201-223, 1998.

Gorski JP, Griffin D, Dudley G, Stanford C, Thomas R, Huang C, Lai E, Karr B, Solursh M: Bone acidic glycoprotein-75 is a major synthetic product of osteoblastic cells and localized as 75- and/or 50-kDa forms in mineralized phases of bone and growth plate and in serum. *Journal of Biological Chemistry,* 265(25): 14956-14963, 1990.

Gorski JP, Kremer EA, Chen Y: Bone acidic glycoprotein-75 self-associates to form large macromolecular complexes. *Connective Tissue Research,* 35(1-4):137-143, 1996.

Gorski JP, Kremer EA, Chen Y, Ryan S, Fullenkamp C, Delviscio J, Jensen K, McKee MD: Bone acidic glycoprotein-75 self-associates to form macromolecular complexes in vitro and in vivo with the potential to sequester phosphate ions. *Journal of Cellular Biochemistry,* 64(4):547-564, 1997.

Gorski JP, Kremer E, Ruiz-Perez J, Wise GE, Artigues A: Conformational analyses on soluble and surface bound osteopontin. *Annals of the New York Academy of Sciences,* 760:12-23, 1995.

Gotoh Y, Gerstenfeld LC, Glimcher MJ: Identification and characterization of the major chicken bone phosphoprotein. Analysis of its synthesis by cultured embryonic chick osteoblasts. *European Journal of Biochemistry,* 187(1):49-58, 1990.

Gotoh Y, Pierschbacher MD, Grzesiak JJ, Gerstenfeld L, Glimcher MJ: Comparison of two phosphoproteins in chicken bone and their similarities to the mammalian bone proteins, osteopontin and bone sialoprotein II. *Biochemical and Biophysical Research Communications,* 173(1):471-479, 1990.

Gotoh Y, Salih E, Glimcher MJ, Gerstenfeld LC: Characterization of the major non-collagenous proteins of chicken bone: Identification of a novel 60 kDa non-collagenous phosphoprotein. *Biochemical and Biophysical Research Communications,* 208(2):863-870, 1995.

Gould SJ, Keller GA, Hosken N, Wilkinson J, Subramani S: A conserved tripeptide sorts proteins to peroxisomes. *Journal of Cellular Biology,* 108:1657, 1989.

Gow J, Behan WM, Simpson K, McGarry F, Keir S, Behan PO: Studies on enterovirus in patients with chronic fatigue syndrome. *Clinical Infectious Diseases,* 18(Suppl 1):S126-S129, 1994.

Graf K, Do YS, Ashizawa N, Meehan WP, Giachelli CM, Marboe CC, Fleck E, Hsueh WA: Myocardial osteopontin expression is associated with left ventricular hypertrophy. *Circulation,* 96(9):3063-3071, 1997.

Grainger DJ, Witchell CM, Metcalfe JC: Tamoxifen elevates transforming growth factor-beta and suppresses diet-induced formation of lipid lesions in mouse aorta. *Nature Medicine,* 1(10):1067-1073, 1995.

Grano M, Zigrino P, Colucci S, Zambonin G, Trusolino L, Serra M, Baldini N, Teti A, Marchisio PC, Zallone AZ: Adhesion properties and integrin expression of cultured human osteoclast-like cells. *Experimental Cell Research,* 212(2):209-218, 1994.

Grantham JJ: Mechanisms of progression in autosomal dominant polycystic kidney disease. *Kidney International Supplement,* 63:S93-S97, 1997.

Grayston JT: Chlamydial diseases: 159: *Chlamydia pneumoniae (TWAR).* Vol. 2, Part III, Section C, In *Principles and Practice in Infectious Diseases,* Mandell GL, Bennet JE, Dolin R, eds. Churchill Livingstone, New York, pp. 1696-1701, 1995.

Green RS, Lieb ME, Weintraub AS, Gacheru SN, Rosenfield CL, Shah S, Kagan HM, Taubman MB: Identification of lysyl oxidase and other platelet-derived growth factor-inducible genes in vascular smooth muscle cells by differential screening. *Laboratory Investigation,* 73(4):476-482, 1995.

Grigoriadis AE, Schellander K, Wang ZQ, Wagner EF: Osteoblasts are target cells for transformation in c-fos transgenic mice. *Journal of Cellular Biology,* 122(3): 685-701, 1993.

Gronthos S, Zannettino AC, Graves SE, Ohta S, Hay SJ, Simmons PJ: Differential cell surface expression of the STRO-1 and alkaline phosphatase antigens on discrete developmental stages in primary cultures of human bone cells. *Journal of Bone Minerals Research,* 14(1):47-56, 1999.

Gross C, Krishnan AV, Malloy PJ, Eccleshall TR, Zhao XY, Feldman D: The vitamin D receptor gene start codon polymorphism: A functional analysis of FokI variants. *Journal of Bone Minerals Research,* 13(11):1691-1699, 1998.

Groves MG, Osterman JV: Host defenses in experimental scrub typhus: Genetics of natural resistance to infection. *Infection and Immunity,* 19(2):583-588, 1978.

Groves MG, Rosenstreich DL, Taylor BA, Osterman JV: Host defenses in experimental scrub typhus: Mapping the gene that controls natural resistance in mice. *Journal of Immunology,* 125:1395-1400, 1980.

Gruber R, Mayer C, Bobacz K, Krauth MT, Graninger W, Luyten FP, Erlacher L: Effects of cartilage-derived morphogenetic proteins and osteogenic protein-1 on osteochondrogenic differentiation of periosteum-derived cells. *Endocrinology,* 142(5):2087-2094, 2001.

Grzesik WJ: Integrins and bone-cell adhesion and beyond. *Archives of Immunology and Therapeutics Experimental (Warsz),* 45(4):271-275, 1997.

Grzesik WJ, Robey PG: Bone matrix RGD glycoproteins: Immunolocalization and interaction with human primary osteoblastic bone cells in vitro. *Journal of Bone Mineral Research,* 9(4):487-496, 1994.

Guidon PT Jr, Salvatori R, Bockman RS: Gallium nitrate regulates rat osteoblast expression of osteocalcin protein and mRNA levels. *Journal of Bone Minerals Research,* 8(1):103-112, 1993.

Gunnersen JM, Spirkoska V, Smith PE, Danks RA, Tan SS: Growth and migration markers of rat C6 glioma cells identified by serial analysis of gene expression. *Glia,* 32(2):146-154, 2000.

Guo H, Cai CQ, Schroeder RA, Kuo PC: Osteopontin is a negative feedback regulator of nitric oxide synthesis in murine macrophages. *Journal of Immunology,* 166(2):1079-1086, 2001.

Guo X, Zhang YP, Mitchell DA, Denhardt DT, Chambers AF: Identification of a ras-activated enhancer in the mouse osteopontin promoter and its interaction with a putative ETS-related transcription factor whose activity correlates with the metastatic potential of the cell. *Molecular and Cellular Biology,* 15(1):476-487, 1995.

Gura TA, Wright KL, Veis A, Webb CL: Identification of specific calcium-binding noncollagenous proteins associated with glutaraldehyde-preserved bovine pericardium in the rat subdermal model. *Journal of Biomedical Materials Research,* 35(4):483-495, 1997.

Hadley TJ, Klotz FW, Miller LH: Invasion of erythrocytes by malaria parasites: A cellular and molecular overview. *Annual Reviews of Microbiology,* 40:451, 1986.

Hahn CN, Kerry DM, Omdahl JL, May BK: Identification of a vitamin D responsive element in the promoter of the rat cytochrome P450(24) gene. *Nucleic Acids Research,* 22(12):2410-2416, 1994.

Hai T, Liu F, Allegretto E, Karin M, Green MR: A family of immunologically related transcription factors that include multiple forms of ATF and AP-1. *Genes and Development,* 2(10):1216-1226, 1988.

Hakki SS, Berry JE, Somerman MJ: The effect of enamel matrix protein derivative on follicle cells in vitro. *Journal of Periodontology,* 72(5):679-687, 2001.

Halasy-Nagy J, Hofstetter W: Expression of colony-stimulating factor-1 in vivo during the formation of osteoclasts. *Journal of Bone Minerals Research,* 13(8):1267-1274, 1998.

Hall TJ, Chambers TJ: Molecular aspects of osteoclast function. *Inflammation Research,* 45(1):1-9, 1996.

Hang LM, Aguado MT, Dixon FJ, Theofilopoulos AN: Induction of severe autoimmune disease in normal mice by simultaneous action of multiple immunostimulators. *Journal of Experimental Medicine,* 161(2):423-428, 1985.

Hanks SK, Quinn AM, Hunter T: The protein kinase family: Conserved features and deduced phylogeny of the catalytic domains. *Science,* 241(4861):42-52, 1988.

Hao H, Hirota S, Tsukamoto Y, Imakita M, Ishibashi-Ueda H, Yutani C: Alterations of bone matrix protein mRNA expression in rat aorta in vitro. *Arteriosclerosis and Thrombosis Vascular Biology,* 15(9):1474-1480, 1995.

Hara A, Ikeda T, Nomura S, Yagita H, Okumura K, Yamauchi Y: In vivo implantation of human osteosarcoma cells in nude mice induces bones with human-derived osteoblasts and mouse-derived osteocytes. *Laboratory Investigations,* 75(5):707-717, 1996.

Harada H, Miki R, Masushige S, Kato S: Gene expression of retinoic acid receptors, retinoid-X receptors, and cellular retinol-binding protein I in bone and its regulation by vitamin A. *Endocrinology,* 136(12):5329-5335, 1995.

Harada H, Tagashira S, Fujiwara M, Ogawa S, Katsumata T, Yamaguchi A, Komori T, Nakatsuka M: Cbfa1 isoforms exert functional differences in osteoblast differentiation. *Journal of Biological Chemistry,* 274(11):6972-6878, 1999.

Harada N, Mizoi T, Kinouchi M, Hoshi K, Ishii S, Shiiba K, Sasaki I, Matsuno S: Introduction of antisense CD44S CDNA down-regulates expression of overall CD44 isoforms and inhibits tumor growth and metastasis in highly metastatic colon carcinoma cells. *International Journal of Cancer,* 91(1):67-75, 2001.

Harant H, Spinner D, Reddy GS, Lindley IJ: Natural metabolites of 1alpha,25-dihydroxyvitamin D(3) retain biologic activity mediated through the vitamin D receptor. *Journal of Cellular Biochemistry,* 78(1):112-120, 2000.

Harle J, Salih V, Mayia F, Knowles JC, Olsen I: Effects of ultrasound on the growth and function of bone and periodontal ligament cells in vitro. *Ultrasound Medicine and Biology,* 27(4):579-586, 2001.

Harris SA, Enger RJ, Riggs BL, Spelsberg TC: Development and characterization of a conditionally immortalized human fetal osteoblastic cell line. *Journal of Bone Minerals Research,* 10(2):178-186, 1995.

Harris SE, Bonewald LF, Harris MA, Sabatini M, Dallas S, Feng JQ, Ghosh-Choudhury N, Wozney J, Mundy GR: Effects of transforming growth factor beta on bone nodule formation and expression of bone morphogenetic protein 2, osteocalcin, osteopontin, alkaline phosphatase, and type I collagen mRNA in long-term cultures of fetal rat calvarial osteoblasts. *Journal of Bone Minerals Research,* 9(6):855-863, 1994.

Harris SE, Sabatini M, Harris MA, Feng JQ, Wozney J, Mundy GR: Expression of bone morphogenetic protein messenger RNA in prolonged cultures of fetal rat calvarial cells. *Journal of Bone Minerals Research,* 9(3):389-394, 1994.

Harter LV, Hruska KA, Duncan RL: Human osteoblast-like cells respond to mechanical strain with increased bone matrix protein production independent of hormonal regulation. *Endocrinology,* 136(2):528-535, 1995.

Hartner A, Porst M, Gauer S, Prols F, Veelken R, Hilgers KF: Glomerular osteopontin expression and macrophage infiltration in glomerulosclerosis of doca-salt rats. *American Journal of Kidney Diseases,* 38(1):153-164, 2001.

Hashimoto F, Kobayashi Y, Kobayashi ET, Sakai E, Kobayashi K, Shibata M, Kato Y, Sakai H: Expression and localization of MGP in rat tooth cementum. *Archives of Oral Biology,* 46(7):585-592, 2001.

Hashimoto Y, Tajima O, Hashiba H, Nose K, Kuroki T: Elevated expression of secondary, but not early, responding genes to phorbol ester tumor promoters in papillomas and carcinomas of mouse skin. *Molecular Carcinogenesis,* 3(5):302-308, 1990.

Haussler MR, Haussler CA, Jurutka PW, Thompson PD, Hsieh JC, Remus LS, Selznick SH, Whitfield GK: The vitamin D hormone and its nuclear receptor: Molecular actions and disease states. *Journal of Endocrinology,* 154(Suppl):S57-S73, 1997.

Haussler MR, Jurutka PW, Hsieh JC, Thompson PD, Selznick SH, Haussler CA, Whitfield GK: New understanding of the molecular mechanism of receptor-mediated genomic actions of the vitamin D hormone. *Bone,* 17(Suppl 2):33S-38S, 1995.

Hay E, Hott M, Graulet AM, Lomri A, Marie PJ: Effects of bone morphogenetic protein-2 on human neonatal calvaria cell differentiation. *Journal of Cellular Biochemistry,* 72(1):81-93, 1999.

Hayami T, Endo N, Tokunaga K, Yamagiwa H, Hatano H, Uchida M, Takahashi HE: Spatiotemporal change of rat collagenase (MMP-13) mRNA expression in the development of the rat femoral neck. *Journal of Bone Mineral Metabolism,* 18(4):185-193, 2000.

Heath JK, Rodan SB, Yoon K, Rodan GA: Rat calvarial cell lines immortalized with SV-40 large T antigen: Constitutive and retinoic acid-inducible expression of osteoblastic features. *Endocrinology,* 124(6):3060-3068, 1989a.

Heath JK, Rodan SB, Yoon K, Rodan GA: SV-40 large-T immortalization of embryonic bone cells: Establishment of osteoblastic clonal cell lines. *Connective Tissue Research,* 20(1-4):15-21, 1989b.

Hedgepeth RC, Yang L, Resnick MI, Marengo SR: Expression of proteins that inhibit calcium oxalate crystallization in vitro in the urine of normal and stone-forming individuals. *American Journal of Kidney Disease,* 37(1):104-112, 2001.

Heinegard D: Studies of bone matrix molecules give us insights into bone remodelling. *Experientia,* 51(3):195-196, 1995.

Heinegard D, Andersson G, Reinholt FP: Roles of osteopontin in bone remodeling. *Annals of the New York Academy of Sciences,* 760:213-222, 1995.

Heinegard D, Hultenby K, Oldberg A, Reinholt F, Wendel M: Macromolecules in bone matrix. *Connect Tissue Research,* 21(1-4):3-11; discussion 12-14, 1989.

Heinegard D, Oldberg A: Structure and biology of cartilage and bone matrix noncollagenous macromolecules. *FASEB Journal,* 3(9):2042-2051, 1989.

Helder MN, Bronckers AL, Woltgens JH: Dissimilar expression patterns for the extracellular matrix proteins osteopontin (OPN) and collagen type I in dental tissues and alveolar bone of the neonatal rat. *Matrix,* 13(5):415-425, 1993.

Helfrich MH, Nesbitt SA, Dorey EL, Horton MA: Rat osteoclasts adhere to a wide range of RGD (Arg-Gly-Asp) peptide-containing proteins, including the bone sialoproteins and fibronectin, via a beta 3 integrin. *Journal of Bone Mineral Research,* 7(3):335-343, 1992.

Helluin O, Chan C, Vilaire G, Mousa S, DeGrado WF, Bennett JS: The activation state of alphavbeta 3 regulates platelet and lymphocyte adhesion to intact and thrombin-cleaved osteopontin. *Journal of Biological Chemistry,* 275(24):8337-8343, 2000.

Heneine W: Lack of evidence for infection with known human and animal retroviruses in patients with chronic fatigue syndrome. *Clinical Infectious Diseases,* 18(Suppl 1):S121, 1994.

Hennessy T: CFS: A comprehensive approach. May 12, F. Nightingale's birthday. *Annales Internationales de Medécine,* 121:953-959, 1994.

Hession C, Decker JM, Shorblom AP, Kumar S, Yue CC, Mattaliano RJ, Tizard R, Kawashima E, Schmeissner U, Heletky S, et al.: Uromodulin (Tamm-Horsfall glycoprotein): A renal ligand for lymphokines. *Science,* 237(4821):1479-1484, 1987.

Heymann D, Guicheux J, Gouin F, Passuti N, Daculsi G: Cytokines, growth factors and osteoclasts. *Cytokine,* 10(3):155-168, 1998.

Higashi Y, Takenaka A, Takahashi SI, Noguchi T: Effect of protein restriction on the messenger RNA contents of bone-matrix proteins, insulin-like growth factors and insulin-like growth factor binding proteins in femur of ovariectomized rats. *British Journal of Nutrition,* 75(6):811-823, 1996.

Higuchi Y, Ito M, Tajima M, Higuchi S, Miyamoto N, Nishio M, Kawano M, Kusagawa S, Tsurudome M, Sudo A, et al.: Gene expression during osteoclast-like cell formation induced by antifusion regulatory protein-1/CD98/4F2 monoclonal antibodies (MAbs): c-src is selectively induced by anti-FRP-1 MAb. *Bone,* 25(1):17-24, 1999.

Hijiya N, Setoguchi M, Matsuura K, Higuchi Y, Akizuki S, Yamamoto S: Cloning and characterization of the human osteopontin gene and its promoter. *Biochemical Journal,* 303(Pt 1):255-262, 1994.

Hillsley MV, Frangos JA: Alkaline phosphatase in osteoblasts is down-regulated by pulsatile fluid flow. *Calcified Tissue International,* 60(1):48-53, 1997.

Hirakawa K, Hirota S, Ikeda T, Yamaguchi A, Takemura T, Nagoshi J, Yoshiki S, Suda T, Kitamura Y, Nomura S: Localization of the mRNA for bone matrix proteins during fracture healing as determined by in situ hybridization. *Journal of Bone Minerals Research,* 9(10):1551-1557, 1994.

Hirota S, Imakita M, Kohri K, Ito A, Morii E, Adachi S, Kim HM, Kitamura Y, Yutani C, Nomura S: Expression of osteopontin messenger RNA by macrophages in atherosclerotic plaques. A possible association with calcification. *American Journal of Pathology,* 143(4):1003-1008, 1993.

Hirota S, Ito A, Nagoshi J, Takeda M, Kurata A, Takatsuka Y, Kohri K, Nomura S, Kitamura Y: Expression of bone matrix protein messenger ribonucleic acids in human breast cancers. Possible involvement of osteopontin in development of calcifying foci. *Laboratory Investigations,* 72(1):64-69, 1995.

Hirota S, Nakajima Y, Yoshimine T, Kohri K, Nomura S, Taneda M, Hayakawa T, Kitamura Y: Expression of bone-related protein messenger RNA in human meningiomas: Possible involvement of osteopontin in development of psammoma bodies. *Journal of Neuropathology and Experimental Neurology,* 54(5):698-703, 1995.

Hirota S, Takaoka K, Hashimoto J, Nakase T, Takemura T, Morii E, Fukuyama A, Morihana K, Kitamura Y, Nomura S: Expression of mRNA of murine bone-related proteins in ectopic bone induced by murine bone morphogenetic protein-4. *Cell and Tissue Research,* 277(1):27-32, 1994.

Holzman LB, Marks RM, Dixit VM: A novel immediate-early response gene of endothelium is induced by cytokines and encodes a secreted protein. *Molecular and Cellular Biology,* 10:5830-5838, 1990.

Honda M, Yoshioka T, Yamaguchi S, Yoshimura K, Miyake O, Utsunomiya M, Koide T, Okuyama A: Characterization of protein components of human urinary crystal surface binding substance. *Urology Research,* 25(5):355-360, 1997.

Hopp TP, Woods KR: A computer program for predicting protein antigenic determinants. *Molecular Immunology,* 20(4):483-489, 1983.

Horowitz S, Horowitz J, Hou L, Fuchs E, Rager-Zisman B, Jacobs E, Alkan M: Antibodies to *Mycoplasma fermentans* in HIV-positive heterosexual patients: Seroprevalence and association with AIDS. *Journal of Infectious Diseases,* 36(1): 79-84, 1998.

Horton MA, Nesbit MA, Helfrich MH: Interaction of osteopontin with osteoclast integrins. *Annals of the New York Academy of Sciences,* 760:190-200, 1995.

Hoshi K, Ejiri S, Ozawa H: Organic components of crystal sheaths in bones. *Journal of Electron Microscopy (Tokyo),* 50(1):33-40, 2001.

Hoshi K, Komori T, Ozawa H: Morphological characterization of skeletal cells in Cbfa1-deficient mice. *Bone,* 25(6):639-651, 1999.

Hossain MS, Takimoto H, Ninomiya T, Yoshida H, Kishihara K, Matsuzaki G, Kimura G, Nomoto K: Characterization of CD4- CD8- CD3+ T-cell receptor-alphabeta+ T cells in murine cytomegalovirus infection. *Immunology,* 101(1): 19-29, 2000.

Hotta H, Kon S, Katagiri YU, Tosa N, Tsukamoto T, Chambers AF, Uede T: Detection of various epitopes of murine osteopontin by monoclonal antibodies. *Biochemical and Biophysical Research Communications,* 257(1):6-11, 1999.

Hou LT, Liu CM, Chen YJ, Wong MY, Chen KC, Chen J, Thomas HF: Characterization of dental follicle cells in developing mouse molar. *Archives of Oral Biology,* 44(9):759-770, 1999.

Hou LT, Liu CM, Lei JY, Wong MY, Chen JK: Biological effects of cementum and bone extracts on human periodontal fibroblasts. *Journal of Periodontology,* 71(7):1100-1109, 2000.

Hoyer JR: Uropontin in urinary calcium stone formation. *Mineral and Electrolyte Metabolism,* 20(6):385-392, 1994.

Hoyer JR, Asplin JR, Otvos L: Phosphorylated osteopontin peptides suppress crystallization by inhibiting the growth of calcium oxalate crystals. *Kidney International,* 60(1):77-82, 2001.

Hoyer JR, Otvos L Jr, Urge L: Osteopontin in urinary stone formation. *Annals of the New York Academy of Sciences,* 760:257-265, 1995.

Hoyer JR, Pietrzyk RA, Liu H, Whitson PA: Effects of microgravity on urinary osteopontin. *Journal of the American Society of Nephrology,* 10(Suppl 14):S389-S393, 1999.

Hruska KA, Rifas L, Cheng SL, Gupta A, Halstead L, Avioli L: X-linked hypophosphatemic rickets and the murine Hyp homologue. *American Journal of Physiology,* 268(3 Pt 2):F357-F362, 1995.

Hruska KA, Rolnick F, Huskey M, Alvarez U, Cheresh D: Engagement of the osteoclast integrin alpha v beta 3 by osteopontin stimulates phosphatidylinositol 3-hydroxyl kinase activity. *Endocrinology,* 136(7):2984-2992, 1995a.

Hruska KA, Rolnick F, Huskey M, Alvarez U, Cheresh D: Engagement of the osteoclast integrin alpha v beta 3 by osteopontin stimulates phosphatidylinositol 3-hydroxyl kinase activity. *Annals of the New York Academy of Sciences,* 760:151-165, 1995b.

Hsieh JC, Nakajima S, Galligan MA, Jurutka PW, Haussler CA, Whitfield GK, Haussler MR: Receptor mediated genomic action of the 1,25(OH)2D3 hormone: Expression of the human vitamin D receptor in *E. coli. Journal of Steroid Biochemistry and Molecular Biology,* 53(1-6):583-594, 1995.

Hsueh WA, Do YS, Jeyaseelan R: Angiotensin II and cardiac remodeling. *Mount Sinai Journal of Medicine,* 65(2):104-147, 1998.

Hu DD, Hoyer JR, Smith JW: Ca2+ suppresses cell adhesion to osteopontin by attenuating binding affinity for integrin alpha v beta 3. *Journal of Biological Chemistry,* 270(17):9917-9925, 1995a.

Hu DD, Hoyer JR, Smith JW: Characterization of the interaction between integrins and recombinant human osteopontin. *Annals of the New York Academy of Sciences,* 760:312-314, 1995b.

Hu DD, Lin EC, Kovach NL, Hoyer JR, Smith JW: A biochemical characterization of the binding of osteopontin to integrins alpha v beta 1 and alpha v beta 5. *Journal of Biological Chemistry,* 270(44):26232-26238, 1995.

Hu WY, Fukuda N, Satoh C, Jian T, Kubo A, Nakayama M, Kishioka H, Kanmatsuse K: Phenotypic modulation by fibronectin enhances the angiotensin II-generating system in cultured vascular smooth muscle cells. *Arteriosclerosis and Thrombosis Vascular Biology,* 20(6):1500-1505, 2000.

Huang LF, Fukai N, Selby PB, Olsen BR, Mundlos S: Mouse clavicular development: Analysis of wild-type and cleidocranial dysplasia mutant mice. *Development Dynamics,* 210(1):33-40, 1997.

Huang XZ, Wu JF, Ferrando R, Lee JH, Wang YL, Farese RV Jr, Sheppard D: Fatal bilateral chylothorax in mice lacking the integrin alpha9beta1. *Molecular and Cellular Biology,* 20(14):5208-5215, 2000.

Huang YQ, Li JJ, Moscatelli D, Basilico C, Nicolaides A, Zhang WG, Poiesz BJ, Friedman-Kien AE: Expression of int-2 oncogene in Kaposi's sarcoma lesions. *Journal of Clinical Investigation,* 91(3):1191-1197, 1993.

Hudkins KL, Giachelli CM, Cui Y, Couser WG, Johnson RJ, Alpers CE: Osteopontin expression in fetal and mature human kidney. *Journal of the American Society of Nephrology,* 10(3):444-457, 1999.

Hudkins KL, Giachelli CM, Eitner F, Couser WG, Johnson RJ, Alpers CE: Osteopontin expression in human crescentic glomerulonephritis. *Kidney International,* 57(1):105-116, 2000.

Hudkins KL, Lee QC, Segerer S, Johnson RJ, Davis CL, Giachelli CM, Alpers CE: Osteopontin expression in human cyclosponine toxicity. *Kidney International,* 60(2):635-640, 2001.

Hullinger TG, Pan Q, Viswanathan HL, Somerman MJ: TGFbeta and BMP-2 activation of the OPN promoter: Roles of smad- and hox-binding elements. *Experimental Cell Research,* 262(1):69-74, 2001.

Hullinger TG, Taichman RS, Linseman DA, Somerman MJ: Secretory products from PC-3 and MCF-7 tumor cell lines upregulate osteopontin in MC3T3-E1 cells. *Journal of Cellular Biochemistry,* 78(4):607-616, 2000.

Hultenby K, Reinholt FP, Heinegard D, Andersson G, Marks SC Jr: Osteopontin: A ligand for the alpha v beta 3 integrin of the osteoclast clear zone in osteopetrotic (ia/ia) rats. *Annals of the New York Academy of Sciences,* 760:315-318, 1995.

Hultenby K, Reinholt FP, Norgard M, Oldberg A, Wendel M, Heinegard D: Distribution and synthesis of bone sialoprotein in metaphyseal bone of young rats show a distinctly different pattern from that of osteopontin. *European Journal of Cellular Biology,* 63(2):230-239, 1994.

Hultenby K, Reinholt FP, Oldberg A, Heinegard D: Ultrastructural immunolocalization of osteopontin in metaphyseal and cortical bone. *Matrix,* 11(3):206-213, 1991.

Hultgardh-Nilsson A, Cercek B, Wang JW, Naito S, Lovdahl C, Sharifi B, Forrester JS, Fagin JA: Regulated expression of the ets-1 transcription factor in vascular smooth muscle cells in vivo and in vitro. *Circulation Research,* 78(4):589-595, 1996.

Hultgardh-Nilsson A, Lovdahl C, Blomgren K, Kallin B, Thyberg J: Expression of phenotype- and proliferation-related genes in rat aortic smooth muscle cells in primary culture. *Cardiovascular Research,* 34(2):418-430, 1997.

Hulth A, Johnell O, Lindberg L, Heinegard D: Sequential appearance of macromolecules in bone induction in the rat. *Journal of Orthopedics Research,* 11(3):367-378, 1993.

Hunter GK, Goldberg HA: Nucleation of hydroxyapatite by bone sialoprotein. *Proceedings of the National Academy of Sciences of the United States of America,* 90(18):8562-8565, 1993.

Hunter GK, Hauschka PV, Poole AR, Rosenberg LC, Goldberg HA: Nucleation and inhibition of hydroxyapatite formation by mineralized tissue proteins. *Biochemical Journal,* 317(Pt 1):59-64, 1996.

Hunter GK, Kyle CL, Goldberg HA: Modulation of crystal formation by bone phosphoproteins: Structural specificity of the osteopontin-mediated inhibition of hydroxyapatite formation. *Biochemical Journal,* 300(Pt 3):723-728, 1994.

Hwang SM, Lopez CA, Heck DE, Gardner CR, Laskin DL, Laskin JD, Denhardt DT: Osteopontin inhibits induction of nitric oxide synthase gene expression by inflammatory mediators in mouse kidney epithelial cells. *Journal of Biological Chemistry,* 269(1):711-715, 1994.

Hwang SM, Wilson PD, Laskin JD, Denhardt DT: Age and development-related changes in osteopontin and nitric oxide synthase mRNA levels in human kidney proximal tubule epithelial cells: Contrasting responses to hypoxia and reoxygenation. *Journal of Cellular Physiology,* 160(1):61-68, 1994.

Iba K, Chiba H, Sawada N, Hirota S, Ishii S, Mori M: Glucocorticoids induce mineralization coupled with bone protein expression without influence on growth of a human osteoblastic cell line. *Cell Structure and Function,* 20(5):319-330, 1995.

Iba K, Sawada N, Nuka S, Chiba H, Obata H, Isomura H, Satoh M, Ishii S, Mori M: Phase-dependent effects of transforming growth factor beta 1 on osteoblastic markers of human osteoblastic cell line sV-HFO during mineralization. *Bone,* 19(4):363-369, 1996.

Ibaraki K, Termine JD, Whitson SW, Young MF: Bone matrix mRNA expression in differentiating fetal bovine osteoblasts. *Journal of Bone Minerals Research,* 7(7):743-754, 1992.

Ibrahim T, Leong I, Sanchez-Sweatman O, Khokha R, Sodek J, Tenenbaum HC, Ichikawa H, Itota T, Nishitani Y, Torii Y, et al.: Osteopontin-immunoreactive primary sensory neurons in the rat spinal and trigeminal nervous systems. *Brain Research,* 863(1-2):276-281, 2000.

Ichikawa H, Itota T, Nishitani Y, Torii Y, Inoue K, Sugimoto T: Osteopontin-immunoreactive primary sensory neurons in the rat spinal and trigeminal nervous systems. *Brain Research,* 863(1-2):276-281, 2000.

Ichimiya I, Adams JC, Kimura RS: Immunolocalization of Na+, K(+)-ATPase, Ca(++)-ATPase, calcium-binding proteins, and carbonic anhydrase in the guinea pig inner ear. *Acta Otolaryngologica,* 114(2):167-176, 1994.

Iguchi M, Takamura C, Umekawa T, Kurita T, Kohri K: Inhibitory effects of female sex hormones on urinary stone formation in rats. *Kidney International,* 56(2):479-485, 1999.

Ihara H, Denhardt DT, Furuya K, Yamashita T, Muguruma Y, Tsuji K, Hruska KA, Higashio K, Enomoto S, Nifuji A, et al.: Parathyroid hormone-induced bone resorption does not occur in the absence of osteopontin. *Journal of Biological Chemistry,* 276(16):13065-13071, 2001.

Iizuka J: [Relationship between osteopontin expression and autoimmune disease—analysis of osteopontin expressed in transgenic mice]. *Hokkaido Igaku Zasshi,* 73(5):487-495, 1998.

Iizuka J, Katagiri Y, Tada N, Murakami M, Ikeda T, Sato M, Hirokawa K, Okada S, Hatano M, Tokuhisa T, et al.: Introduction of an osteopontin gene confers the increase in B1 cell population and the production of anti-DNA autoantibodies. *Laboratory Investigations,* 78(12):1523-1533, 1998.

Iizuka K, Murakami T, Kawaguchi H: Pure atmospheric pressure promotes an expression of osteopontin in human aortic smooth muscle cells. *Biochemical and Biophysical Research Communications,* 283(2):493-498, 2001.

Ikeda T, Nagai Y, Yamaguchi A, Yokose S, Yoshiki S: Age-related reduction in bone matrix protein mRNA expression in rat bone tissues: Application of histomorphometry to in situ hybridization. *Bone,* 16(1):17-23, 1995.

Ikeda T, Nomura S, Yamaguchi A, Suda T, Yoshiki S: In situ hybridization of bone matrix proteins in undecalcified adult rat bone sections. *Journal of Histochemistry and Cytochemistry,* 40(8):1079-1088, 1992.

Ikeda T, Shirasawa T, Esaki Y, Yoshiki S, Hirokawa K: Osteopontin mRNA is expressed by smooth muscle-derived foam cells in human atherosclerotic lesions of the aorta. *Journal of Clinical Investigation,* 92(6):2814-2820, 1993.

Ikeda T, Yamaguchi A, Yokose S, Nagai Y, Yamato H, Nakamura T, Tsurukami H, Tanizawa T, Yoshiki S: Changes in biological activity of bone cells in ovariectomized rats revealed by in situ hybridization. *Journal of Bone Minerals Research,* 11(6):780-788, 1996.

Ikedo D, Ohishi K, Yamauchi N, Kataoka M, Kido J, Nagata T: Stimulatory effects of phenytoin on osteoblastic differentiation of fetal rat calvaria cells in culture. *Bone,* 25(6):653-660, 1999.

Ikenoue T, Jingushi S, Urabe K, Okazaki K, Iwamoto Y: Inhibitory effects of activin-A on osteoblast differentiation during cultures of fetal rat calvarial cells. *Journal of Cellular Biochemistry,* 75(2):206-214, 1999.

Inada M, Yasui T, Nomura S, Miyake S, Deguchi K, Himeno M, Sato M, Yamagiwa H, Kimura T, Yasui N, et al.: Maturational disturbance of chondrocytes in Cbfa1-deficient mice. *Developmental Dynamics,* 214(4):279-290, 1999.

Ingram RT, Clarke BL, Fisher LW, Fitzpatrick LA: Distribution of noncollagenous proteins in the matrix of adult human bone: Evidence of anatomic and functional heterogeneity. *Journal of Bone Minerals Research,* 8(9):1019-1029, 1993.

Ingram RT, Collazo-Clavell M, Tiegs R, Fitzpatrick LA: Paget's disease is associated with changes in the immunohistochemical distribution of noncollagenous matrix proteins in bone. *Journal of Clinical Endocrinology and Metabolism,* 81(5):1810-1820, 1996.

Ingram RT, Park YK, Clarke BL, Fitzpatrick LA: Age- and gender-related changes in the distribution of osteocalcin in the extracellular matrix of normal male and female bone. Possible involvement of osteocalcin in bone remodeling. *Journal of Clinical Investigation,* 93(3):989-997, 1994.

Inoue H, Nebgen D, Veis A: Changes in phenotypic gene expression in rat mandibular condylar cartilage cells during long-term culture. *Journal of Bone Minerals Research,* 10(11):1691-1697, 1995.

Inouye H, Kirschner DA: Folding and function of the myelin proteins form primary sequence data. *Journal of Neuroscience Research,* 28(1):1-17, 1991.

Irie K, Zalzal S, Ozawa H, McKee MD, Nanci A: Morphological and immunocytochemical characterization of primary osteogenic cell cultures derived from fetal rat cranial tissue. *Anatomy Records,* 252(4):554-567, 1998.

Iseki S, Wilkie AO, Heath JK, Ishimaru T, Eto K, Morriss-Kay GM: Fgfr2 and osteopontin domains in the developing skull vault are mutually exclusive and can be altered by locally applied FGF2. *Development,* 124(17):3375-3384, 1997.

Iseki S, Wilkie AO, Morriss-Kay GM: Fgfr1 and Fgfr2 have distinct differentiation- and proliferation-related roles in the developing mouse skull vault. *Development,* 126(24):5611-5620, 1999.

Ishijima M, Rittling SR, Yamashita T, Tsuji K, Kurosawa H, Nifuji A, Ishizeki K, Nomura S, Takigawa M, Shioji H, et al.: Expression of osteopontin in Meckel's cartilage cells during phenotypic transdifferentiation in vitro, as detected by in situ hybridization and immunocytochemical analysis. *Histochemistry and Cellular Biology,* 110(5):457-466, 1998.

Ishizeki K, Saito H, Shinagawa T, Fujiwara N, Nawa T: Histochemical and immunohistochemical analysis of the mechanism of calcification of Meckel's cartilage during mandible development in rodents. *Journal of Anatomy,* 194(Pt 2):265-277, 1999.

Isogai N, Landis WJ, Mori R, Gotoh Y, Gerstenfeld LC, Upton J, Vacanti JP: Experimental use of fibrin glue to induce site-directed osteogenesis from cultured periosteal cells. *Plastic Reconstruction Surgery,* 105(3):953-963, 2000.

Ito T: [Significance of macrophage and cytokines in expression of stone matrix]. *Nippon Hinyokika Gakkai Zasshi,* 87(5):865-874, 1996.

Itoh Y, Okanoue T: Chemotactic cytokines (chemokines) in human hepatitis and experimental hepatitis models: Which ones play the crucial role? *Journal of Gastroenterology,* 35(9):724-725, 2000.

Ivanovski S, Haase HR, Bartold PM: Expression of bone matrix protein mRNAs by primary and cloned cultures of the regenerative phenotype of human periodontal fibroblasts. *Journal of Dental Research,* 80(7):1665-1671, 2001.

Ivanovski S, Li H, Daley T, Bartold PM: An immunohistochemical study of matrix molecules associated with barrier membrane-mediated periodontal wound healing. *Journal of Periodontal Research,* 35(3):115-126, 2000.

Iwamoto M, Shapiro IM, Yagami K, Boskey AL, Leboy PS, Adams SL, Pacifici M: Retinoic acid induces rapid mineralization and expression of mineralization-related genes in chondrocytes. *Experimental Cell Research,* 207(2):413-420, 1993.

Iwamoto M, Yagami K, Shapiro IM, Leboy PS, Adams SL, Pacifici M: Retinoic acid is a major regulator of chondrocyte maturation and matrix mineralization. *Microscopy Research Techniques,* 28(6):483-491, 1994.

Jaaskelainen T, Itkonen A, Maenpaa PH: Retinoid-X-receptor-alpha-independent binding of vitamin D receptor to its response element from human osteocalcin gene. *European Journal of Biochemistry,* 228(2):222-228, 1995.

Jadin CL: Common clinical and biological windows on CFS and rickettsial diseases. *Journal of Chronic Fatigue Syndrome,* 6:133-146, 2000.

Jadin JB: Origine des maladies Rickettsiennes. [Origin of rickettsial diseases.] *Annales de la Societé Belge de Medécine Tropicale,* Vol. 3, pp. 1 ff., 1953.

Jakob F, Siggelkow H, Homann D, Kohrle J, Adamski J, Schutze N: Local estradiol metabolism in osteoblast- and osteoclast-like cells. *Journal of Steroid Biochemistry and Molecular Biology,* 61(3-6):167-174, 1997.

James IE, Dodds RA, Lee-Rykaczewski E, Eichman CF, Connor JR, Hart TK, Maleeff BE, Lackman RD, Gowen M: Purification and characterization of fully functional human osteoclast precursors. *Journal of Bone Minerals Research,* 11(11):1608-1618, 1996.

Janeway CA Jr, Yagi J, Conrad PJ, Katz ME, James B, Vroegop S, Buxser S: T-cell responses to Mls and bacterial proteins that mimic its behavior. *Immunology Reviews,* 107:61-88, 1989.

Jang A, Hill RP: An examination of the effects of hypoxia, acidosis, and glucose starvation on the expression of metastasis-associated genes in murine tumor cells. *Clinical and Experimental Metastasis,* 15(5):469-483, 1997.

Jenis LG, Lian JB, Stein GS, Baran DT: 1 alpha,25-dihydroxyvitamin D3-induced changes in intracellular pH in osteoblast-like cells modulate gene expression. *Journal of Cellular Biochemistry,* 53(3):234-239, 1993.

Jenis LG, Ongphiphadhanakul B, Braverman LE, Stein GS, Lian JB, Lew R, Baran DT: Responsiveness of gene expression markers of osteoblastic and osteoclastic activity to calcitonin in the appendicular and axial skeleton of the rat in vivo. *Calcified Tissue International,* 54(6):511-515, 1994.

Jenkins JK, Huang H, Ndebele K, Salahudeen AK: Vitamin E inhibits renal mRNA expression of COX II, HO I, TGFbeta, and osteopontin in the rat model of cyclosporine nephrotoxicity. *Transplantation,* 71(2):331-334, 2001.

Jerrells TR, Eismann CS: Role of T lymphocytes in production of antibody to antigens of *Rickettsia tsutsugamushi* and other *Rickettsia* species. *Infection and Immunity,* 41:666-675, 1983.

Jerrells TR, Osterman JV: Host defenses in experimental scrub typhus: Inflammatory response of congenic C3H mice differing at the *Ric* locus. *Infection and Immunity,* 31:1014-1020, 1981.

Jerrells TR, Osterman JV: Role of macrophages in innate and acquired host resistance to experimental scrub typhus infection of inbred mice. *Infection and Immunity,* 39:1066-1074, 1982.

Jiang XJ, Feng T, Chang LS, Kong XT, Wang G, Zhang ZW, Guo YL: Expression of osteopontin mRNA in normal and stone-forming rat kidney. *Urology Research,* 26(6):389-394, 1998.

Jin CH, Miyaura C, Ishimi Y, Hong MH, Sato T, Abe E, Suda T: Interleukin 1 regulates the expression of osteopontin mRNA by osteoblasts. *Molecular and Cellular Endocrinology,* 74(3):221-228, 1990.

Jin CH, Shinki T, Hong MH, Sato T, Yamaguchi A, Ikeda T, Yoshiki S, Abe E, Suda T: 1 alpha,25-dihydroxyvitamin D3 regulates in vivo production of the third component of complement (C3) in bone. *Endocrinology,* 131(5):2468-2475, 1992.

Jin Y, Kuroda N, Kakiuchi S, Yamasaki Y, Miyazaki E, Hayashi Y, Toi M, Naruse K, Hiroi M, Enzan H: Bronchial granular cell tumor with osteopontin and osteonectin expression: A case report. *Pathology International,* 50(5):421-426, 2000.

Johansson CB, Roser K, Bolind P, Donath K, Albrektsson T: Bone-tissue formation and integration of titanium implants: An evaluation with newly developed enzyme and immunohistochemical techniques. *Clinical Implant Dentistry Related Research,* 1(1):33-40, 1999.

Johnson GA, Burghardt RC, Spencer TE, Newton GR, Ott TL, Bazer FW: Ovine osteopontin: II. Osteopontin and alpha(v)beta(3) integrin expression in the uterus and conceptus during the periimplantation period. *Biology and Reproduction,* 61(4):892-899, 1999.

Johnson GA, Spencer TE, Burghardt RC, Bazer FW: Ovine osteopontin: I. Cloning and expression of messenger ribonucleic acid in the uterus during the periimplantation period. *Biology and Reproduction,* 61(4):884-891, 1999.

Johnson GA, Spencer TE, Burghardt RC, Taylor KM, Gray CA, Bazer FW: Progesterone modulation of osteopontin gene expression in the ovine uterus. *Biology and Reproduction,* 62(5):1315-1321, 2000.

Johnson RJ, Gordon KL, Giachelli C, Kurth T, Skelton MM, Cowley AW Jr: Tubulointerstitial injury and loss of nitric oxide synthases parallel the development of hypertension in the Dahl-SS rat. *Journal of Hypertension,* 18(10):1497-1505, 2000.

Johnson RJ, Gordon KL, Suga S, Duijvestijn AM, Griffin K, Bidani A: Renal injury and salt-sensitive hypertension after exposure to catecholamines. *Hypertension,* 34(1):151-159, 1999.

Johnson-Pais TL, Leach RJ: Regulation of osteoblast gene expression in intratypic osteosarcoma hybrid cells. *Experimental Cell Research,* 221(2):370-376, 1995.

Jonassen JA, Cooney R, Kennington L, Gravel K, Honeyman T, Scheid CR: Oxalate-induced changes in the viability and growth of human renal epithelial cells. *Journal of the American Society of Nephrology,* 10 (Suppl 14):S446-S451, 1999.

Jono S, Nishizawa Y, Shioi A, Morii H: 1,25-Dihydroxyvitamin D3 increases in vitro vascular calcification by modulating secretion of endogenous parathyroid hormone-related peptide. *Circulation,* 98(13):1302-1306, 1998.

Jono S, Peinado C, Giachelli CM: Phosphorylation of osteopontin is required for inhibition of vascular smooth muscle cell calcification. *Journal of Biological Chemistry,* 275(26):20197-20203, 2000.

Jonsson K, McDevitt D, McGavin MH, Patti JM, Hook M: Staphylococcus aureus expresses a major histocompatibility complex class II analog. *Journal of Biological Chemistry,* 270(37):21457-21460, 1995.

Josephs SF, Henry B, Balachandran N, Strayer D, Peterson D, Komaroff AL, Ablashi DV: HHV-6 reactivation in chronic fatigue syndrome. *Lancet,* 337(8753):1346-1347, 1991.

Ju WK, Kim KY, Cha JH, Kim IB, Lee MY, Oh SJ, Chung JW, Chun MH: Ganglion cells of the rat retina show osteopontin-like immunoreactivity. *Brain Research,* 852(1):217-220, 2000.

Juntunen K, Rochel N, Moras D, Vihko P: Large-scale expression and purification of the human vitamin D receptor and its ligand-binding domain for structural studies. *Biochemical Journal,* 344(Pt 2):297-303, 1999.

Kaartinen MT, Pirhonen A, Linnala-Kankkunen A, Maenpaa PH: Transglutaminase-catalyzed cross-linking of osteopontin is inhibited by osteocalcin. *Journal of Biological Chemistry,* 272(36):22736-22741, 1997.

Kaartinen MT, Pirhonen A, Linnala-Kankkunen A, Maenpaa PH: Cross-linking of osteopontin by tissue transglutaminase increases its collagen binding properties. *Journal of Biological Chemistry,* 274(3):1729-1735, 1999.

Kadena T, Matsuzaki G, Fujise S, Kishihara K, Takimoto H, Sasaki M, Beppu M, Nakamura S, Nomoto K: TCR alpha beta+ CD4- CD8- T cells differentiate extrathymically in an lck-independent manner and participate in early response against *Listeria monocytogenes* infection through interferon-gamma production. *Immunology,* 91(4):511-519, 1997.

Kadono H, Kido J, Kataoka M, Yamauchi N, Nagata T: Inhibition of osteoblastic cell differentiation by lipopolysaccharide extract from *Porphyromonas gingivalis*. *Infection and Immunity,* 67(6):2841-2846, 1999.

Kaji H, Sugimoto T, Kanatani M, Fukase M, Kumegawa M, Chihara K: Retinoic acid induces osteoclast-like cell formation by directly acting on hemopoietic blast cells and stimulates osteopontin mRNA expression in isolated osteoclasts. *Life Scientist,* 56(22):1903-1913, 1995.

Kaji H, Sugimoto T, Kanatani M, Fukase M, Kumegawa M, Chihara K: Prostaglandin E2 stimulates osteoclast-like cell formation and bone-resorbing activity via osteoblasts: Role of cAMP-dependent protein kinase. *Journal of Bone Minerals Research,* 11(1):62-71, 1996.

Kaji H, Sugimoto T, Miyauchi A, Fukase M, Tezuka K, Hakeda Y, Kumegawa M, Chihara K: Calcitonin inhibits osteopontin mRNA expression in isolated rabbit osteoclasts. *Endocrinology,* 135(1):484-487, 1994.

Kajikawa H: [The influence of dietary lipids on nephrolithiasis in rats]. *Nippon Hinyokika Gakkai Zasshi,* 89(12):931-938, 1998.

Kaneto H, Morrissey J, McCracken R, Reyes A, Klahr S: Osteopontin expression in the kidney during unilateral ureteral obstruction. *Mineral and Electrolyte Metabolism,* 24(4):227-237, 1998.

Kang DH, Anderson S, Kim YG, Mazzalli M, Suga S, Jefferson JA, Gordon KL, Oyama TT, Hughes J, Hugo C, et al.: Impaired angiogenesis in the aging kidney: Vascular endothelial growth factor and thrombospondin-1 in renal disease. *American Journal of Kidney Diseases,* 37(3):601-611, 2001.

Kang DH, Hughes J, Mazzali M, Schreiner GF, Johnson RJ: Impaired angiogenesis in the remnant kidney model: II. Vascular endothelial growth factor administration reduces renal fibrosis and stabilizes renal function. *Journal of the American Society of Nephrology,* 12(7):1448-1457, 2001.

Kang DH, Kim YG, Andoh TF, Gordon KL, Suga S, Mazzali M, Jefferson JA, Hughes J, Bennett W, Schreiner GF, et al.: Post-cyclosporine-mediated hypertension and nephropathy: Amelioration by vascular endothelial growth factor. *American Journal of Physiology and Renal Physiology,* 280(4):F727-F736, 2001.

Kang TC, Jeon GS, Kim HJ, Shin DH, Lee KH, Lee HY, Yoo YB, Lee BL, Cho SS: Rat osteopontin antibody is cross-reactive to a novel myelin-associated protein in chick. *Brain Research,* 818(2):527-530, 1999.

Kasahara S, Nishikawa S, Ishida H, Nagata T, Yamauchi N, Ohishi K, Wakano Y, Inoue H: The role of 5'-methylthioadenosine on rat calvaria cell differentiation. *Biochemical and Biophysical Research Communications,* 182(2):817-823, 1992.

Kasprowicz DJ, Kohm AP, Berton MT, Chruscinski AJ, Sharpe A, Sanders VM: Stimulation of the B cell receptor, CD86 (B7-2), and the beta 2-adrenergic receptor intrinsically modulates the level of IgGI and IgE produced per B cell. *Journal of Immunology,* 165(2):680-690, 2000.

Kasugai S, Nagata T, Sodek J: Temporal studies on the tissue compartmentalization of bone sialoprotein (BSP), osteopontin (OPN), and SPARC protein during bone formation in vitro. *Journal of Cellular Physiology,* 152(3):467-477, 1992.

Kasugai S, Todescan R Jr, Nagata T, Yao KL, Butler WT, Sodek J: Expression of bone matrix proteins associated with mineralized tissue formation by adult rat bone marrow cells in vitro: Inductive effects of dexamethasone on the osteoblastic phenotype. *Journal of Cellular Physiology,* 147(1):111-120, 1991.

Kasugai S, Zhang Q, Overall CM, Wrana JL, Butler WT, Sodek J: Differential regulation of the 55 and 44 kDa forms of secreted phosphoprotein 1 (SPP-1, osteopontin) in normal and transformed rat bone cells by osteotropic hormones, growth factors and a tumor promoter. *Bone Minerals,* 13(3):235-250, 1991.

Katagiri Y, Mori K, Hara T, Tanaka K, Murakami M, Uede T: Functional analysis of the osteopontin molecule. *Annals of the New York Academy of Sciences,* 760:371-374, 1995.

Katagiri YU, Murakami M, Mori K, Iizuka J, Hara T, Tanaka K, Jia WY, Chambers AF, Uede T: Non-RGD domains of osteopontin promote cell adhesion without involving alpha v integrins. *Journal of Cellular Biochemistry,* 62(1):123-131, 1996.

Katagiri YU, Sleeman J, Fujii H, Herrlich P, Hotta H, Tanaka K, Chikuma S, Yagita H, Okumura K, Murakami M, et al.: CD44 variants but not CD44s cooperate with beta1-containing integrins to permit cells to bind to osteopontin independently of arginine-glycine-aspartic acid, thereby stimulating cell motility and chemotaxis. *Cancer Research,* 59(1):219-226, 1999.

Katagiri YU, Uede T: [Functional domain and its receptor of osteopontin]. *Seikagaku,* 70(4):253-264, 1998.

Katayama Y, Celic S, Nagata N, Martin TJ, Findlay DM: Nonenzymatic glycation of type I collagen modifies interaction with UMR 201-10B preosteoblastic cells. *Bone,* 21(3):237-242, 1997.

Katayama Y, House CM, Udagawa N, Kazama JJ, McFarland RJ, Martin TJ, Findlay DM: Casein kinase 2 phosphorylation of recombinant rat osteopontin enhances adhesion of osteoclasts but not osteoblasts. *Journal of Cellular Physiology,* 176(1):179-187, 1998.

Kato Y, Windle JJ, Koop BA, Mundy GR, Bonewald LF: Establishment of an osteocyte-like cell line, MLO-Y4. *Journal of Bone Minerals Research,* 12(12):2014-2023, 1997.

Kawano H, Cody RJ, Graf K, Goetze S, Kawano Y, Schnee J, Law RE, Hsueh WA: Angiotensin II enhances integrin and alpha-actinin expression in adult rat cardiac fibroblasts. *Hypertension,* 35(1 Pt 2):273-279, 2000.

Kawashima R, Mochida S, Matsui A, YouLuTuZ Y, Ishikawa K, Toshima K, Yamanobe F, Inao M, Ikeda H, Ohno A, et al.: Expression of osteopontin in Kupffer cells and hepatic macrophages and Stellate cells in rat liver after carbon tetrachloride intoxication: A possible factor for macrophage migration into hepatic necrotic areas. *Biochemical and Biophysical Research Communications,* 256(3):527-531, 1999.

Keeting PE, Scott RE, Colvard DS, Anderson MA, Oursler MJ, Spelsberg TC, Riggs BL: Development and characterization of a rapidly proliferating, well-differentiated cell line derived from normal adult human osteoblast-like cells transfected with SV40 large T antigen. *Journal of Bone Minerals Research,* 7(2):127-136, 1992.

Kennedy JH, Henrion D, Wassef M, Shanahan CM, Bloch G, Tedgui A: Osteopontin expression and calcium content in human aortic valves. *Journal of Thoracic and Cardiovascular Surgery,* 120(2):427, 2000.

Kerr JM, Fisher LW, Termine JD, Young MF: The cDNA cloning and RNA distribution of bovine osteopontin. *Gene,* 108(2):237-243, 1991.

Khan AS, Heinene W, Chapman LE, Gary HE, Woods TC, Folks TM, Schonberger LB: Assessment of a retrovirus sequence and other possible risk factors for the chronic fatigue syndrome in adults. *Annals of Internal Medicine,* 118(4):241-245, 1993.

Khan SR: Animal models of kidney stone formation: An analysis. *World Journal of Urology,* 15(4):236-243, 1997.

Khan SR, Thamilselvan S: Nephrolithiasis: A consequence of renal epithelial cell exposure to oxalate and calcium oxalate crystals. *Molecular Urology,* 4(4):305-312, 2000.

Khanna C, Prehn J, Yeung C, Caylor J, Tsokos M, Helman L: An orthotopic model of murine osteosarcoma with clonally related variants differing in pulmonary metastatic potential. *Clinical and Experimental Metastasis,* 18(3):261-271, 2000.

Khoury R, Ridall AL, Norman AW, Farach-Carson MC: Target gene activation by 1,25-dihydroxyvitamin D3 in osteosarcoma cells is independent of calcium influx. *Endocrinology,* 135(6):2446-2453, 1994.

Kido J, Kasahara C, Ohishi K, Nishikawa S, Ishida H, Yamashita K, Kitamura S, Kohri K, Nagata T: Identification of osteopontin in human dental calculus matrix. *Archives of Oral Biology,* 40(10):967-972, 1995.

Kido J, Nishikawa S, Ishida H, Yamashita K, Kitamura S, Kohri K, Nagata T: Identification of calprotectin, a calcium binding leukocyte protein, in human dental calculus matrix. *Journal of Periodontal Research,* 32(4):355-361, 1997.

Kido J, Yamauchi N, Ohishi K, Kataoka M, Nishikawa S, Nakamura T, Kadono H, Ikedo D, Ueno A, Nonomura N, et al.: Inhibition of osteoblastic cell differentiation by conditioned medium derived from the human prostatic cancer cell line PC-3 in vitro. *Journal of Cellular Biochemistry,* 67(2):248-256, 1997.

Kiefer MC, Bauer DM, Barr PJ: The cDNA and derived amino acid sequence for human osteopontin. *Nucleic Acids Research,* 17(8):3306, 1989.

Kikukawa I: [Characterization of rat periodontal ligament cells in culture]. *Kokubyo Gakkai Zasshi,* 63(2):296-312, 1996.

Kim CH, Cheng SL, Kim GS: Lack of autocrine effects of IL-6 on human bone marrow stromal osteoprogenitor cells. *Endocrinology Research,* 23(3):181-190, 1997.

Kim IS, Otto F, Zabel B, Mundlos S: Regulation of chondrocyte differentiation by Cbfa1. *Mechanics and Development,* 80(2):159-170, 1999.

Kim RH, Sodek J: Transcription of the bone sialoprotein gene is stimulated by v-Src acting through an inverted CCAAT box. *Cancer Research,* 59(3):565-571, 1999.

Kim YW, Park YK, Lee J, Ko SW, Yang MH: Expression of osteopontin and osteonectin in breast cancer. *Journal of Korean Medical Sciences,* 13(6):652-657, 1998.

Kimber SJ: Molecular interactions at the maternal-embryonic interface during the early phase of implantation. *Seminars in Reproductive Medicine,* 18(3):237-253, 2000.

Kimbro KS, Saavedra RA: The Puerap motif in the promoter of the mouse osteopontin gene. *Annals of the New York Academy of Sciences,* 760:319-320, 1995.

Kimmel-Jehan C, Darwish HM, Strugnell SA, Jehan F, Wiefling B, DeLuca HF: DNA bending is induced by binding of vitamin D receptor-retinoid X receptor heterodimers to vitamin D response elements. *Journal of Cellular Biochemistry,* 74(2):220-228, 1999.

Kimmel-Jehan C, Jehan F, DeLuca HF: Salt concentration determines 1,25-dihydroxyvitamin D3 dependency of vitamin D receptor-retinoid X receptor-vitamin D-responsive element complex formation. *Archives of Biochemistry and Biophysics,* 341(1):75-80, 1997.

Kinoshita S, Finnegan M, Bucholz RW, Mizuno K: Three-dimensional collagen gel culture promotes osteoblastic phenotype in bone marrow derived cells. *Kobe Journal of Medical Sciences,* 45(5):201-211, 1999.

Kitani T, Kuratsune H, Fuke I, Nakamura Y, Nakaya T, Asahi S, Tobiume M, Yamaguti M, Machii T, Inagi R, et al.: Possible correlation between borna disease virus infection and Japanese patients with chronic fatigue syndrome. *Microbiology and Immunology,* 40(6):459-462, 1996.

Kitano Y, Kurihara H, Kurihara Y, Maemura K, Ryo Y, Yazaki Y, Harii K: Gene expression of bone matrix proteins and endothelin receptors in endothelin-1-deficient mice revealed by in situ hybridization. *Journal of Bone Minerals Research,* 13(2):237-244, 1998.

Kitazawa S, Kitazawa R, Maeda S: In situ hybridization with polymerase chain reaction-derived single-stranded DNA probe and S1 nuclease. *Histochemistry and Cell Biology,* 111(1):7-12, 1999.

Klahr S: Urinary tract obstruction. *Seminars in Nephrology,* 21(2):133-145, 2001.

Klahr S, Morrissey JJ: The role of vasoactive compounds, growth factors and cytokines in the progression of renal disease. *Kidney International,* 57(Suppl 75):S7-S14, 2000.

Kleinerman ES, Schroit AJ, Fogler WE, Fidler IJ: Tumoricidal activity of human monocytes activated in vitro by free and liposome-encapsulated human lymphokines. *Journal of Clinical Investigation,* 72:304, 1983.

Kleinman JG, Beshensky A, Worcester EM, Brown D: Expression of osteopontin, a urinary inhibitor of stone mineral crystal growth, in rat kidney. *Kidney International,* 47(6):1585-1596, 1995.

Kleinman JG, Worcester EM, Beshensky AM, Sheridan AM, Bonventre JV, Brown D: Upregulation of osteopontin expression by ischemia in rat kidney. *Annals of the New York Academy of Sciences,* 760:321-323, 1995.

Klein-Nulend J, Roelofsen J, Semeins CM, Bronckers AL, Burger EH: Mechanical stimulation of osteopontin mRNA expression and synthesis in bone cell cultures. *Journal of Cellular Physiology,* 170(2):174-181, 1997.

Klinman DM, Ishigatsubo Y, Steinberg AS: Acquisition and maturation of expressed B-cell repertoires in normal and autoimmune mice. *Journal of Immunology,* 141:801, 1988.

Klinman DM, Steinberg AD: Systemic autoimmune disease arises from polyclonal B-cell activation. *Journal of Experimental Medicine,* 165:1755, 1987.

Klonoff DC: Chronic fatigue syndrome. *Clinical Infectious Diseases,* 15:812, 1992.

Knoll A, Stratil A, Cepica S, Dvorak J: Length polymorphism in an intron of the porcine osteopontin (SPP1) gene is caused by the presence or absence of a SINE (PRE-1) element. *Animal Genetics,* 30(6):466, 1999.

Knopov V, Hadash D, Hurwitz S, Leach RM, Pines M: Gene expression during cartilage differentiation in turkey tibial dyschondroplasia, evaluated by in situ hybridization. *Avian Diseases,* 41(1):62-72, 1997.

Knopov V, Leach RM, Barak-Shalom T, Hurwitz S, Pines M: Osteopontin gene expression and alkaline phosphatase activity in avian tibial dyschondroplasia. *Bone,* 16(Suppl 4):329S-334S, 1995a.

Knopov V, Leach RM, Barak-Shalom T, Hurwitz S, Pines M: Osteopontin gene expression in avian tibial dyschondroplasia. *Annals of the New York Academy of Sciences,* 760:350-353, 1995b.

Koch AE, Polverini PJ, Kunkel SL, Harlow LA, DiPrieto LA, Elner VM, Strieter RM: Interleukin-8 as a macrophage-derived mediator of angiogenesis. *Science,* 258:1798, 1992.

Kockx M, McCabe L, Stein JL, Lian JB, Stein GS: Influence of DNA replication inhibition on expression of cell growth and tissue-specific genes in osteoblasts and osteosarcoma cells. *Journal of Cellular Biochemistry,* 54(1):47-55, 1994.

Koeneman KS, Yeung F, Chung LW: Osteomimetic properties of prostate cancer cells: A hypothesis supporting the predilection of prostate cancer metastasis and growth in the bone environment. *Prostate,* 39(4):246-261, 1999.

Kohm AP, Tang Y, Sanders VM, Jones SB: Activation of antigen-specific $CD4^+$ Th2 cells and B cells in vivo increases norepinephrine release in the spleen and bone marrow. *Journal of Immunology,* 165(2):725-733, 2000.

Kohri K, Nomura S, Kitamura Y, Nagata T, Yoshioka K, Iguchi M, Yamate T, Umekawa T, Suzuki Y, Sinohara H, et al.: Structure and expression of the mRNA encoding urinary stone protein (osteopontin). *Journal of Biological Chemistry,* 268(20):15180-15184, 1993.

Kohri K, Suzuki Y, Yoshida K, Yamamoto K, Amasaki N, Yamate T, Umekawa T, Iguchi M, Sinohara H, Kurita T: Molecular cloning and sequencing of cDNA encoding urinary stone protein, which is identical to osteopontin. *Biochemical and Biophysical Research Communications,* 184(2):859-864, 1992.

Koistinen P, Pulli T, Uitto VJ, Nissinen L, Hyypia T, Heino J: Depletion of alphaV integrins from osteosarcoma cells by intracellular antibody expression induces bone differentiation marker genes and suppresses gelatinase (MMP-2) synthesis. *Matrix Biology,* 18(3):239-251, 1999.

Koka RM, Huang E, Lieske JC: Adhesion of uric acid crystals to the surface of renal epithelial cells. *American Journal of Physiology and Renal Physiology,* 278(6):F989-F998, 2000.

Komaroff AL, Buchwald D: Symptoms and signs of chronic fatigue syndrome. *Review of Infectious Diseases,* 13(Suppl 1):S8, 1991.

Komori T, Yagi H, Nomura S, Yamaguchi A, Sasaki K, Deguchi K, Shimizu Y, Bronson RT, Gao YH, Inada M, et al.: Targeted disruption of Cbfa1 results in a complete lack of bone formation owing to maturational arrest of osteoblasts. *Cell,* 89(5):755-764, 1997.

Kon S, Maeda M, Segawa T, Hagiwara Y, Horikoshi Y, Chikuma S, Tanaka K, Rashid MM, Inobe M, Chambers AF, et al.: Antibodies to different peptides in osteopontin reveal complexities in the various secreted forms. *Journal of Cellular Biochemistry,* 77(3):487-498, 2000.

Kondo H, Ohyama T, Ohya K, Kasugai S: Temporal changes of mRNA expression of matrix proteins and parathyroid hormone and parathyroid hormone-related protein (PTH/PTHrP) receptor in bone development. *Journal of Bone Minerals Research,* 12(12):2089-2097, 1997.

Konttinen YT, Li TF, Mandelin J, Ainola M, Lassus J, Virtanen I, Santavirta S, Tammi, M, Tammi R: Hyaluronan synthases, hyaluronan, and its CD44 receptor in tissue around loosened total hip prostheses. *Journal of Pathology,* 194(3):384-390, 2001.

Koszewski NJ, Reinhardt TA, Horst RL: Vitamin D receptor interactions with the murine osteopontin response element. *Journal of Steroid Biochemistry and Molecular Biology,* 59(5-6):377-388, 1996.

Koszewski NJ, Reinhardt TA, Horst RL: Differential effects of 20-epi vitamin D analogs on the vitamin D receptor homodimer. *Journal of Bone Minerals Research,* 14(4):509-517, 1999.

Kraft M, Cassell GH, Henson JE, Watson H, Williamson J, Marmion BP, Gaydos CA, Martin RJ: Detection of *Mycoplasma pneumoniae* in the airways of adults with chronic asthma. *American Journal of Respiration and Critical Care Medicine,* 158(3):998-1001, 1998.

Kraichely DM, MacDonald PN: Transcriptional activation through the vitamin D receptor in osteoblasts. *Frontiers in Bioscience,* 3:D821-D833, 1998.

Krause SW, Rehli M, Kreutz M, Schwarzfischer L, Paulauskis JD, Andreesen R: Differential screening identifies genetic markers of monocyte to macrophage maturation. *Journal of Leukocyte Biology,* 60(4):540-545, 1996.

Kremer EA, Chen Y, Suzuki K, Nagase H, Gorski JP: Hydroxyapatite induces autolytic degradation and inactivation of matrix metalloproteinase-1 and -3. *Journal of Bone Minerals Research,* 13(12):1890-1902, 1998.

Kroenke K, Wood DR, Mangelsdorff AD, Meier NJ, Powell JB: Chronic fatigue in primary care. Prevalence, patient characteristics and outcome. *Journal of the American Medical Association,* 260(7):929-934, 1988.

Krook A, Rapoport MJ, Anderson S, Pross H, Zhou YC, Denhardt DT, Delovitch TL, Haliotis T: p21ras and protein kinase C function in distinct and interdependent signaling pathways in C3H 10T1/2 fibroblasts. *Molecular and Cellular Biology,* 13(3):1471-1479, 1993.

Kubota T, Yamauchi M, Onozaki J, Sato S, Suzuki Y, Sodek J: Influence of an intermittent compressive force on matrix protein expression by ROS 17/2.8 cells, with selective stimulation of osteopontin. *Archives of Oral Biology,* 38(1):23-30, 1993.

Kubota T, Yamauchi M, Ueda R, Yoneyama T, Saito C, Sato S, Suzuki Y: Molecular mechanism of mechanical stress in bone and periodontium. *Bulletin of the Kanagawa Dentistry College,* 18(2):127-133, 1990.

Kubota T, Zhang Q, Wrana JL, Ber R, Aubin JE, Butler WT, Sodek J: Multiple forms of SppI (secreted phosphoprotein, osteopontin) synthesized by normal and transformed rat bone cell populations: Regulation by TGF-beta. *Biochemical and Biophysical Research Communications,* 162(3):1453-1459, 1989.

Kumar CS, James IE, Wong A, Mwangi V, Feild JA, Nuthulaganti P, Connor JR, Eichman C, Ali F, Hwang SM, et al.: Cloning and characterization of a novel integrin beta3 subunit. *Journal of Biological Chemistry,* 272(26):16390-16397, 1997.

Kunicki TJ, Annis DS, Felding-Habermann B: Molecular determinants of arg-gly-asp ligand specificity for beta3 integrins. *Journal of Biological Chemistry,* 272(7):4103-4107, 1997.

Kuno H, Kurian SM, Hendy GN, White J, deLuca HF, Evans CO, Nanes MS: Inhibition of 1,25-dihydroxyvitamin D3 stimulated osteocalcin gene transcription by tumor necrosis factor-alpha: Structural determinants within the vitamin D response element. *Endocrinology,* 134(6):2524-2531, 1994.

Kupfahl C, Pink D, Friedrich K, Zurbrugg HR, Neuss M, Warnecke C, Fielitz J, Graf K, Fleck E, Regitz-Zagrosek V: Angiotensin II directly increases transforming growth factor beta1 and osteopontin and indirectly affects collagen mRNA expression in the human heart. *Cardiovascular Research,* 46(3):463-475, 2000.

Kusafuka K, Yamaguchi A, Kayano T, Takemura T: Expression of bone matrix proteins, osteonectin and osteopontin, in salivary pleomorphic adenomas. *Pathology Research and Practice,* 195(11):733-739, 1999.

Kusumi T, Nishi T, Tanaka M, Tsuchida S, Kudo H: A murine osteosarcoma cell line with a potential to develop ossification upon transplantation. *Japanese Journal of Cancer Research,* 92(6):649-658, 2001.

Kuykindoll RJ, Nishimura H, Thomason DB, Nishimoto SK: Osteopontin expression in spontaneously developed neointima in fowl *(Gallus gallus). Journal of Experimental Biology,* 203 (Pt 2):273-282, 2000.

Kwon HM, Hong BK, Kang TS, Kwon K, Kim HK, Jang Y, Choi D, Park HY, Kang SM, Cho SY, et al.: Expression of osteopontin in calcified coronary atherosclerotic plaques. *Journal of Korean Medical Sciences,* 15(5):485-493, 2000.

Kyte J, Doolittle RF: A simple method for displaying the hydropathic character of a protein. *Journal of Molecular Biology,* 157:105-112, 1982.

Lafage-Proust MH, Wesolowski G, Ernst M, Rodan GA, Rodan SB: Retinoic acid effects on an SV-40 large T antigen immortalized adult rat bone cell line. *Journal of Cellular Physiology,* 179(3):267-275, 1999.

Lai CF, Chaudhary L, Fausto A, Halstead LR, Ory DS, Avioli LV, Cheng SL: Erk is essential for growth, differentiation, integrin expression, and cell function in human osteoblastic cells. *Journal of Biological Chemistry,* 276(17):14443-14450, 2001.

Lampe MA, Patarca R, Iregui MV, Cantor H: Polyclonal B cell activation by the Eta-1 cytokine and its relationship to the development of systemic autoimmune disease in MRL/l mice. *Journal of Immunology,* 147(9):2902-2906, 1991.

Lan HY, Yu XQ, Yang N, Nikolic-Paterson DJ, Mu W, Pichler R, Johnson RJ, Atkins RC: De novo glomerular osteopontin expression in rat crescentic glomerulonephritis. *Kidney International,* 53(1):136-145, 1998.

Landay AL, Jessop C, Lennette ET, Levy JA: Chronic fatigue syndrome, clinical condition associated with immune activation. *Lancet,* 338(8769):707-712, 1991.

Landis WJ, Hodgens KJ, McKee MD, Nanci A, Song MJ, Kiyonaga S, Arena J, McEwen B: Extracellular vesicles of calcifying turkey leg tendon characterized by immunocytochemistry and high voltage electron microscopic tomography and 3-D graphic image reconstruction. *Bone Minerals,* 17(2):237-241, 1992.

Langub MC, Herman JP, Malluche HH, Koszewski NJ: Evidence of functional vitamin D receptors in rat hippocampus. *Neuroscience,* 104(1):49-56, 2001.

Lanske B, Divieti P, Kovacs CS, Pirro A, Landis WJ, Krane SM, Bringhurst FR, Kronenberg HM: The parathyroid hormone (PTH)/PTH-related peptide receptor mediates actions of both ligands in murine bone. *Endocrinology,* 139(12):5194-5204, 1998.

Lasa M, Chang PL, Prince CW, Pinna LA: Phosphorylation of osteopontin by Golgi apparatus casein kinase. *Biochemical and Biophysical Research Communications,* 240(3):602-605, 1997.

Lavelin I, Meiri N, Pines M: New insight in eggshell formation. *Poultry Sciences,* 79(7):1014-1017, 2000.

Lavelin I, Yarden N, Ben-Bassat S, Bar A, Pines M: Regulation of osteopontin gene expression during egg shell formation in the laying hen by mechanical strain. *Matrix Biology,* 17(8-9):615-623, 1998.

Lawton DM, Andrew JG, Marsh DR, Hoyland JA, Freemont AJ: Expression of the gene encoding the matrix gla protein by mature osteoblasts in human fracture non-unions. *Molecular Pathology,* 52(2):92-96, 1999.

Leboy PS, Beresford JN, Devlin C, Owen ME: Dexamethasone induction of osteoblast mRNAs in rat marrow stromal cell cultures. *Journal of Cellular Physiology,* 146(3):370-378, 1991.

Lecanda F, Avioli LV, Cheng SL: Regulation of bone matrix protein expression and induction of differentiation of human osteoblasts and human bone marrow stromal cells by bone morphogenetic protein-2. *Journal of Cellular Biochemistry,* 67(3):386-396, 1997.

Lecanda F, Towler DA, Ziambaras K, Cheng SL, Koval M, Steinberg TH, Civitelli R: Gap junctional communication modulates gene expression in osteoblastic cells. *Molecular Biology of the Cell,* 9(8):2249-2258, 1998.

Lecrone V, Li W, Devoll RE, Logothetis C, Farach-Carson MC: Calcium signals in prostate cancer cells: Specific activation by bone-matrix proteins. *Cellular Calcium,* 27(1):35-42, 2000.

Lee KL, Aubin JE, Heersche JN: beta-Glycerophosphate-induced mineralization of osteoid does not alter expression of extracellular matrix components in fetal rat calvarial cell cultures. *Journal of Bone Minerals Research,* 7(10):1211-1219, 1992.

Lee M, Na S, Jeon D, Kim H, Choi Y, Baik M: Induction of osteopontin gene expression during mammary gland involution and effects of glucocorticoid on its expression in mammary epithelial cells. *Bioscience, Biotechnology and Biochemistry,* 64(10):2225-2228, 2000.

Lee MS, Lowe GN, Strong DD, Wergedal JE, Glackin CA: TWIST, a basic helix-loop-helix transcription factor, can regulate the human osteogenic lineage. *Journal of Cellular Biochemistry,* 75(4):566-577, 1999.

Lee MY, Shin SL, Choi YS, Kim EJ, Cha JH, Chun MH, Lee SB, Kim SY: Transient upregulation of osteopontin mRNA in hippocampus and striatum following global forebrain ischemia in rats. *Neuroscience Letters,* 271(2):81-84, 1999.

Lee SK, Park JY, Chung SJ, Yang WS, Kim SB, Park SK, Park JS: Chemokines, osteopontin, ICAM-1 gene expression in cultured rat mesangial cells. *Journal of Korean Medical Sciences,* 13(2):165-170, 1998.

Lefebvre V, Garofalo S, de Crombrugghe B: Type X collagen gene expression in mouse chondrocytes immortalized by a temperature-sensitive simian virus 40 large tumor antigen. *Journal of Cellular Biology,* 128(1-2):239-245, 1995.

Lehenkari PP, Horton MA: Single integrin molecule adhesion forces in intact cells measured by atomic force microscopy. *Biochemical and Biophysical Research Communications,* 259(3):645-650, 1999.

Lehninger AL: *Biochemistry,* Second edition, Worth Publishers, New York, p. 220, 1975.

Leibovich SJ, Polverini PJ, Sheperd HM, Wiseman DM, Shively V, Nuseir N: Macrophage-induced angiogenesis is mediated by tumor necrosis factor-alpha. *Nature,* 329:630-632, 1987.

Lekic PC, Rajshankar D, Chen H, Tenenbaum H, McCulloch CA: Transplantation of labeled periodontal ligament cells promotes regeneration of alveolar bone. *Anatomy Records,* 262(2):193-202, 2001.

Lekic PC, Rojas J, Birek C, Tenenbaum H, McCulloch CA: Phenotypic comparison of periodontal ligament cells in vivo and in vitro. *Journal of Periodontal Research,* 36(2):71-79, 2001.

Lekic PC, Rubbino I, Krasnoshtein F, Cheifetz S, McCulloch CA, Tenenbaum H: Bisphosphonate modulates proliferation and differentiation of rat periodontal ligament cells during wound healing. *Anatomy Records,* 247(3):329-340, 1997.

Lekic PC, Sodek J, McCulloch CA: Osteopontin and bone sialoprotein expression in regenerating rat periodontal ligament and alveolar bone. *Anatomy Records,* 244(1):50-58, 1996a.

Lekic PC, Sodek J, McCulloch CA: Relationship of cellular proliferation to expression of osteopontin and bone sialoprotein in regenerating rat periodontium. *Cell and Tissue Research,* 285(3):491-500, 1996b.

Lemire JM, Covin CW, White S, Giachelli CM, Schwartz SM: Characterization of cloned aortic smooth muscle cells from young rats. *American Journal of Pathology,* 144(5):1068-1081, 1994.

Lemon BD, Freedman LP: Selective effects of ligands on vitamin D3 receptor- and retinoid X receptor-mediated gene activation in vivo. *Molecular and Cellular Biology,* 16(3):1006-1016, 1996.

Lemonnier J, Delannoy P, Hott M, Lomri A, Modrowski D, Marie PJ: The Ser252Trp fibroblast growth factor receptor-2 (FGFR-2) mutation induces PKC-independent downregulation of FGFR-2 associated with premature calvaria osteoblast differentiation. *Experimental Cell Research,* 256(1):158-167, 2000.

Levine PH, Jacobson S, Pocinki AG, Cheney P, Peterson D, Connelly PR, Weil R, Robinson SM, Ablashi DV, Salahuddin SZ, et al.: Clinical, epidemiological, and virological studies in four clusters of the chronic fatigue syndrome. *Archives of Internal Medicine,* 152(8):1611-1616, 1992.

Levy J: Viral studies of chronic fatigue syndrome, introduction. *Clinical Infectious Diseases,* 18(Suppl 1):S117, 1994.

Lewington AJ, Padanilam BJ, Martin DR, Hammerman MR: Expression of CD44 in kidney after acute ischemic injury in rats. *American Journal of Physiology, Regulation, and Integrative Comparative Physiology,* 278(1):R247-R254, 2000.

Li G, Chen YF, Kelpke SS, Oparil S, Thompson JA: Estrogen attenuates integrin-beta(3)-dependent adventitial fibroblast migration after inhibition of osteopontin production in vascular smooth muscle cells. *Circulation,* 101(25):2949-2955, 2000.

Li H, Bartold PM, Young WG, Xiao Y, Waters MJ: Growth hormone induces bone morphogenetic proteins and bone-related proteins in the developing rat periodontium. *Journal of Bone Minerals Research,* 16(6):1068-1076, 2001.

Li IW, Cheifetz S, McCulloch CA, Sampath KT, Sodek J: Effects of osteogenic protein-1 (OP-1, BMP-7) on bone matrix protein expression by fetal rat calvarial cells are differentiation stage specific. *Journal of Cellular Physiology,* 169(1):115-125, 1996.

Li JJ, Kim RH, Zhang Q, Ogata Y, Sodek J: Characteristics of vitamin D3 receptor (VDR) binding to the vitamin D response element (VDRE) in rat bone sialoprotein gene promoter. *European Journal of Oral Sciences,* 106(Suppl 1):408-417, 1998.

Li JQ, Zhang JT: [Effects of age and ginsenoside RG1 on membrane fluidity of cortical cells in rats]. *Yao Xue Xue Bao,* 32(1):23-27, 1997.

Li Z, Zhou Z, Yellowley CE, Donahue HJ: Inhibiting gap junctional intercellular communication alters expression of differentiation markers in osteoblastic cells. *Bone,* 25(6):661-666, 1999.

Lian JB, Shalhoub V, Aslam F, Frenkel B, Green J, Hamrah M, Stein GS, Stein JL: Species-specific glucocorticoid and 1,25-dihydroxyvitamin D responsiveness in mouse MC3T3-E1 osteoblasts: Dexamethasone inhibits osteoblast differentiation and vitamin D down-regulates osteocalcin gene expression. *Endocrinology,* 138(5):2117-2127, 1997.

Liang CT, Barnes J: Renal expression of osteopontin and alkaline phosphatase correlates with BUN levels in aged rats. *American Journal of Physiology,* 269 (3 Pt 2):F398-F404, 1995.

Liang CT, Barnes J, Seedor JG, Quartuccio HA, Bolander M, Jeffrey JJ, Rodan GA: Impaired bone activity in aged rats: Alterations at the cellular and molecular levels. *Bone,* 13(6):435-441, 1992.

Liao H, Wurtz T, Li J: Influence of titanium ion on mineral formation and properties of osteoid nodules in rat calvaria cultures. *Journal of Biomedical Materials Research,* 47(2):220-227, 1999.

Liaw L, Almeida M, Hart CE, Schwartz SM, Giachelli CM: Osteopontin promotes vascular cell adhesion and spreading and is chemotactic for smooth muscle cells in vitro. *Circulation Research,* 74(2):214-224, 1994.

Liaw L, Birk DE, Ballas CB, Whitsitt JS, Davidson JM, Hogan BL: Altered wound healing in mice lacking a functional osteopontin gene (spp1). *Journal of Clinical Investigation,* 101(7):1468-1478, 1998.

Liaw L, Crawford HC: Functions of the extracellular matrix and matrix degrading proteases during tumor progression. *Brazilian Journal of Medical Biology Research,* 32(7):805-812, 1999.

Liaw L, Lindner V, Schwartz SM, Chambers AF, Giachelli CM: Osteopontin and beta 3 integrin are coordinately expressed in regenerating endothelium in vivo and stimulate Arg-Gly-Asp-dependent endothelial migration in vitro. *Circulation Research,* 77(4):665-672, 1995.

Liaw L, Lombardi DM, Almeida MM, Schwartz SM, deBlois D, Giachelli CM: Neutralizing antibodies directed against osteopontin inhibit rat carotid neointimal thickening after endothelial denudation. *Arteriosclerosis and Thrombosis Vascular Biology,* 17(1):188-193, 1997.

Liaw L, Skinner MP, Raines EW, Ross R, Cheresh DA, Schwartz SM, Giachelli CM: The adhesive and migratory effects of osteopontin are mediated via distinct cell surface integrins. Role of alpha v beta 3 in smooth muscle cell migration to osteopontin in vitro. *Journal of Clinical Investigation,* 95(2):713-724, 1995.

Lieske JC, Hammes MS, Hoyer JR, Toback FG: Renal cell osteopontin production is stimulated by calcium oxalate monohydrate crystals. *Kidney International,* 51(3):679-686, 1997.

Lieske JC, Norris R, Toback FG: Adhesion of hydroxyapatite crystals to anionic sites on the surface of renal epithelial cells. *American Journal of Physiology,* 273(2 Pt 2):F224-F233, 1997.

Lin DG, Kenny DJ, Barrett EJ, Lekic P, McCulloch CA: Storage conditions of avulsed teeth affect the phenotype of cultured human periodontal ligament cells. *Journal of Periodontal Research,* 35(1):42-50, 2000.

Lin WL, Chien HH, Cho MI: N-cadherin expression during periodontal ligament cell differentiation in vitro. *Journal of Periodontology,* 70(9):1039-1045, 1999.

Lin YH, Huang CJ, Chao JR, Chen ST, Lee SF, Yen JJ, Yang-Yen HF: Coupling of osteopontin and its cell surface receptor CD44 to the cell survival response elicited by interleukin-3 or granulocyte-macrophage colony-stimulating factor. *Molecular and Cellular Biology,* 20(8):2734-2742, 2000.

Lin YS, Green MR: Interaction of a common cellular transcription factor, ATF, with regulatory elements in both E1a- and cyclic AMP-inducible promoters. *Proceedings of the National Academy of Sciences of the United States of America,* 85:3396, 1988.

Lincoln TM, Dey NB, Boerth NJ, Cornwell TL, Soff GA: Nitric oxide—cyclic GMP pathway regulates vascular smooth muscle cell phenotypic modulation: Implications in vascular diseases. *Acta Physiologica Scandinavica,* 164(4):507-515, 1998.

Lisignoli G, Grassi F, Piacentini A, Cocchini B, Remiddi G, Bevilacqua C, Facchini A: Hyaluronan does not affect cytokine and chemokine expression in osteoarthritic chondrocytes and synoviocytes. *Osteoarthritis and Cartilage,* 9(2):161-168, 2001.

Liu F, Malaval L, Aubin JE: The mature osteoblast phenotype is characterized by extensive plasticity. *Experimental Cell Research,* 232(1):97-105, 1997.

Liu F, Malaval L, Gupta AK, Aubin JE: Simultaneous detection of multiple bone-related mRNAs and protein expression during osteoblast differentiation: Polymerase chain reaction and immunocytochemical studies at the single cell level. *Developmental Biology,* 166(1):220-234, 1994.

Liu M, Freedman LP: Transcriptional synergism between the vitamin D3 receptor and other nonreceptor transcription factors. *Molecular Endocrinology,* 8(12):1593-1604, 1994.

Liu Y, Watanabe H, Nifuji A, Yamada Y, Olson EN, Noda M: Overexpression of a single helix-loop-helix-type transcription factor, scleraxis, enhances aggrecan gene expression in osteoblastic osteosarcoma ROS17/2.8 cells. *Journal of Biological Chemistry,* 272(47):29880-29885, 1997.

Liu YK, Uemura T, Nemoto A, Yabe T, Fujii N, Ushida T, Tateishi T: Osteopontin involvement in integrin-mediated cell signaling and regulation of expression of alkaline phosphatase during early differentiation of UMR cells. *FEBS Letters,* 420(1):112-116, 1997.

Ljusberg J, Ek-Rylander B, Andersson G: Tartrate-resistant purple acid phosphatase is synthesized as a latent proenzyme and activated by cysteine proteinases. *Biochemical Journal,* 343 (Pt 1):63-69, 1999.

Lloyd A, Hickie I, Wakefield D, Boughton C, Dwyer J: A double-blind, placebo-controlled trial of intravenous immunoglobin therapy in patients with chronic fatigue syndrome. *American Journal of Medicine,* 89:561-568, 1990.

Loeser RF: Integrin-mediated attachment of articular chondrocytes to extracellular matrix proteins. *Arthritis and Rheumatism,* 36(8):1103-1110, 1993.

Loeser RF: Chondrocyte integrin expression and function. *Biorheology,* 37(1-2):109-116, 2000.

Lombardi DM, Viswanathan M, Vio CP, Saavedra JM, Schwartz SM, Johnson RJ: Renal and vascular injury induced by exogenous angiotensin II is AT1 receptor-dependent. *Nephron,* 87(1):66-74, 2001.

Loo P, Menier J: Psychose intermittente et rickettsie. [Intermittent psychosis and rickettsias.] *Annales de Medécine Psychologique,* 120(1):820-824, 1962.

Loo P, Menier J: Les rickettsies et nec-rickettsies en neuro-psychiatrie. [The rickettsias and nec-rickettsias in neuropsychiatry.] *Annales de Medécine Psychologique,* 119(2):732-740, 1993.

Lopez CA, Davis RL, Mou K, Denhardt DT: Activation of a signal transduction pathway by osteopontin. *Annals of the New York Academy of Sciences,* 760:324-326, 1995.

Lopez CA, Hoyer JR, Wilson PD, Waterhouse P, Denhardt DT: Heterogeneity of osteopontin expression among nephrons in mouse kidneys and enhanced expression in sclerotic glomeruli. *Laboratory Investigations,* 69(3):355-363, 1993.

Lopez CA, Olson ES, Adams JC, Mou K, Denhardt DT, Davis RL: Osteopontin expression detected in adult cochleae and inner ear fluids. *Hearing Research,* 85 (1-2):210-222, 1995.

Losch A, Koch-Brandt C: Dithiothreitol treatment of Madin-Darby canine kidney cells reversibly blocks export from the endoplasmic reticulum but does not affect vectorial targeting of secretory proteins. *Journal of Biological Chemistry,* 270(19):11543-11548, 1995.

Luan Y, Praul CA, Gay CV: Confocal imaging and timing of secretion of matrix proteins by osteoblasts derived from avian long bone. *Comparative Biochemistry, Physiology and Molecular Integrative Physiology,* 126(2):213-221, 2000.

Luka J, Okano M, Thiele G: Isolation of human herpesvirus-6 from clinical specimens using human fibroblast cultures. *Journal of Clinical Laboratory Analysis,* 4(6):483-486, 1990.

Lutz W, Burritt MF, Nixon DE, Kao PC, Kumar R: Zinc increases the activity of vitamin D-dependent promoters in osteoblasts. *Biochemical and Biophysical Research Communications,* 271(1):1-7, 2000.

Lynch MP, Stein JL, Stein GS, Lian JB: The influence of type I collagen on the development and maintenance of the osteoblast phenotype in primary and passaged rat calvarial osteoblasts: Modification of expression of genes supporting cell growth, adhesion, and extracellular matrix mineralization. *Experimental Cell Research,* 216(1):35-45, 1995.

MacDonald KL, Osterholm MT, Le Dell KH, White KE, Schenck CH, Chao CC, Persing DH, Johnson RC, Barker JM, Peterson PK: A case-control study to assess possible triggers and cofactors in chronic fatigue syndrome. *American Journal of Medicine,* 100(5):548-554, 1996.

MacDougall M: Refined mapping of the human dentin sialophosphoprotein (DSPP) gene within the critical dentinogenesis imperfecta type II and dentin dysplasia type II loci. *European Journal of Oral Sciences,* 106(Suppl 1):227-233, 1998.

MacDougall M, Gu TT, Simmons D: Dentin matrix protein-1, a candidate gene for dentinogenesis imperfecta. *Connective Tissue Research,* 35(1-4):267-272, 1996.

Machtey I: *Chlamydia pneumoniae* antibodies in myalgia of unknown cause (including fibromyalgia). *British Journal of Rheumatology,* 36(10):1134, 1997.

Mackie PS, Fisher JL, Zhou H, Choong PF: Bisphosphonates regulate cell growth and gene expression in the UMR 106-01 clonal rat osteosarcoma cell line. *British Journal of Cancer,* 84(7):951-958, 2001.

MacNeil RL, Berry J, D'Errico J, Strayhorn C, Piotrowski B, Somerman MJ: Role of two mineral-associated adhesion molecules, osteopontin and bone sialoprotein, during cementogenesis. *Connective Tissue Research,* 33(1-3):1-7, 1995.

MacNeil RL, Berry J, D'Errico J, Strayhorn C, Somerman MJ: Localization and expression of osteopontin in mineralized and nonmineralized tissues of the periodontium. *Annals of the New York Academy of Sciences,* 760:166-176, 1995.

MacNeil RL, D'Errico JA, Ouyang H, Berry J, Strayhorn C, Somerman MJ: Isolation of murine cementoblasts: Unique cells or uniquely-positioned osteoblasts? *European Journal of Oral Sciences,* 106(Suppl 1):350-356, 1998.

Madsen KM, Zhang L, Abu Shamat AR, Siegfried S, Cha JH: Ultrastructural localization of osteopontin in the kidney: Induction by lipopolysaccharide. *Journal of the American Society of Nephrology,* 8(7):1043-1053, 1997.

Maeda H, Kukita T, Akamine A, Kukita A, Iijima T: Localization of osteopontin in resorption lacunae formed by osteoclast-like cells: A study by a novel monoclonal antibody which recognizes rat osteopontin. *Histochemistry,* 102(4):247-254, 1994.

Maeda S, Wu S, Juppner H, Green J, Aragay AM, Fagin JA, Clemens TL: Cell-specific signal transduction of parathyroid hormone (PTH)-related protein through stably expressed recombinant PTH/PTHrP receptors in vascular smooth muscle cells. *Endocrinology,* 137(8):3154-3162, 1996.

Magil AB, Pichler RH, Johnson RJ: Osteopontin in chronic puromycin aminonucleoside nephrosis. *Journal of the American Society of Nephrology,* 8(9):1383-1390, 1997.

Mahmoodian F, Gosiewska A, Peterkofsky B: Regulation and properties of bone alkaline phosphatase during vitamin C deficiency in guinea pigs. *Archives of Biochemistry and Biophysics,* 336(1):86-96, 1996.

Majeska RJ, Port M, Einhorn TA: Attachment to extracellular matrix molecules by cells differing in the expression of osteoblastic traits. *Journal of Bone Minerals Research,* 8(3):277-289, 1993.

Majeska RJ, Ryaby JT, Einhorn TA: Direct modulation of osteoblastic activity with estrogen. *Journal of Bone Joint Surgery of America,* 76(5):713-721, 1994.

Maki M, Hirota S, Kaneko Y, Morohoshi T: Expression of osteopontin messenger RNA by macrophages in ovarian serous papillary cystadenocarcinoma: A possible association with calcification of psammoma bodies. *Pathology International,* 50(7):531-535, 2000.

Makiishi-Shimobayashi C, Tsujimura T, Sugihara A, Iwasaki T, Yamada N, Malam-Souley R, Seye C, Gadeau AP, Loirand G, Pillois X, et al.: Nucleotide receptor P2u partially mediates ATP-induced cell cycle progression of aortic smooth muscle cells. *Journal of Cellular Physiology,* 166(1):57-65, 1996.

Malaval L, Gupta AK, Aubin JE: Leukemia inhibitory factor inhibits osteogenic differentiation in rat calvaria cell cultures. *Endocrinology,* 136(4):1411-1418, 1995.

Malaval L, Liu F, Roche P, Aubin JE: Kinetics of osteoprogenitor proliferation and osteoblast differentiation in vitro. *Journal of Cellular Biochemistry,* 74(4):616-627, 1999.

Malaval L, Modrowski D, Gupta AK, Aubin JE: Cellular expression of bone-related proteins during in vitro osteogenesis in rat bone marrow stromal cell cultures. *Journal of Cellular Physiology,* 158(3):555-572, 1994.

Malyankar UM, Almeida M, Johnson RJ, Pichler RH, Giachelli CM: Osteopontin regulation in cultured rat renal epithelial cells. *Kidney International,* 51(6):1766-1773, 1997.

Malyankar UM, Hanson R, Schwartz SM, Ridall AL, Giachelli CM: Upstream stimulatory factor 1 regulates osteopontin expression in smooth muscle cells. *Experimental Cell Research,* 250(2):535-547, 1999.

Malyankar UM, Scatena M, Suchland KL, Yun TJ, Clark EA, Giachelli CM: Osteoprotegerin is an alpha v beta 3-induced, NF-kappa B-dependent survival factor for endothelial cells. *Journal of Biological Chemistry,* 275(28):20959-20962, 2000.

Manji SS, Ng KW, Martin TJ, Zhou H: Transcriptional and posttranscriptional regulation of osteopontin gene expression in preosteoblasts by retinoic acid. *Journal of Cellular Physiology,* 176(1):1-9, 1998.

Manzano VM, Munoz JC, Jimenez JR, Puyol MR, Puyol DR, Kitamura M, Cazana FJ: Human renal mesangial cells are a target for the anti-inflammatory action of 9-cis retinoic acid. *British Journal of Pharmacology,* 131(8):1673-1683, 2000.

Manzano VM, Puyol MR, Puyol DR, Cazana FJ: Tretinoin prevents age-related renal changes and stimulates antioxidant defenses in cultured renal mesangial cells. *Journal of Pharmacology and Experimental Therapeutics,* 289(1):123-132, 1999.

Maor G, Hochberg Z, von der Mark K, Heinegard D, Silbermann M: Human growth hormone enhances chondrogenesis and osteogenesis in a tissue culture system of chondroprogenitor cells. *Endocrinology,* 125(3):1239-1245, 1989.

Marcinkiewicz C, Taooka Y, Yokosaki Y, Calvete JJ, Marcinkiewicz MM, Lobb RR, Niewiarowski S, Sheppard D: Inhibitory effects of MLDG-containing heterodimeric disintegrins reveal distinct structural requirements for interaction of the integrin alpha 9beta 1 with VCAM-1, tenascin-C, and osteopontin. *Journal of Biological Chemistry,* 275(41):31930-31937, 2000.

Margerie D, Flechtenmacher J, Buttner FH, Karbowski A, Puhl W, Schleyerbach R, Bartnik E: Complexity of IL-1 beta induced gene expression pattern in human articular chondrocytes. *Osteoarthritis and Cartilage,* 5(2):129-138, 1997.

Mark MP, Butler WT, Prince CW, Finkelman RD, Ruch JV: Developmental expression of 44-kDa bone phosphoprotein (osteopontin) and bone gamma-carboxyglutamic acid (Gla)-containing protein (osteocalcin) in calcifying tissues of rat. *Differentiation,* 37(2):123-136, 1988.

Mark MP, Prince CW, Gay S, Austin RL, Bhown M, Finkelman RD, Butler WT: A comparative immunocytochemical study on the subcellular distributions of 44 kDa bone phosphoprotein and bone gamma-carboxyglutamic acid (Gla)-containing protein in osteoblasts. *Journal of Bone Minerals Research,* 2(4):337-346, 1987.

Mark MP, Prince CW, Gay S, Austin RL, Butler WT: 44-kDal bone phosphoprotein (osteopontin) antigenicity at ectopic sites in newborn rats: Kidney and nervous tissues. *Cell Tissue Research,* 251(1):23-30, 1988.

Mark MP, Prince CW, Oosawa T, Gay S, Bronckers AL, Butler WT: Immunohistochemical demonstration of a 44-KDa phosphoprotein in developing rat bones. *Journal of Histochemistry and Cytochemistry,* 35(7):707-715, 1987.

Markert JM, Fuller CM, Gillespie GY, Bubien JK, McLean LA, Hong RL, Lee K, Gullans SR, Mapstone TB, Benos DJ: Differential gene expression profiling in human brain tumors. *Physiological Genomics,* 5(1):21-33, 2001.

Marks SC Jr, Mackowiak S, Shaloub V, Lian JB, Stein GS: Proliferation and differentiation of osteoblasts in osteopetrotic rats: Modification in expression of genes encoding cell growth and extracellular matrix proteins. *Connective Tissue Research,* 21(1-4):107-113; discussion 114-116, 1989.

Marmion BP, Shannon M: Post Q fever syndrome. *Lancet,* 347:977-978, 1996.

Marshall-Heyman H, Engel G, Ljungdahl S, Shoshan MC, Svensson C, Wasylyk B, Linder S: Tumorigenic and metastatic properties of two ras-oncogene transfected rat fibrosarcoma cell lines defective in c-jun. *Oncogene,* 9(12):3655-3663, 1994.

Martin I, Jakob M, Schafer D, Dick W, Spagnoli G, Heberer M: Quantitative analysis of gene expression in human articular cartilage from normal and osteoarthritic joints. *Osteoarthritis and Cartilage,* 9(2):112-118, 2001.

Martin WJ: Detection of RNA sequences in cultures of a stealth virus isolated from the cerebrospinal fluid of a health care worker with chronic fatigue syndrome. Case report. *Pathobiology,* 65(1):57-60, 1997.

Marusic A, Grcevic D, Katavic V, Kovacic N, Lukic IK, Kalajzic I, Lorenzo JA: Role of B lymphocytes in new bone formation. *Laboratory Investigations,* 80(11):1761-1774, 2000.

Marzia M, Sims NA, Voit S, Migliaccio S, Taranta A, Bernardini S, Faraggiana T, Yoneda T, Mundy GR, Boyce BF, et al.: Decreased c-Src expression enhances osteoblast differentiation and bone formation. *Journal of Cellular Biology,* 151(2):311-320, 2000.

Masbernard A: Les localizations neurologiques des rickettsioses. [The neurological localizations of rickettsial infections.] *Bulletin de Societé des Pathologies Exotiques,* 56:714-740, 1963.

Maslamani S, Glenton PA, Khan SR: Changes in urine macromolecular composition during processing. *Journal of Urology,* 164(1):230-236, 2000.

Masuda K, Takahashi N, Tsukamoto Y, Honma H, Kohri K: N-glycan structures of an osteopontin from human bone. *Biochemical and Biophysical Research Communications,* 268(3):814-817, 2000.

Mathieu E, Meheus L, Raymackers J, Merregaert J: Characterization of the osteogenic stromal cell line MN7: Identification of secreted MN7 proteins using two-dimensional polyacrylamide gel electrophoresis, western blotting, and microsequencing. *Journal of Bone Minerals Research,* 9(6):903-913, 1994.

Mathieu E, Merregaert J: Characterization of the stromal osteogenic cell line MN7: mRNA steady-state level of selected osteogenic markers depends on cell density and is influenced by 17 beta-estradiol. *Journal of Bone Minerals Research,* 9(2):183-192, 1994.

Matkovits T, Christakos S: Variable in vivo regulation of rat vitamin D-dependent genes (osteopontin, Ca,Mg-adenosine triphosphatase, and 25-hydroxyvitamin D3 24-hydroxylase): Implications for differing mechanisms of regulation and involvement of multiple factors. *Endocrinology,* 136(9):3971-3982, 1995.

Matsue M, Kageyama R, Denhardt DT, Noda M: Helix-loop-helix-type transcription factor (HES-1) is expressed in osteoblastic cells, suppressed by 1,25(OH)2 vitamin D3, and modulates 1,25(OH)2 vitamin D3 enhancement of osteopontin gene expression. *Bone,* 20(4):329-334, 1997.

Matsumoto HN, Tamura M, Denhardt DT, Obinata M, Noda M: Establishment and characterization of bone marrow stromal cell lines that support osteoclastogenesis. *Endocrinology,* 136(9):4084-4091, 1995.

Matsumoto M, Sakao Y, Akira S: Inducible expression of nuclear factor IL-6 increases endogenous gene expression of macrophage inflammatory protein-1 alpha, osteopontin and CD14 in a monocytic leukemia cell line. *International Immunology*, 10(12):1825-1835, 1998.

Matsumura S, Hiranuma H, Deguchi A, Maeda T, Jikko A, Fuchihata H: Changes in phenotypic expression of osteoblasts after X irradiation. *Radiation Research*, 149(5):463-471, 1998.

Matsuzaka K, Inoue T, Nashimoto M, Takemoto K, Ishikawa H, Asaka M, Shimono M, Fujikawa M, Noma H: A case of an ameloblastic fibro-odontoma arising from a calcifying odontogenic cyst. *Bulletin of the Tokyo Dental College* 42(1):51-55, 2001.

Maxian SH, Di Stefano T, Melican MC, Tiku ML, Zawadsky JP: Bone cell behavior on Matrigel-coated Ca/P coatings of varying crystallinities. *Journal of Biomedical Materials Research*, 40(2):171-179, 1998.

May LT, Torcia G, Cozzolino F, Ray A, Tatter SB, Santhanam U, Seghal PB, Stern D: Interleukin-6 gene expression in human endothelial cells: RNA start sites, multiple IL-6 proteins and inhibition of proliferation. *Biochemical and Biophysical Research Communications*, 159:991, 1989.

Mazzali M, Kim YG, Suga S, Gordon KL, Kang DH, Jefferson JA, Hughes J, McCabe LR, Last TJ, Lynch M, et al.: Expression of cell growth and bone phenotypic genes during the cell cycle of normal diploid osteoblasts and osteosarcoma cells. *Journal of Cellular Biochemistry*, 56(2):274-282, 1994.

McCabe LR, Last TJ, Lynch M, Lian J, Stein J, Stein G: Expression of cell growth on bone phenotypic genes during the cell cycle of normal diploid osteoblasts and osteosarcomal cells. *Journal of Cellular Biochemistry*, 56(2):274-282, 1994.

McDevitt TC, Nelson KE, Stayton PS: Constrained cell recognition peptides engineered into streptavidin. *Biotechnology Progress*, 15(3):391-396, 1999.

McFarland RJ, Garza S, Butler WT, Hook M: The mutagenesis of the RGD sequence of recombinant osteopontin causes it to lose its cell adhesion ability. *Annals of the New York Academy of Sciences*, 760:327-331, 1995.

McGregor NR, Butt HL, Zerbes M, Klineberg IJ, Dunstan RH, Roberts TK: Assessment of pain (distribution and onset), symptoms, SCL-90R inventory responses and the association with infectious events in patients with chronic orofacial pain. *Journal of Orofacial Pain*, 10:339-350, 1996.

McKee MD, Farach-Carson MC, Butler WT, Hauschka PV, Nanci A: Ultrastructural immunolocalization of noncollagenous (osteopontin and osteocalcin) and plasma (albumin and alpha 2HS-glycoprotein) proteins in rat bone. *Journal of Bone Minerals Research*, 8(4):485-496, 1993.

McKee MD, Glimcher MJ, Nanci A: High-resolution immunolocalization of osteopontin and osteocalcin in bone and cartilage during endochondral ossification in the chicken tibia. *Anatomy Records*, 234(4):479-492, 1992.

McKee MD, Nanci A: Osteopontin and the bone remodeling sequence. Colloidal-gold immunocytochemistry of an interfacial extracellular matrix protein. *Annals of the New York Academy of Sciences*, 760:177-189, 1995a.

McKee MD, Nanci A: Postembedding colloidal-gold immunocytochemistry of noncollagenous extracellular matrix proteins in mineralized tissues. *Microscopy Research Technqiues*, 31(1):44-62, 1995b.

McKee MD, Nanci A: Osteopontin: An interfacial extracellular matrix protein in mineralized tissues. *Connective Tissue Research,* 35(1-4):197-205, 1996a.

McKee MD, Nanci A: Osteopontin at mineralized tissue interfaces in bone, teeth, and osseointegrated implants: Ultrastructural distribution and implications for mineralized tissue formation, turnover, and repair. *Microscopy Research Techniques,* 33(2):141-164, 1996b.

McKee MD, Nanci A: Osteopontin deposition in remodeling bone: An osteoblast mediated event. *Journal of Bone Minerals Research,* 11(6):873-875, 1996c.

McKee MD, Nanci A: Secretion of osteopontin by macrophages and its accumulation at tissue surfaces during wound healing in mineralized tissues: A potential requirement for macrophage adhesion and phagocytosis. *Anatomy Records,* 245(2):394-409, 1996d.

McKee MD, Nanci A, Khan SR: Ultrastructural immunodetection of osteopontin and osteocalcin as major matrix components of renal calculi. *Journal of Bone Minerals Research,* 10(12):1913-1929, 1995.

McKee MD, Nanci A, Landis WJ, Gotoh Y, Gerstenfeld LC, Glimcher MJ: Effects of fixation and demineralization on the retention of bone phosphoprotein and other matrix components as evaluated by biochemical analyses and quantitative immunocytochemistry. *Journal of Bone Minerals Research,* 6(9):937-945, 1991.

McKee MD, Zalzal S, Nanci A: Extracellular matrix in tooth cementum and mantle dentin: Localization of osteopontin and other noncollagenous proteins, plasma proteins, and glycoconjugates by electron microscopy. *Anatomy Records,* 245(2): 293-312, 1996.

Meazzini MC, Toma CD, Schaffer JL, Gray ML, Gerstenfeld LC: Osteoblast cytoskeletal modulation in response to mechanical strain in vitro. *Journal of Orthopedics Research,* 16(2):170-180, 1998.

Medcalf RL, Ruegg M, Schleuning WD: A DNA motif related to the camp-responsive element and an exon-located activator protein-2 binding site in the human tissue-type plasminogen activator gene promoter cooperate in basal expression and convey activation by phorbol ester and camp. *Journal of Biological Chemistry,* 265:14618, 1990.

Medico E, Gentile A, Lo Celso C, Williams TA, Gambarotta G, Trusolino L, Comoglio PM: Osteopontin is an autocrine mediator of hepatocyte growth factor-induced invasive growth. *Cancer Research,* 61(15):5861-5868, 2001.

Meleti Z, Shapiro IM, Adams CS: Inorganic phosphate induces apoptosis of osteoblast-like cells in culture. *Bone,* 27(3):359-366, 2000.

Merry K, Dodds R, Littlewood A, Gowen M: Expression of osteopontin mRNA by osteoclasts and osteoblasts in modelling adult human bone. *Journal of Cellular Sciences,* 104(Pt 4):1013-1020, 1993.

Metzler DE: *Biochemistry: The Chemical Reactions of Living Cells.* Academic Press, New York, p. 381, 1977.

Mezey E, Palkovits M: Localization of targets for anti-ulcer drugs in cells of the immune system. *Science,* 258(5088):1662-1665, 1992.

Mezzano SA, Droguett MA, Burgos ME, Ardiles LG, Aros CA, Caorsi I, Egido J: Overexpression of chemokines, fibrogenic cytokines, and myofibroblasts in human membranous nephropathy. *Kidney International,* 57(1):147-158, 2000.

Mickos H, Sundberg K, Luning B: Synthesis, NMR spectra and function of peptides with alpha-methylserine attached to the RGD sequence of osteopontin. *Acta Chemica Scandinavica,* 46(10):989-993, 1992.

Midura RJ, McQuillan DJ, Benham KJ, Fisher LW, Hascall VC: A rat osteogenic cell line (UMR 106-01) synthesizes a highly sulfated form of bone sialoprotein. *Journal of Biological Chemistry,* 265(9):5285-5291, 1990.

Mignatti P, Tsubi R, Robbins E, Rifkin DB: In vitro angiogenesis on the human amniotic membrane: Requirement for basic fibroblast growth factor-induced proteinases. *Journal of Cell Biology,* 108:671-682, 1989.

Miles RR, Turner CH, Santerre R, Tu Y, McClelland P, Argot J, DeHoff BS, Mundy CW, Rosteck PR Jr, Bidwell J, et al.: Analysis of differential gene expression in rat tibia after an osteogenic stimulus in vivo: Mechanical loading regulates osteopontin and myeloperoxidase. *Journal of Cellular Biochemistry,* 68(3):355-365, 1998.

Min W, Shiraga H, Chalko C, Goldfarb S, Krishna GG, Hoyer JR: Quantitative studies of human urinary excretion of uropontin. *Kidney International,* 53(1):189-193, 1998.

Miyamoto Y, Shinki T, Ohyama Y, Kasama T, Iwasaki H: Regulation of vitamin D-responsive gene expression by fluorinated analogs of calcitriol in rat osteoblastic ROB-C26 cells. *Journal of Biochemistry (Tokyo),* 118(5):1068-1076, 1995.

Miyauchi A, Alvarez J, Greenfield EM, Teti A, Grano M, Colucci S, Zambonin-Zallone A, Ross FP, Teitelbaum SL, Cheresh D, et al.: Recognition of osteopontin and related peptides by an alpha v beta 3 integrin stimulates immediate cell signals in osteoclasts. *Journal of Biological Chemistry,* 266(30):20369-20374, 1991.

Miyauchi A, Alvarez J, Greenfield EM, Teti A, Grano M, Colucci S, Zambonin-Zallone A, Ross FP, Teitelbaum SL, Cheresh D, et al.: Binding of osteopontin to the osteoclast integrin alpha v beta 3. *Osteoporosis International,* 3(Suppl 1):132-135, 1993.

Miyaura C, Suda T: [Vitamin D]. *Nippon Rinsho,* 51(4):893-900, 1993.

Miyazaki Y, Setoguchi M, Yoshida S, Higuchi Y, Akizuki S, Yamamoto S: The mouse osteopontin gene. Expression in monocytic lineages and complete nucleotide sequence. *Journal of Biological Chemistry,* 265(24):14432-14438, 1990.

Miyazaki Y, Tashiro T, Higuchi Y, Setoguchi M, Yamamoto S, Nagai H, Nasu M, Vassalli P: Expression of osteopontin in a macrophage cell line and in transgenic mice with pulmonary fibrosis resulting from the lung expression of a tumor necrosis factor-alpha transgene. *Annals of the New York Academy of Sciences,* 760:334-341, 1995.

Mizuno M, Fujisawa R, Kuboki Y: Type I collagen-induced osteoblastic differentiation of bone-marrow cells mediated by collagen-alpha2beta1 integrin interaction. *Journal of Cellular Physiology,* 184(2):207-213, 2000.

Mizuno M, Kuboki Y: Osteoblast-related gene expression of bone marrow cells during the osteoblastic differentiation induced by type I collagen. *Journal of Biochemistry (Tokyo),* 129(1):133-138, 2001.

Mocetti P, Ballanti P, Zalzal S, Silvestrini G, Bonucci E, Nanci A: A histomorphometric, structural, and immunocytochemical study of the effects of diet-induced hypocalcemia on bone in growing rats. *Journal of Histochemistry and Cytochemistry,* 48(8):1059-1078, 2000.

Mohler ER III, Adam LP, McClelland P, Graham L, Hathaway DR: Detection of osteopontin in calcified human aortic valves. *Arteriosclerosis and Thrombosis Vascular Biology,* 17(3):547-552, 1997.

Moiseeva EP, Javed Q, Spring EL, de Bono DP: Galectin 1 is involved in vascular smooth muscle cell proliferation. *Cardiovascular Research,* 45(2):493-502, 2000.

Monsonego E, Baumbach WR, Lavelin I, Gertler A, Hurwitz S, Pines M: Generation of growth hormone binding protein by avian growth plate chondrocytes is dependent on cell differentiation. *Molecular and Cellular Endocrinology,* 135(1):1-10, 1997.

Monsonego E, Halevy O, Gertler A, Hurwitz S, Pines M: Growth hormone inhibits differentiation of avian epiphyseal growth-plate chondrocytes. *Molecular and Cellular Endocrinology,* 114(1-2):35-42, 1995.

Montminy MR, Sevarino KA, Wagner JA, Mandel G, Goodman RH: Identification of a cyclic-AMP-responsive element within the rat somatostatin gene. *Proceedings of the National Academy of Sciences of the United States of America,* 83:6682, 1986.

Montrucchio G, Lupia E, Battaglia E, Passerini G, Bussolino F, Emanuelli G, Camussi G: Tumor necrosis factor-α-induced angiogenesis depends on in situ platelet-activating factor biosynthesis. *Journal of Experimental Medicine,* 180:377-382, 1994.

Moore MA, Gotoh Y, Rafidi K, Gerstenfeld LC: Characterization of a cDNA for chicken osteopontin: Expression during bone development, osteoblast differentiation, and tissue distribution. *Biochemistry,* 30(9):2501-2508, 1991.

Mori K: [Studies on expression and function of Eta-1(early T lymphocyte activation-1) in autoimmune prone MRL/Mp-lpr/lpr mice]. *Hokkaido Igaku Zasshi,* 69(4):708-717, 1994.

Mori K, Kobayashi S, Inobe M, Jia WY, Tamakoshi M, Miyazaki T, Uede T: In vivo cytokine gene expression in various T cell subsets of the autoimmune MRL/Mp-lpr/lpr mouse. *Autoimmunity,* 17(1):49-57, 1994.

Mori S, Saito Y: Cytokine and atherosclerosis: A possible role of osteopontin in development in diabetic macroangiopathy. *Nihon Rinsho Meneki Gakkai Kaishi,* 23(6):613-617, 2000.

Morris VL, Tuck AB, Wilson SM, Percy D, Chambers AF: Tumor progression and metastasis in murine D2 hyperplastic alveolar nodule mammary tumor cell lines. *Clinical and Experimental Metastasis,* 11(1):103-112, 1993.

Morrison JD: Fatigue as a presenting complaint in family practice. *Journal of Family Practice,* 10:795-801, 1980.

Morriss-Kay GM, Iseki S, Johnson D: Genetic control of the cell proliferation-differentiation balance in the developing skull vault: Roles of fibroblast growth factor receptor signaling pathways. *Novartis Foundation Symposia,* 232:102-116; discussion 116-121, 2001.

Mosely B, Beckmann MP, March CJ, Idzerda RL, Gimpel SD, Van den Bos T, Friend D, Alpert A, Anderson D, Jackson S, et al.: The murine interleukin 4 receptor: Molecular cloning and characterization of secreted and membrane bound forms. *Cell,* 59:335-343, 1989.

Motomura K, Ohtsuru A, Enomoto H, Tsukazaki T, Namba H, Tsuji Y, Yamashita S: Osteogenic action of parathyroid hormone-related peptide (1-141) in rat ROS cells. *Endocrinology Journal,* 43(5):527-535, 1996.

Moursi AM, Damsky CH, Lull J, Zimmerman D, Doty SB, Aota S, Globus RK: Fibronectin regulates calvarial osteoblast differentiation. *Journal of Cellular Sciences,* 109(Pt 6):1369-1380, 1996.

Mueller SM, Mizuno S, Gerstenfeld LC, Glowacki J: Medium perfusion enhances osteogenesis by murine osteosarcoma cells in three-dimensional collagen sponges. *Journal of Bone Minerals Research,* 14(12):2118-2126, 1999.

Mukherjee BB, Nemir M, Beninati S, Cordella-Miele E, Singh K, Chackalaparampil I, Shanmugam V, DeVouge MW, Mukherjee AB: Interaction of osteopontin with fibronectin and other extracellular matrix molecules. *Annals of the New York Academy of Sciences,* 760:201-212, 1995.

Muller GA, Strutz FM: Renal fibroblast heterogeneity. *Kidney International Supplement,* 50:S33-S36, 1995.

Mundy GR: Regulation of bone formation by bone morphogenetic proteins and other growth factors. *Clinical Orthopedics,* (324):24-28, 1996.

Murata M, Kawamura A: Restoration of the infectivity of *Rickettsia tsutsugamushi* to susceptible animals by passage in a thymic nude mice. *Japanese Journal of Experimental Medicine,* 47(5):385-391, 1977.

Murry CE, Giachelli CM, Schwartz SM, Vracko R: Macrophages express osteopontin during repair of myocardial necrosis. *American Journal of Pathology,* 145(6):1450-1462, 1994.

Nacy CA, Groves MG: Macrophages in resistance to rickettsial infections: Early host defense mechanisms in experimental scrub typhus. *Infection and Immunity,* 31:1239, 1981.

Nagai S, Hashimoto S, Yamashita T, Toyoda N, Satoh T, Suzuki T, Matsushima K: Comprehensive gene expression profile of human activated T(h)1- and T(h)2-polarized cells. *International Immunology,* 13(3):367-376, 2001.

Nagasaki T, Ishimura E, Koyama H, Shioi A, Jono S, Inaba M, Hasuma T, Yokoyama M, Nishizawa Y, Morii H, et al.: Alphav integrin regulates TNF-alpha-induced nitric oxide synthesis in rat mesangial cells—possible role of osteopontin. *Nephrology, Dialysis, and Transplantation,* 14(8):1861-1866, 1999.

Nagasaki T, Ishimura E, Shioi A, Jono S, Inaba M, Nishizawa Y, Morii H, Otani S: Osteopontin gene expression and protein synthesis in cultured rat mesangial cells. *Biochemical and Biophysical Research Communications,* 233(1):81-85, 1997.

Nagasawa Y, Takenaka M, Kaimori J, Matsuoka Y, Akagi Y, Tsujie M, Imai E, Nagata T, Bellows CG, Kasugai S, et al.: Biosynthesis of bone proteins [SPP-1 (secreted phosphoprotein-1, osteopontin), BSP (bone sialoprotein) and SPARC (osteonectin)] in association with mineralized-tissue formation by fetal-rat calvarial cells in culture. *Biochemical Journal,* 274(Pt 2):513-520, 1991.

Nagata T, Goldberg HA, Zhang Q, Domenicucci C, Sodek J: Biosynthesis of bone proteins by fetal porcine calvariae in vitro. Rapid association of sulfated sialoproteins (secreted phosphoprotein-1 and bone sialoprotein) and chondroitin sulfate proteoglycan (CS-PGIII) with bone mineral. *Matrix,* 11(2):86-100, 1991.

Nagata T, Kaho K, Nishikawa S, Shinohara H, Wakano Y, Ishida H: Effect of prostaglandin E2 on mineralization of bone nodules formed by fetal rat calvarial cells. *Calcified Tissue International,* 55(6):451-457, 1994.

Nagata T, Todescan R, Goldberg HA, Zhang Q, Sodek J: Sulphation of secreted phosphoprotein I (SPPI, osteopontin) is associated with mineralized tissue formation. *Biochemical and Biophysical Research Communications,* 165(1):234-240, 1989.

Nagata T, Yokota M, Nishikawa S, Ishida H, Wakano Y: Osteopontin expression in clonal dental pulp cells. *Annals of the New York Academy of Sciences,* 760:342-345, 1995.

Nagata T, Yokota M, Ohishi K, Nishikawa S, Shinohara H, Wakano Y, Ishida H: 1 alpha,25-dihydroxyvitamin D3 stimulation of osteopontin expression in rat clonal dental pulp cells. *Archives of Oral Biology,* 39(9):775-782, 1994.

Nagoshi J, Nomura S, Uchida N, Hirota S, Ito A, Nakase T, Hirakawa K, Shiozaki H, Mori T, Kitamura Y: Expression of genes encoding connective tissue proteins in androgen-dependent SC115 tumors after androgen removal. *Laboratory Investigations,* 70(2):210-216, 1994.

Nakajima Y, Shimokawa H, Terai K, Onoue H, Seino Y, Tanaka H, Sobue S, Kitamura Y, Nomura S: Identification of the cell type origin of odontoma-like cell masses in microphthalmic (mi/mi) mice by in situ hybridization. *Pathology International,* 46(10):743-750, 1996.

Nakama K, Miyazaki Y, Nasu M: Immunophenotyping of lymphocytes in the lung interstitium and expression of osteopontin and interleukin-2 mRNAs in two different murine models of pulmonary fibrosis. *Experimental Lung Research,* 24(1):57-70, 1998.

Nakase T, Sugimoto M, Sato M, Kaneko M, Tomita T, Sugamoto K, Nomura S, Kitamura Y, Yoshikawa H, Yasui N, et al.: Switch of osteonectin and osteopontin mRNA expression in the process of cartilage-to-bone transition during fracture repair. *Acta Histochemica,* 100(3):287-295, 1998.

Nakase T, Takaoka K, Hirakawa K, Hirota S, Takemura T, Onoue H, Takebayashi K, Kitamura Y, Nomura S: Alterations in the expression of osteonectin, osteopontin and osteocalcin mRNAs during the development of skeletal tissues in vivo. *Bone Minerals,* 26(2):109-122, 1994.

Nakaya T, Kuratsune H, Kitani T, Ikuta K: Demonstration of borna disease virus in patients with chronic fatigue syndrome. *Nippon Rinsho—Japanese Journal of Clinical Medicine,* 55(11):3064-3071, 1997.

Nakaya T, Takahashi H, Nakamura Y, Asahi S, Tobiume M, Kuratsune H, Kitani T, Yamanishi K, Ikuta K: Demonstration of borna disease virus RNA in peripheral blood mononuclear cells derived from Japanese patients with chronic fatigue syndrome. *FEBS Letters,* 378(2):145-149, 1996.

Nakaya T, Takahashi H, Nakamura Y, Huratsune H, Kitani T, Machii T, Yamanishi K, Ikuta K: Borna disease virus infection in two family clusters of patients with chronic fatigue syndrome. *Microbiology and Immunology,* 43(7):679-689, 1999.

Nam TJ, Busby WH Jr, Rees C, Clemmons DR: Thrombospondin and osteopontin bind to insulin-like growth factor (IGF)-binding protein-5 leading to an alteration in IGF-I-stimulated cell growth. *Endocrinology,* 141(3):1100-1106, 2000.

Nambi P, Gellai M, Wu HL, Prabhakar U: Upregulation of osteopontin in ischemia-induced renal failure in rats: A role for ET-1? *Biochemical and Biophysical Research Communications,* 241(1):212-214, 1997.

Namen AE, Lupton SZ, Hjerrild K, Wignall J, Mochizuki DY, Schmierer A, Mosely B, March CJ, Urdal D, Gillis S, et al.: Stimulation of B-cell progenitors by cloned murine interleukin-7. *Nature,* 333(6173):571-573, 1988.

Nanci A: Content and distribution of noncollagenous matrix proteins in bone and cementum: Relationship to speed of formation and collagen packing density. *Journal of Structural Biology,* 126(3):256-269, 1999.

Nanci A, Zalzal S, Gotoh Y, McKee MD: Ultrastructural characterization and immunolocalization of osteopontin in rat calvarial osteoblast primary cultures. *Microscopy Research Techniques,* 33(2):214-231, 1996.

Nangaku M, Pippin J, Couser WG: Complement membrane attack complex (C5b-9) mediates interstitial disease in experimental nephrotic syndrome. *Journal of the American Society of Nephrology,* 10(11):2323-2331, 1999.

Naot D, Sionov RV, Ish-Shalom D: CD44: Structure, function, and association with the malignant process. *Advances in Cancer Research,* 71:241-319, 1997.

Narayanan K, Srinivas R, Ramachandran A, Hao J, Quinn B, George A: Differentiation of embryonic mesenchymal cells to odontoblast-like cells by overexpression of dentin matrix protein 1. *Proceedings of the National Academy of Sciences of the United States of America,* 98(8):4516-4521, 2001.

Narita I, Nakayama H, Goto S, Takeda T, Sakatsume M, Saito A, Nakagawa Y, Arakawa M: Identification of genes specifically expressed in chronic and progressive glomerulosclerosis. *Kidney International Supplement,* 63:S215-S217, 1997.

Nasu K, Ishida T, Setoguchi M, Higuchi Y, Akizuki S, Yamamoto S: Expression of wild-type and mutated rabbit osteopontin in *Escherichia coli,* and their effects on adhesion and migration of P388D1 cells. *Biochemical Journal,* 307(Pt 1):257-265, 1995.

Nau GJ, Chupp GL, Emile JF, Jouanguy E, Berman JS, Casanova JL, Young RA: Osteopontin expression correlates with clinical outcome in patients with mycobacterial infection. *American Journal of Pathology,* 157(1):37-42, 2000.

Nau GJ, Guilfoile P, Chupp GL, Berman JS, Kim SJ, Kornfeld H, Young RA: A chemoattractant cytokine associated with granulomas in tuberculosis and silicosis. *Proceedings of the National Academy of Sciences of the United States of America,* 94(12):6414-6419, 1997.

Nau GJ, Liaw L, Chupp GL, Berman JS, Hogan BL, Young RA: Attenuated host resistance against *Mycobacterium* bovis BCG infection in mice lacking osteopontin. *Infection and Immunity,* 67(8):4223-4230, 1999.

Neame PJ, Butler WT: Posttranslational modification in rat bone osteopontin. *Connective Tissue Research,* 35(1-4):145-150, 1996.

Nemeth A, Penneys N: Factor XIIIa is expressed by fibroblasts in fibrovascuolar tumors. *Journal of Cutaneous Pathology,* 16:266-271, 1989.

Nemir M, Bhattacharyya D, Li X, Singh K, Mukherjee AB, Mukherjee BB: Targeted inhibition of osteopontin expression in the mammary gland causes abnormal morphogenesis and lactation deficiency. *Journal of Biological Chemistry,* 275(2):969-976, 2000.

Nemir M, DeVouge MW, Mukherjee BB: Normal rat kidney cells secrete both phosphorylated and nonphosphorylated forms of osteopontin showing different physiological properties. *Journal of Biological Chemistry,* 264(30):18202-18208, 1989.

Nemoto A, Uemura T: [Integrin signal transduction via FAK in osteoblasts—early differentiation triggered by osteopontin]. *Seikagaku,* 71(2):140-145, 1999.

Nemoto H, Rittling SR, Yoshitake H, Furuya K, Amagasa T, Tsuji K, Nifuji A, Denhardt DT, Noda M: Osteopontin deficiency reduces experimental tumor cell metastasis to bone and soft tissues. *Journal of Bone Minerals Research,* 16(4): 652-659, 2001.

Newman CM, Bruun BC, Mistry PK, Weissberg PL, Shanahan CM: High expression of osteopontin mRNA in human macrophages but not human vascular smooth muscle cells in culture. *Annals of the New York Academy of Sciences,* 760:381-382, 1995.

Newman CM, Bruun BC, Porter KE, Mistry PK, Shanahan CM, Weissberg PL: Osteopontin is not a marker for proliferating human vascular smooth muscle cells. *Arteriosclerosis and Thrombosis Vascular Biology,* 15(11):2010-2018, 1995.

Nguyen L, Lekic P, McCulloch CA: Collagen implants do not preserve periodontal ligament homeostasis in periodontal wounds. *Journal of Periodontal Research,* 32(5):419-429, 1997.

Nicolson GL: Chronic infections as a common etiology for many patients with chronic fatigue syndrome, Fibromyalgia syndrome and Gulf War illnesses. *International Journal of Medicine,* 1:42-46, 1998.

Nicolson GL, Nasralla MY, Franco AR, De Meirleir K, Nicolson NL, Ngwenya R, Haier J: Role of mycoplasmal infections in fatigue illnesses: Chronic fatigue and fibromyalgia syndromes, Gulf War illness, and rheumatoid arthritis. *Journal of Chronic Fatigue Syndrome,* 6(3/4):23-39, 2000.

Nicolson GL, Nasralla M, Haier J: Diagnosis and treatment of mycoplasmal infections in fibromyalgia and chronic fatigue. *Biomedical Therapy,* 16:266-269, 1998.

Nicolson GL, Nasralla MY, Haier J: Mycoplasmal infections in chronic illnesses: Fybromyalgia and chronic fatigue syndromes, Gulf War illness, HIV-AIDS and rheumatoid arthritis. *Medical Sentinel,* 5:172-176, 1999.

Ninomiya JT, Struve JA, Stelloh CT, Toth JM, Crosby KE: Effects of hydroxyapatite particulate debris on the production of cytokines and proteases in human fibroblasts. *Journal of Orthopedic Research,* 19(4):621-628, 2001.

Nishida T, Nakanishi T, Asano M, Shimo T, Takigawa M: Effects of CTGF/Hcs24, a hypertrophic chondrocyte-specific gene product, on the proliferation and differentiation of osteoblastic cells in vitro. *Journal of Cellular Physiology,* 184(2): 197-206, 2000.

Nishikawa J, Kitaura M, Matsumoto M, Imagawa M, Nishihara T: Difference and similarity of DNA sequence recognized by VDR homodimer and VDR/RXR heterodimer. *Nucleic Acids Research,* 22(15):2902-2907, 1994.

Nishikawa J, Matsumoto M, Sakoda K, Kitaura M, Imagawa M, Nishihara T: Vitamin D receptor zinc finger region binds to a direct repeat as a dimer and discriminates the spacing number between each half-site. *Journal of Biological Chemistry,* 268(26):19739-19743, 1993.

Nishio K, Neo M, Akiyama H, Nishiguchi S, Kim HM, Kokubo T, Nakamura T: The effect of alkali- and heat-treated titanium and apatite-formed titanium on osteoblastic differentiation of bone marrow cells. *Journal of Biomedical Materials Research,* 52(4):652-661, 2000.

Nishio K, Neo M, Akiyama H, Okada Y, Kokubo T, Nakamura T: Effects of apatite and wollastonite containing glass-ceramic powder and two types of alumina powder in composites on osteoblastic differentiation of bone marrow cells. *Journal of Biomedical Materials Research,* 55(2):164-176, 2001.

Nishio S, Hatanaka M, Takeda H, Aoki K, Iseda T, Iwata H, Yokoyama M: Calcium phosphate crystal-associated proteins: alpha2-HS-glycoprotein, prothrombin F1, and osteopontin. *Molecular Urology,* 4(4):383-390, 2000.

Nishio S, Hatanaka M, Takeda H, Iseda T, Iwata H, Yokoyama M: Analysis of urinary concentrations of calcium phosphate crystal-associated proteins: alpha2-HS-glycoprotein, prothrombin F1, and osteopontin. *Journal of the American Society of Nephrology,* 10(Suppl 14):S394-S396, 1999.

Nishio S, Iseda T, Takeda H, Iwata H, Yokoyama M: Inhibitory effect of calcium phosphate-associated proteins on calcium oxalate crystallization: alpha2-HS-glycoprotein, prothrombin-F1 and osteopontin. *BJU International,* 86(4):543-548, 2000.

Noble BS, Reeve J: Osteocyte function, osteocyte death and bone fracture resistance. *Molecular and Cellular Endocrinology,* 159(1-2):7-13, 2000.

Noda M, Denhardt DT: Regulation of osteopontin gene expression in osteoblasts. *Annals of the New York Academy of Sciences,* 760:242-248, 1995.

Noda M, Rodan GA: Transcriptional regulation of osteopontin production in rat osteoblast-like cells by parathyroid hormone. *Journal of Cellular Biology,* 108(2):713-718, 1989a.

Noda M, Rodan GA: Type beta transforming growth factor regulates expression of genes encoding bone matrix proteins. *Connective Tissue Research,* 21(1-4):71-75, 1989b.

Noda M, Vogel RL, Craig AM, Prahl J, DeLuca HF, Denhardt DT: Identification of a DNA sequence responsible for binding of the 1,25-dihydroxyvitamin D3 receptor and 1,25-dihydroxyvitamin D3 enhancement of mouse secreted phosphoprotein 1 (SPP-1 or osteopontin) gene expression. *Proceedings of the National Academy of Sciences of the United States of America,* 87(24):9995-9999, 1990.

Noda M, Vogel RL, Hasson DM, Rodan GA: Leukemia inhibitory factor suppresses proliferation, alkaline phosphatase activity, and type I collagen messenger ribonucleic acid level and enhances osteopontin mRNA level in murine osteoblast-like (MC3T3E1) cells. *Endocrinology,* 127(1):185-190, 1990.

Noda M, Yoon K, Prince CW, Butler WT, Rodan GA: Transcriptional regulation of osteopontin production in rat osteosarcoma cells by type beta transforming growth factor. *Journal of Biological Chemistry,* 263(27):13916-13921, 1988.

Nohutcu RM, McCauley LK, Koh AJ, Somerman MJ: Expression of extracellular matrix proteins in human periodontal ligament cells during mineralization in vitro. *Journal of Periodontology,* 68(4):320-327, 1997.

Nohutcu RM, McCauley LK, Shigeyama Y, Somerman MJ: Expression of mineral-associated proteins by periodontal ligament cells: In vitro vs. ex vivo. *Journal of Periodontal Research,* 31(5):369-372, 1996.

Noiri E, Dickman K, Miller F, Romanov G, Romanov VI, Shaw R, Chambers AF, Rittling SR, Denhardt DT, Goligorsky MS: Reduced tolerance to acute renal ischemia in mice with a targeted disruption of the osteopontin gene. *Kidney International,* 56(1):74-82, 1999.

Nomura S, Takano-Yamamoto T: Molecular events caused by mechanical stress in bone. *Matrix Biology,* 19(2):91-96, 2000.

Nomura S, Wills AJ, Edwards DR, Heath JK, Hogan BL: Developmental expression of 2ar (osteopontin) and SPARC (osteonectin) RNA as revealed by in situ hybridization. *Journal of Cellular Biology,* 106(2):441-450, 1988.

Nomura S, Wills AJ, Edwards DR, Heath JK, Hogan BL: Expression of genes for non-collagenous proteins during embryonic bone formation. *Connective Tissue Research,* 21(1-4):31-35; discussion 36-39, 1989.

Nordahl J, Mengarelli-Widholm S, Hultenby K, Reinholt FP: Ultrastructural immunolocalization of fibronectin in epiphyseal and metaphyseal bone of young rats. *Calcified Tissue International,* 57(6):442-449, 1995.

Norman AW, Manchand PS, Uskokovic MR, Okamura WH, Takeuchi JA, Bishop JE, Hisatake JI, Koeffler HP, Peleg S: Characterization of a novel analogue of 1alpha,25(OH)(2)-vitamin D(3) with two side chains: Interaction with its nuclear receptor and cellular actions. *Journal of Medical Chemistry,* 43(14):2719-2730, 2000.

Nose K, Saito H, Kuroki T: Isolation of a gene sequence induced later by tumor-promoting 12-O-tetradecanoylphorbol-13-acetate in mouse osteoblastic cells (MC3T3-E1) and expressed constitutively in ras-transformed cells. *Cellular Growth and Differentiation,* 1(11):511-518, 1990.

Noti JD: Adherence to osteopontin via alphavbeta3 suppresses phorbol ester-mediated apoptosis in MCF-7 breast cancer cells that overexpress protein kinase C-alpha. *International Journal of Oncology,* 17(6):1237-1243, 2000.

Nunohiro T, Ashizawa N, Graf K, Do YS, Hsueh WA, Yano K: Angiotensin II promotes remodelling-related events in cardiac fibroblasts. *Heart Vessels,* 12(Suppl):201-204, 1997.

Nunohiro T, Ashizawa N, Graf K, Hsueh WA, Yano K: Angiotensin II promotes integrin-mediated collagen gel contraction by adult rat cardiac fibroblasts. *Japanese Heart Journal,* 40(4):461-469, 1999.

Oates AJ, Barraclough R, Rudland PS: The identification of osteopontin as a metastasis-related gene product in a rodent mammary tumour model. *Oncogene,* 13(1):97-104, 1996.

Oates AJ, Barraclough R, Rudland PS: The role of osteopontin in tumorigenesis and metastasis. *Invasion Metastasis,* 17(1):1-15, 1997.

O'Brien ER, Garvin MR, Stewart DK, Hinohara T, Simpson JB, Schwartz SM, Giachelli CM: Osteopontin is synthesized by macrophage, smooth muscle, and endothelial cells in primary and restenotic human coronary atherosclerotic plaques. *Arteriosclerosis and Thrombosis,* 14(10):1648-1656, 1994.

O'Brien KD, Kuusisto J, Reichenbach DD, Ferguson M, Giachelli C, Alpers CE, Otto CM: Osteopontin is expressed in human aortic valvular lesions. *Circulation,* 92(8):2163-2168, 1995.

Ogawa T, Tokuda M, Tomizawa K, Matsui H, Itano T, Konishi R, Nagahata S, Hatase O: Osteoblastic differentiation is enhanced by rapamycin in rat osteoblast-like osteosarcoma (ROS 17/2.8) cells. *Biochemical and Biophysical Research Communications,* 249(1):226-230, 1998.

Ohishi K, Ishida H, Nagata T, Yamauchi N, Tsurumi C, Nishikawa S, Wakano Y: Thyroid hormone suppresses the differentiation of osteoprogenitor cells to osteoblasts, but enhances functional activities of mature osteoblasts in cultured rat calvaria cells. *Journal of Cellular Physiology,* 161(3):544-552, 1994.

Ohishi K, Nishikawa S, Nagata T, Yamauchi N, Shinohara H, Kido J, Ishida H: Physiological concentrations of retinoic acid suppress the osteoblastic differentiation of fetal rat calvaria cells in vitro. *European Journal of Endocrinology,* 133(3):335-341, 1995.

Ohishi M, Horibe M, Ikedo D, Miyazaki M, Ohishi K, Kataoka M, Kido J, Nagata T: Effect of retinoic acid on osteopontin expression in rat clonal dental pulp cells. *Journal of Endodontics,* 25(10):683-685, 1999.

Ohma N, Takagi Y, Takano Y: Distribution of non-collagenous dentin matrix proteins and proteoglycans, and their relation to calcium accumulation in bisphosphonate-affected rat incisors. *European Journal of Oral Sciences,* 108(3):222-232, 2000.

Ohmura T: [The expression of osteoblastic features in a SV40 large T antigen immortalized mouse calvarial cell line]. *Kokubyo Gakkai Zasshi,* 60(3):359-371, 1993.

Ohsawa K, Neo M, Matsuoka H, Akiyama H, Ito H, Kohno H, Nakamura T: The expression of bone matrix protein mRNAs around beta-TCP particles implanted into bone. *Journal of Biomedical Materials Research,* 52(3):460-466, 2000.

Ohsawa K, Neo M, Matsuoka H, Akiyama H, Ito H, Nakamura T: Tissue responses around polymethylmethacrylate particles implanted into bone: Analysis of expression of bone matrix protein mRNAs by in situ hybridization. *Journal of Biomedical Materials Research,* 54(4):501-508, 2001.

Ohta S, Yamamuro T, Lee K, Okumura H, Kasai R, Hiraki Y, Ikeda T, Iwasaki R, Kikuchi H, Konishi J, et al.: Fracture healing induces expression of the proto-oncogene c-fos in vivo. Possible involvement of the Fos protein in osteoblastic differentiation. *FEBS Letters,* 284(1):42-45, 1991.

Ohtsuki T, Furuya S, Yamada T, Nomura S, Hata J, Yabe Y, Hosoda Y: Gene expression of noncollagenous bone matrix proteins in the limb joints and intervertebral disks of the twy mouse. *Calcified Tissue International,* 63(2):167-172, 1998.

Ohyama Y, Ozono K, Uchida M, Shinki T, Kato S, Suda T, Yamamoto O, Noshiro M, Kato Y: Identification of a vitamin D-responsive element in the 5'-flanking region of the rat 25-hydroxyvitamin D3 24-hydroxylase gene. *Journal of Biological Chemistry,* 269(14):10545-10550, 1994.

Okada H, Moriwaki K, Kalluri R, Takenaka T, Imai H, Ban S, Takahama M, Suzuki H: Osteopontin expressed by renal tubular epithelium mediates interstitial monocyte infiltration in rats. *American Journal of Physiology and Renal Physiology,* 278(1):F110-F121, 2000.

Okada H, Moriwaki K, Konishi K, Kobayashi T, Sugahara S, Nakamoto H, Saruta T, Suzuki H: Tubular osteopontin expression in human glomerulonephritis and renal vasculitis. *American Journal of Kidney Diseases,* 36(3):498-506, 2000.

Oldberg A, Franzen A, Heinegard D: Cloning and sequence analysis of rat bone sialoprotein (osteopontin) cDNA reveals an Arg-Gly-Asp cell-binding sequence. *Proceedings of the National Academy of Sciences of the United States of America,* 83(23):8819-8823, 1986.

Oldberg A, Franzen A, Heinegard D, Pierschbacher MD, Ruoshlati E: Identification of a bone sialoprotein receptor in osteosarcoma cells. *Journal of Biological Chemistry,* 263(36):19433-19436, 1988.

Omigbodun A, Daiter E, Walinsky D, Fisher L, Young M, Hoyer J, Coutifaris C: Regulated expression of osteopontin in human trophoblasts. *Annals of the New York Academy of Sciences,* 760:346-349, 1995.

Omigbodun A, Ziolkiewicz P, Tessler C, Hoyer JR, Coutifaris C: Progesterone regulates osteopontin expression in human trophoblasts: A model of paracrine control in the placenta? *Endocrinology,* 138(10):4308-4315, 1997.

O'Neal RB, Sauk JJ, Somerman MJ: Biological requirements for material integration. *Journal of Oral Implantology,* 18(3):243-255, 1992.

Ongphiphadhanakul B, Jenis LG, Braverman LE, Alex S, Stein GS, Lian JB, Baran DT: Etidronate inhibits the thyroid hormone-induced bone loss in rats assessed by bone mineral density and messenger ribonucleic acid markers of osteoblast and osteoclast function. *Endocrinology,* 133(6):2502-2507, 1993.

Ono M, Yamamoto T, Nose M: Allelic difference in the nucleotide sequence of the Eta-1/Op gene transcript. *Molecular Immunology,* 32(6):447-448, 1995.

Onyia JE, Hale LV, Miles RR, Cain RL, Tu Y, Hulman JF, Hock JM, Santerre RF: Molecular characterization of gene expression changes in ROS 17/2.8 cells cultured in diffusion chambers in vivo. *Calcified Tissue International,* 65(2):133-138, 1999.

Ophascharoensuk V, Giachelli CM, Gordon K, Hughes J, Pichler R, Brown P, Liaw L, Schmidt R, Shankland SJ, Alpers CE, et al.: Obstructive uropathy in the mouse: Role of osteopontin in interstitial fibrosis and apoptosis. *Kidney International,* 56(2):571-580, 1999.

Ophascharoensuk V, Pippin JW, Gordon KL, Shankland SJ, Couser WG, Johnson RJ: Role of intrinsic renal cells versus infiltrating cells in glomerular crescent formation. *Kidney International,* 54(2):416-425, 1998.

O'Regan A, Berman JS: Osteopontin: A key cytokine in cell-mediated and granulomatous inflammation. *International Journal of Experimental Pathology,* 81(6):373-390, 2000.

O'Regan AW, Chupp GL, Lowry JA, Goetschkes M, Mulligan N, Berman JS: Osteopontin is associated with T cells in sarcoid granulomas and has T cell adhesive and cytokine-like properties in vitro. *Journal of Immunology,* 162(2):1024-1031, 1999.

O'Regan AW, Hayden JM, Berman JS: Osteopontin augments CD3-mediated interferon-gamma and CD40 ligand expression by T cells, which results in IL-12 production from peripheral blood mononuclear cells. *Journal of Leukocyte Biology,* 68(4):495-502, 2000.

O'Regan AW, Nau GJ, Chupp GL, Berman JS: Osteopontin (Eta-1) in cell-mediated immunity: Teaching an old dog new tricks. *Immunology Today,* 21(10):475-478, 2000.

Otawara-Hamamoto Y: [Biochemistry of bone matrix]. *Nippon Rinsho,* 48(12):2729-2735, 1990.

Otawara-Hamamoto Y: [Biochemistry of bone matrix]. *Nippon Rinsho,* 52(9):2239-2245, 1994.

Owan I, Burr DB, Turner CH, Qiu J, Tu Y, Onyia JE, Duncan RL: Mechanotransduction in bone: Osteoblasts are more responsive to fluid forces than mechanical strain. *American Journal of Physiology,* 273(3 Pt 1):C810-C815, 1997.

Owen TA, Aronow MS, Barone LM, Bettencourt B, Stein GS, Lian JB: Pleiotropic effects of vitamin D on osteoblast gene expression are related to the proliferative and differentiated state of the bone cell phenotype: Dependency upon basal levels of gene expression, duration of exposure, and bone matrix competency in normal rat osteoblast cultures. *Endocrinology,* 128(3):1496-1504, 1991.

Owen TA, Aronow M, Shalhoub V, Barone LM, Wilming L, Tassinari MS, Kennedy MB, Pockwinse S, Lian JB, Stein GS: Progressive development of the rat osteoblast phenotype in vitro: Reciprocal relationships in expression of genes associated with osteoblast proliferation and differentiation during formation of the bone extracellular matrix. *Journal of Cellular Physiology,* 143(3):420-430, 1990.

Oyajobi BO, Lomri A, Hott M, Marie PJ: Isolation and characterization of human clonogenic osteoblast progenitors immunoselected from fetal bone marrow stroma using STRO-1 monoclonal antibody. *Journal of Bone Minerals Research,* 14(3):351-361, 1999.

Oyama T, Iijima K, Takei H, Horiguchi J, Iino Y, Nakajima T, Koerner F: Atypical cystic lobule of the breast: An early stage of low-grade ductal carcinoma in-situ. *Breast Cancer,* 7(4):326-331, 2000.

Oyama Y, Kurabayashi M, Akuzawa N, Nagai R: Troglitazone, a PPARgamma ligand, inhibits osteopontin gene expression in human monocytes/macrophage THP-1 cells. *Journal of Atherosclerosis and Thrombosis,* 7(2):77-82, 2000.

Ozawa H, Amizuka N: [Structure and function of bone cells]. *Nippon Rinsho,* 52(9):2246-2254, 1994.

Ozawa S, Kasugai S: Evaluation of implant materials (hydroxyapatite, glass-ceramics, titanium) in rat bone marrow stromal cell culture. *Biomaterials,* 17(1):23-29, 1996.

Pacifici R, Carano A, Santoro SA, Rifas L, Jeffrey JJ, Malone JD, McCracken R, Avioli LV: Bone matrix constituents stimulate interleukin-1 release from human blood mononuclear cells. *Journal of Clinical Investigation,* 87(1):221-228, 1991.

Padanilam BJ, Martin DR, Hammerman MR: Insulin-like growth factor I-enhanced renal expression of osteopontin after acute ischemic injury in rats. *Endocrinology,* 137(5):2133-2140, 1996.

Paddenberg R, Weber A, Wulf S, Mannherz HG: Mycoplasma nucleases able to induce internucleosomal DNA degradation in cultures cells possess many characteristics of eukaryotic apoptotic nucleases. *Cell Death and Differentiation,* 5(6):517-528, 1998.

Padrines M, Rohanizadeh R, Damiens C, Heymann D, Fortun Y: Inhibition of apatite formation by vitronectin. *Connective Tissue Research,* 41(2):101-108, 2000.

Palmer G, Zhao J, Bonjour J, Hofstetter W, Caverzasio J: In vivo expression of transcripts encoding the Glvr-1 phosphate transporter/retrovirus receptor during bone development. *Bone,* 24(1):1-7, 1999.

Panda D, Kundu GC, Lee BI, Peri A, Fohl D, Chackalaparampil I, Mukherjee BB, Li XD, Mukherjee DC, Seides S, et al.: Potential roles of osteopontin and alphaVbeta3 integrin in the development of coronary artery restenosis after angioplasty. *Proceedings of the National Academy of Sciences of the United States of America,* 94(17):9308-9313, 1997.

Pandey A, Shao H, Marks RM, Polverini PJ, Dixit VM: Role of B61, the ligand for the Eck receptor tyrosine kinase, in TNF-α-induced angiogenesis. *Science,* 268:567-569, 1995.

Panheleux M, Bain M, Fernandez MS, Morales I, Gautron J, Arias JL, Solomon SE, Hincke M, Nys Y: Organic matrix composition and ultrastructure of eggshell: A comparative study. *British Poultry Sciences,* 40(2):240-252, 1999.

Paniccia R, Colucci S, Grano M, Serra M, Zallone AZ, Teti A: Immediate cell signal by bone-related peptides in human osteoclast-like cells. *American Journal of Physiology,* 265(5 Pt 1):C1289-C1297, 1993.

Panzer U, Thaiss F, Zahner G, Barth P, Reszka M, Reinking RR, Wolf G, Helmchen U, Stahl RA: Monocyte chemoattractant protein-1 and osteopontin differentially regulate monocytes recruitment in experimental glomerulonephritis. *Kidney International,* 59(5):1762-1769, 2001.

Park CK, Ishimi Y, Ohmura M, Yamaguchi M, Ikegami S: Vitamin A and carotenoids stimulate differentiation of mouse osteoblastic cells. *Journal of Nutrition Sciences and Vitaminology (Tokyo),* 43(3):281-296, 1997.

Park MH, Shin HI, Choi JY, Nam SH, Kim YJ, Kim HJ, Ryoo HM: Differential expression patterns of Runx2 isoforms in cranial suture morphogenesis. *Journal of Bone Minerals Research,* 16(5):885-892, 2001.

Parkar MH, Kuru L, O'Hare M, Newman HN, Hughes F, Olsen I: Retroviral transduction of human periodontal cells with a temperature-sensitive SV40 large T antigen. *Archives of Oral Biology,* 44(10):823-834, 1999.

Parrish AR, Ramos KS: Osteopontin mRNA expression in a chemically-induced model of atherogenesis. *Annals of the New York Academy of Sciences,* 760:354-356, 1995.

Parrish AR, Ramos KS: Differential processing of osteopontin characterizes the proliferative vascular smooth muscle cell phenotype induced by allylamine. *Journal of Cellular Biochemistry,* 65(2):267-275, 1997.

Parrish AR, Weber TJ, Ramos KS: Osteopontin overexpression in vascular smooth muscle cells transfected with the c-Ha-rasEJ oncogene. *In Vitro Cell Developmental Biology of Animals,* 33(8):584-587, 1997.

Partridge NC, Bloch SR, Pearman AT: Signal transduction pathways mediating parathyroid hormone regulation of osteoblastic gene expression. *Journal of Cellular Biochemistry,* 55(3):321-327, 1994.

Pasquali-Ronchetti I, Baccarani-Contri M: Elastic fiber during development and aging. *Microscopy Research Techniques,* 38(4):428-435, 1997.

Patarca R: *Concise Encyclopedia of Chronic Fatigue Syndrome.* Haworth Press, Inc., Binghamton, NY, pp. 1 ff. (1999).

Patarca R, Freeman GJ, Singh RP, Wei FY, Durfee T, Blattner F, Regnier DC, Kozak CA, Mock BA, Morse HC III, et al.: Structural and functional studies of the early T lymphocyte activation 1 (Eta-1) gene. Definition of a novel T cell-dependent response associated with genetic resistance to bacterial infection. *Journal of Experimental Medicine,* 170(1):145-161, 1989.

Patarca R, Saavedra RA, Cantor H: Molecular and cellular basis of genetic resistance to bacterial infection: The role of the early T-lymphocyte activation-1/osteopontin gene. *Critical Reviews in Immunology,* 13(3-4):225-246, 1993.

Patarca R, Sandler D, Maher K, Hutto C, Martin NL, Klimas NG, Scott GB, Fletcher MA: Immunological correlates of disease severity in pediatric slow progressors with human immunodeficiency virus type 1 infection. *AIDS Research and Human Retroviruses,* 12(11):1063-1068, 1996.

Patarca R, Singh RP, Wei F-Y, Iregui MV, Singh P, Schwartz J, Cantor H: Alternative pathways of T-cell activation and positive clonal selection. *Immunology Reviews,* 116:85-100, 1990.

Patarca R, Wei FY, Singh P, Morasso MI, Cantor H: Dysregulated expression of the T cell cytokine Eta-1 in CD4-8- lymphocytes during the development of murine autoimmune disease. *Journal of Experimental Medicine,* 172(4):1177-1183, 1990.

Patel SR, Koenig RJ, Hsu CH: Effect of Schiff base formation on the function of the calcitriol receptor. *Kidney International,* 50(5):1539-1545, 1996.

Patel SR, Xu Y, Koenig RJ, Hsu CH: Effect of glucose on the function of the calcitriol receptor and vitamin D metabolism. *Kidney International,* 52(1):79-86, 1997a.

Patel SR, Xu Y, Koenig RJ, Hsu CH: Effect of glyoxylate on the function of the calcitriol receptor and vitamin D metabolism. *Kidney International,* 52(1):39-44, 1997b.

Pavlin D, Bedalov A, Kronenberg MS, Kream BE, Rowe DW, Smith CL, Pike JW, Lichtler AC: Analysis of regulatory regions in the COL1A1 gene responsible for 1,25-dihydroxyvitamin D3-mediated transcriptional repression in osteoblastic cells. *Journal of Cellular Biochemistry,* 56(4):490-501, 1994.

Pawar S, Kartha S, Toback FG: Differential gene expression in migrating renal epithelial cells after wounding. *Journal of Cellular Physiology,* 165(3):556-565, 1995.

Pearson RB, Woodgett JR, Cohen P, Kemp BE: Substrate specificity of a multifunctional calmodulin-dependent protein kinase. *Journal of Biological Chemistry,* 260:14471, 1985.

Peleg S, Sastry M, Collins ED, Bishop JE, Norman AW: Distinct conformational changes induced by 20-epi analogues of 1 alpha,25-dihydroxyvitamin D3 are associated with enhanced activation of the vitamin D receptor. *Journal of Biological Chemistry,* 270(18):10551-10558, 1995.

Penttila IA, Harris RJ, Storm P, Haynes D, Worsick DA, Marmion BP: Cytokine dysregulation in the post-Q-fever fatigue syndrome. *Quarterly Journal of Medicine,* 91(8):549-560, 1998.

Penttila JM, Anttila M, Varkila K, Puolakkainen M, Sarvas M, Makela PH, Rautonen M: Depletion of CD8+ cells abolishes memory in acquired immunity against *Chlamydia pneumoniae* in BALB/c mice. *Immunology,* 97(3):490-496, 1999.

Persy VP, Verstrepen WA, Ysebaert DK, De Greef KE, De Broe ME: Differences in osteopontin up-regulation between proximal and distal tubules after renal ischemia/reperfusion. *Kidney International,* 56(2):601-611, 1999.

Petrow PK, Hummel KM, Schedel J, Franz JK, Klein CL, Muller-Ladner U, Kriegsmann J, Chang PL, Prince CW, Gay RE, et al.: Expression of osteopontin messenger RNA and protein in rheumatoid arthritis: Effects of osteopontin on the release of collagenase 1 from articular chondrocytes and synovial fibroblasts. *Arthritis and Rheumatism,* 43(7):1597-1605, 2000.

Petterson M, Schaffner W: A purine-rich DNA sequence motif present in SV40 and lymphotropic papovavirus binds a lymphoid-specific factor and contributes to enhancer activity in lymphoid cells. *Genes and Development,* 1(9):962-972, 1987.

Pettersson E, Luning B, Mickos H, Heinegard D: Synthesis, NMR and function of an O-phosphorylated peptide, comprising the RGD-adhesion sequence of osteopontin. *Acta Chemica Scandinavica,* 45(6):604-608, 1991.

Phillips BW, Belmonte N, Vernochet C, Ailhaud G, Dani C: Compactin enhances osteogenesis in murine embryonic stem cells. *Biochemical and Biophysical Research Communications,* 284(2):478-484, 2001.

Pichler RH, Franceschini N, Young BA, Hugo C, Andoh TF, Burdmann EA, Shankland SJ, Alpers CE, Bennett WM, Couser WG, et al.: Pathogenesis of cyclosporine nephropathy: Roles of angiotensin II and osteopontin. *Journal of the American Society of Nephrology,* 6(4):1186-1196, 1995.

Pichler R, Giachelli CM, Lombardi D, Pippin J, Gordon K, Alpers CE, Schwartz SM, Johnson RJ: Tubulointerstitial disease in glomerulonephritis. Potential role of osteopontin (uropontin). *American Journal of Pathology,* 144(5):915-926, 1994.

Pichler R, Giachelli C, Young B, Alpers CE, Couser WG, Johnson RJ: The pathogenesis of tubulointerstitial disease associated with glomerulonephritis: The glomerular cytokine theory. *Mineral and Electrolyte Metabolism,* 21(4-5):317-327, 1995.

Pinero GJ, Farach-Carson MC, Devoll RE, Aubin JE, Brunn JC, Butler WT: Bone matrix proteins in osteogenesis and remodelling in the neonatal rat mandible as studied by immunolocalization of osteopontin, bone sialoprotein, alpha 2HS-glycoprotein and alkaline phosphatase. *Archives of Oral Biology,* 40(2):145-155, 1995.

Pines M, Knopov V, Bar A: Involvement of osteopontin in egg shell formation in the laying chicken. *Matrix Biology,* 14(9):765-771, 1995.

Pines M, Knopov V, Genina O, Hurwitz S, Faerman A, Gerstenfeld LC, Leach RM: Development of avian tibial dyschondroplasia: Gene expression and protein synthesis. *Calcified Tissue International,* 63(6):521-527, 1998.

Pinna LA, Donella-Deana A, Meggio F: Structural features determining the site specificity of a rat liver camp-independent protein kinase. *Biochemical and Biophysical Research Communications,* 87:114-119, 1979.

Pockwinse SM, Lawrence JB, Singer RH, Stein JL, Lian JB, Stein GS: Gene expression at single cell resolution associated with development of the bone cell phenotype: Ultrastructural and in situ hybridization analysis. *Bone,* 14(3):347-352, 1993.

Pockwinse SM, Stein JL, Lian JB, Stein GS: Developmental stage-specific cellular responses to vitamin D and glucocorticoids during differentiation of the osteoblast phenotype: Interrelationship of morphology and gene expression by in situ hybridization. *Experimental Cell Research,* 216(1):244-260, 1995.

Pockwinse SM, Wilming LG, Conlon DM, Stein GS, Lian JB: Expression of cell growth and bone specific genes at single cell resolution during development of bone tissue-like organization in primary osteoblast cultures. *Journal of Cellular Biochemistry,* 49(3):310-323, 1992.

Poliard A, Lamblin D, Marie PJ, Buc-Caron MH, Kellermann O: Commitment of the teratocarcinoma-derived mesodermal clone C1 toward terminal osteogenic differentiation. *Journal of Cellular Sciences,* 106(Pt 2):503-511, 1993.

Pollack SB, Linnemeyer PA, Gill S: Induction of osteopontin mRNA expression during activation of murine NK cells. *Journal of Leukocyte Biology,* 55(3):398-400, 1994.

Pounds JG, Long GJ, Rosen JF: Cellular and molecular toxicity of lead in bone. *Environmental Health Perspectives,* 91:17-32, 1991.

Pramanik R, Ueno A, Nishikawa H, Nagata T, Inoue H, Islam MR: Osteotropic factor-stimulated synthesis of thrombospondin in rat dental pulp cells. *FEBS Letters,* 393(2-3):193-196, 1996.

Prince CW: Secondary structure predictions for rat osteopontin. *Connective Tissue Research,* 21(1-4):15-20, 1989.

Prince CW, Butler WT: 1,25-Dihydroxyvitamin D3 regulates the biosynthesis of osteopontin, a bone-derived cell attachment protein, in clonal osteoblast-like osteosarcoma cells. *Collagen Related Research,* 7(4):305-313, 1987.

Prince CW, Dickie D, Krumdieck CL: Osteopontin, a substrate for transglutaminase and factor XIII activity. *Biochemical and Biophysical Research Communications,* 177(3):1205-1210, 1991.

Prince CW, Oosawa T, Butler WT, Tomana M, Bhown AS, Bhown M, Schroehenloher RE: Isolation, characterization and biosynthesis of a phosphorylated glycoprotein from rat bone. *Journal of Biological Chemistry,* 262(6):2900-2907, 1987.

Prols F, Heidgress D, Rupprecht HD, Marx M: Regulation of osteopontin expression in rat mesangial cells. *FEBS Letters,* 422(1):15-18, 1998.

Prols F, Loser B, Marx M: Differential expression of osteopontin, PC4, and CEC5, a novel mRNA species, during in vitro angiogenesis. *Experimental Cell Research,* 239(1):1-10, 1998.

Proudfoot D, Shanahan CM, Weissberg PL: Vascular calcification: New insights into an old problem. *Journal of Pathology,* 185(1):1-3, 1998.

Proudfoot D, Skepper JN, Shanahan CM, Weissberg PL: Calcification of human vascular cells in vitro is correlated with high levels of matrix Gla protein and low levels of osteopontin expression. *Arteriosclerosis and Thrombosis Vascular Biology,* 18(3):379-388, 1998.

Prud'homme GJ, Park CL, Fieser TM, Kofler R, Dixon FJ, Theofilopoulos AN: Identification of a B-cell differentiation factor(s) spontaneously produced by proliferating T cells in murine lupus strains of the lpr/lpr genotype. *Journal of Experimental Medicine,* 157(2):730-742, 1983.

Puleo DA, Nanci A: Understanding and controlling the bone-implant interface. *Biomaterials,* 20(23-24):2311-2321, 1999.

Puleo DA, Preston KE, Shaffer JB, Bizios R: Examination of osteoblast-orthopaedic biomaterial interactions using molecular techniques. *Biomaterials,* 14(2):111-114, 1993.

Pullig O, Weseloh G, Gauer S, Swoboda B: Osteopontin is expressed by adult human osteoarthritic chondrocytes: Protein and mRNA analysis of normal and osteoarthritic cartilage. *Matrix Biology,* 19(3):245-255, 2000.

Qin C, Brunn JC, Jones J, George A, Ramachandran A, Gorski JP, Butler WT: A comparative study of sialic acid-rich proteins in rat bone and dentin. *European Journal of Oral Sciences,* 109(2):133-141, 2001.

Qiu Q, Sayer M, Kawaja M, Shen X, Davies JE: Attachment, morphology, and protein expression of rat marrow stromal cells cultured on charged substrate surfaces. *Journal of Biomed Materials Research,* 42(1):117-127, 1998.

Qu Q, Perala-Heape M, Kapanen A, Dahllund J, Salo J, Vaananen HK, Harkonen P: Estrogen enhances differentiation of osteoblasts in mouse bone marrow culture. *Bone,* 22(3):201-209, 1998.

Quarto R, Thomas D, Liang CT: Bone progenitor cell deficits and the age-associated decline in bone repair capacity. *Calcified Tissue International,* 56(2):123-129, 1995.

Quelo I, Kahlen JP, Rascle A, Jurdic P, Carlberg C: Identification and characterization of a vitamin D3 response element of chicken carbonic anhydrase-II. *DNA and Cell Biology,* 13(12):1181-1187, 1994.

Qu-Hong T, Brown LF, Dvorak HF, Dvorak AM: Ultrastructural immunogold localization of osteopontin in human gastric mucosa. *Journal of Histochemistry and Cytochemistry,* 45(1):21-33, 1997.

Qu-Hong T, Brown LF, Senger DR, Geng LL, Dvorak HF, Dvorak AM: Ultrastructural immunogold localization of osteopontin in human gallbladder epithelial cells. *Journal of Histochemistry and Cytochemistry,* 42(3):351-361, 1994.

Qu-Hong T, Dvorak AM: Ultrastructural localization of osteopontin immunoreactivity in phagolysosomes and secretory granules of cells in human intestine. *Histochemical Journal,* 29(11-12):801-812, 1997.

Raab-Cullen DM, Thiede MA, Petersen DN, Kimmel DB, Recker RR: Mechanical loading stimulates rapid changes in periosteal gene expression. *Calcified Tissue International,* 55(6):473-478, 1994.

Rabb H, Barroso-Vicens E, Adams R, Pow-Sang J, Ramirez G: Alpha-V/beta-3 and alpha-V/beta-5 integrin distribution in neoplastic kidney. *American Journal of Nephrology,* 16(5):402-408, 1996.

Rafidi K, Simkina I, Johnson E, Moore MA, Gerstenfeld LC: Characterization of the chicken osteopontin-encoding gene. *Gene,* 140(2):163-169, 1994.

Rajshankar D, McCulloch CA, Tenenbaum HC, Lekic PC: Osteogenic inhibition by rat periodontal ligament cells: Modulation of bone morphogenic protein-7 activity in vivo. *Cell and Tissue Research,* 294(3):475-483, 1998.

Ramakrishnan PR, Lin WL, Sodek J, Cho MI: Synthesis of noncollagenous extracellular matrix proteins during development of mineralized nodules by rat periodontal ligament cells in vitro. *Calcified Tissue International,* 57(1):52-59, 1995.

Ramamurthy N, Bain S, Liang CT, Barnes J, Llavaneras A, Liu Y, Puerner D, Strachan MJ, Golub LM: A combination of subtherapeutic doses of chemically modified doxycycline (CMT-8) and a bisphosphonate (clodronate) inhibits bone loss in the ovariectomized rat: A dynamic histomorphometric and gene expression study. *Current Medical Chemistry,* 8(3):295-303, 2001.

Ramos KS: Redox regulation of c-Ha-ras and osteopontin signaling in vascular smooth muscle cells: Implications in chemical atherogenesis. *Annual Reviews of Pharmacology and Toxicology,* 39:243-265, 1999.

Rangan GK, Wang Y, Harris DC: Pharmacologic modulators of nitric oxide exacerbate tubulointerstitial inflammation in proteinuric rats. *Journal of the American Society of Nephrology,* 12(8):1696-1705, 2001.

Raval-Pandya M, Freedman LP, Li H, Christakos S: Thyroid hormone receptor does not heterodimerize with the vitamin D receptor but represses vitamin D receptor-mediated transactivation. *Molecular Endocrinology,* 12(9):1367-1379, 1998.

Ray PE, Suga S, Liu XH, Huang X, Johnson RJ: Chronic potassium depletion induces renal injury, salt sensitivity, and hypertension in young rats. *Kidney International,* 59(5):1850-1858, 2001.

Raynal C, Delmas PD, Chenu C: Bone sialoprotein stimulates in vitro bone resorption. *Endocrinology,* 137(6):2347-2354, 1996.

Reckless J, Rubin EM, Verstuyft JB, Metcalfe JC, Grainger DJ: A common phenotype associated with atherogenesis in diverse mouse models of vascular lipid lesions. *Journal of Vascular Research,* 38(3):256-265, 2001.

Reed J, Hull WE, von der Lieth CW, Kuebler D, Suhai S, Kinzel V: Secondary structure of the Arg-Gly-Asp recognition site in proteins involved in cell-surface adhesion. *European Journal of Biochemistry,* 178(1):141-154, 1988.

Reiff DA, Kelpke S, Rue L 3rd, Thompson JA: Acidic fibroblast growth factor attenuates the cytotoxic effects of peroxynitrite in primary human osteoblast precursors. *Journal of Trauma,* 50(3):433-438; discussion 439, 2001.

Reinholt FP, Hultenby K, Heinegard D, Marks SC Jr, Norgard M, Anderson G: Extensive clear zone and defective ruffled border formation in osteoclasts of osteopetrotic (ia/ia) rats: Implications for secretory function. *Experimental Cell Research,* 251(2):477-491, 1999.

Reinholt FP, Hultenby K, Oldberg A, Heinegard D: Osteopontin—a possible anchor of osteoclasts to bone. *Proceedings of the National Academy of Sciences of the United States of America,* 87(12):4473-4475, 1990.

Remaley AT, Schumacher UK, Amouzadeh HR, Brewer HB Jr, Hoeg JM: Identification of novel differentially expressed hepatic genes in cholesterol-fed rabbits by a non-targeted gene approach. *Journal of Lipid Research,* 36(2):308-314, 1995.

Remy-Martin JP, Marandin A, Challier B, Bernard G, Deschaseaux M, Herve P, Wei Y, Tsuji T, Auerbach R, Dennis JE, et al.: Vascular smooth muscle differentiation of murine stroma: A sequential model. *Experimental Hematology,* 27(12):1782-1795, 1999.

Ricardo SD, Franzoni DF, Roesener CD, Crisman JM, Diamond JR: Angiotensinogen and AT(1) antisense inhibition of osteopontin translation in rat proximal tubular cells. *American Journal of Physiology and Renal Physiology,* 278(5):F708-F716, 2000.

Rich KA, George FWIV, Law JL, Martin WJ: Cell-adhesive motif in region II of malarial circumsporozoite protein. *Science,* 249(4976):1574-1577, 1990.

Rickard DJ, Kassem M, Hefferan TE, Sarkar G, Spelsberg TC, Riggs BL: Isolation and characterization of osteoblast precursor cells from human bone marrow. *Journal of Bone Minerals Research,* 11(3):312-324, 1996.

Rickard DJ, Sullivan TA, Shenker BJ, Leboy PS, Kazhdan I: Induction of rapid osteoblast differentiation in rat bone marrow stromal cell cultures by dexamethasone and BMP-2. *Developmental Biology,* 161(1):218-228, 1994.

Ridall AL, Daane EL, Dickinson DP, Butler WT: Characterization of the rat osteopontin gene. Evidence for two vitamin D response elements. *Annals of the New York Academy of Sciences,* 760:59-66, 1995.

Rifas L, Cheng S, Halstead LR, Gupta A, Hruska KA, Avioli LV: Skeletal casein kinase activity defect in the HYP mouse. *Calcified Tissue International,* 61(3): 256-259, 1997.

Riminucci M, Fisher LW, Shenker A, Spiegel AM, Bianco P, Gehron Robey P: Fibrous dysplasia of bone in the McCune-Albright syndrome: Abnormalities in bone formation. *American Journal of Pathology,* 151(6):1587-1600, 1997.

Ringbom-Anderson T, Sandberg M, Andersson G, Akerman KE: Phenotypic modification of human osteosarcoma cells with the phorbol ester 12-O-tetradecanoylphorbol-13-acetate. *Cellular Growth and Differentiation,* 6(4):457-464, 1995.

Ritchie HH, Hou H, Veis A, Butler WT: Cloning and sequence determination of rat dentin sialoprotein, a novel dentin protein. *Journal of Biological Chemistry,* 269(5):3698-3702, 1994.

Ritter NM, Farach-Carson MC, Butler WT: Evidence for the formation of a complex between osteopontin and osteocalcin. *Journal of Bone Minerals Research,* 7(8):877-885, 1992.

Rittling SR, Denhardt DT: Osteopontin function in pathology: Lessons from osteopontin-deficient mice. *Experimental Nephrology,* 7(2):103-113, 1999.

Rittling SR, Feng F: Detection of mouse osteopontin by western blotting. *Biochemical and Biophysical Research Communications,* 250(2):287-292, 1998.

Rittling SR, Matsumoto HN, McKee MD, Nanci A, An XR, Novick KE, Kowalski AJ, Noda M, Denhardt DT: Mice lacking osteopontin show normal development and bone structure but display altered osteoclast formation in vitro. *Journal of Bone Minerals Research,* 13(7):1101-1111, 1998.

Rittling SR, Novick KE: Osteopontin expression in mammary gland development and tumorigenesis. *Cellular Growth and Differentiation,* 8(10):1061-1069, 1997.

Roach HI: Trans-differentiation of hypertrophic chondrocytes into cells capable of producing a mineralized bone matrix. *Bone Minerals,* 19(1):1-20, 1992.

Roach HI: Why does bone matrix contain non-collagenous proteins? The possible roles of osteocalcin, osteonectin, osteopontin and bone sialoprotein in bone mineralisation and resorption. *Cellular Biology International,* 18(6):617-628, 1994.

Roach HI, Erenpreisa J: The phenotypic switch from chondrocytes to bone-forming cells involves asymmetric cell division and apoptosis. *Connective Tissue Research,* 35(1-4):85-91, 1996.

Rochet N, Dubousset J, Mazeau C, Zanghellini E, Farges MF, de Novion HS, Chompret A, Delpech B, Cattan N, Frenay M, et al.: Establishment, characterisation and partial cytokine expression profile of a new human osteosarcoma cell line (CAL 72). *International Journal of Cancer,* 82(2):282-285, 1999.

Rodan GA: Osteopontin overview. *Annals of the New York Academy of Sciences,* 760:1-5, 1995.

Rodan GA, Noda M: Gene expression in osteoblastic cells. *Critical Reviews in Eukaryotic Gene Expression,* 1(2):85-98, 1991.

Rodan SB, Rodan GA: Integrin function in osteoclasts. *Journal of Endocrinology,* 154(Suppl):S47-S56, 1997.

Rodan SB, Wesolowski G, Yoon K, Rodan GA: Opposing effects of fibroblast growth factor and pertussis toxin on alkaline phosphatase, osteopontin, osteocalcin, and type I collagen mRNA levels in ROS 17/2.8 cells. *Journal of Biological Chemistry,* 264(33):19934-19941, 1989.

Rodriguez CM, Day JR, Killian GJ: Osteopontin gene expression in the Holstein bull reproductive tract. *Journal of Andrology,* 21(3):414-420, 2000.

Roedel J, Woytas M, Groh A, Schmidt KH, Hartmann M, Lehmann M, Straube E: Production of basic fibroblast growth factor and interleukin 6 by human smooth muscle cells following infection with *Chlamydia pneumoniae. Infection and Immunity,* 68(6):3635-3641, 2000.

Roehlecke C, Witt M, Kasper M, Schulze E, Wolf C, Hofer A, Funk RW: Synergistic effect of titanium alloy and collagen type I on cell adhesion, proliferation and differentiation of osteoblast-like cells. *Cells, Tissues and Organs,* 168(3):178-187, 2001.

Rogers SA, Padanilam BJ, Hruska KA, Giachelli CM, Hammerman MR: Metanephric osteopontin regulates nephrogenesis in vitro. *American Journal of Physiology,* 272(4 Pt 2):F469-F476, 1997.

Rollo EE, Denhardt DT: Differential effects of osteopontin on the cytotoxic activity of macrophages from young and old mice. *Immunology,* 88(4):642-647, 1996.

Rollo EE, Laskin DL, Denhardt DT: Osteopontin inhibits nitric oxide production and cytotoxicity by activated RAW264.7 macrophages. *Journal of Leukocyte Biology,* 60(3):397-404, 1996.

Rosati R, Horan GS, Pinero GJ, Garofalo S, Keene DR, Horton WA, Vuorio E, de Crombrugghe B, Behringer RR: Normal long bone growth and development in type X collagen-null mice. *Nature Genetics,* 8(2):129-135, 1994.

Rosenstreich DL, Weinblatt AC, O'Brien AD: Genetic control of resistance to infection in mice. *CRC Critical Reviews in Immunology,* 3:263-285, 1982.

Roser K, Johansson CB, Donath K, Albrektsson T: A new approach to demonstrate cellular activity in bone formation adjacent to implants. *Journal of Biomedical Materials Research,* 51(2):280-291, 2000.

Ross FP, Chappel J, Alvarez JI, Sander D, Butler WT, Farach-Carson MC, Mintz KA, Robey PG, Teitelbaum SL, Cheresh DA: Interactions between the bone matrix proteins osteopontin and bone sialoprotein and the osteoclast integrin alpha v beta 3 potentiate bone resorption. *Journal of Biological Chemistry,* 268(13):9901-9907, 1993.

Roth JA, Kim BG, Lin WL, Cho MI: Melatonin promotes osteoblast differentiation and bone formation. *Journal of Biological Chemistry,* 274(31):22041-22047, 1999.

Rottenberg ME, Gigliotti Rothfuchs A, Gigliotti D, Ceausu M, Une C, Levitsky V, Wigzell H: Regulation and role of IFN-γ in the innate resistance to infection with *Chlamydia pneumoniae. Journal of Immunology,* 164(9):4812-4818, 2000.

Rovin BH, Phan LT: Chemotactic factors and renal inflammation. *American Journal of Kidney Diseases,* 31(6):1065-1084, 1998.

Rowatt E, Sorensen ES, Triffit J, Viess A, Williams RJ: An examination of the binding of aluminum to protein and mineral components of bone and teeth. *Journal of Inorganic Biochemistry,* 68(4):235-238, 1997.

Rudzki Z, Jothy S: CD44 and the adhesion of neoplastic cells. *Molecular Pathology,* 50(2):57-71, 1997.

Ruohslahti E, Pierschbacher MD: Arg-Gly-Asp: A versatile cell recognition signal. *Cell,* 44(4):517-518, 1986.

Ryall RL: Glycosaminoglycans, proteins, and stone formation: Adult themes and child's play. *Pediatric Nephrology,* 10(5):656-666, 1996.

Ryden C, Yacoub AI, Maxe I, Heinegard D, Oldberg A, Franzen A, Ljungh A, Rubin K: Specific binding of bone sialoprotein to *Staphylococcus aureus* isolated from patients with osteomyelitis. *European Journal of Biochemistry,* 184(2):331-336, 1989.

Saavedra RA: The roles of autophosphorylation and phosphorylation in the life of osteopontin. *Bioessays,* 16(12):913-918, 1994.

Saavedra RA, Kimbro SK, Stern DN, Schnuer J, Ashkar S, Glimcher MJ, Ljubetic CI: Gene expression and phosphorylation of mouse osteopontin. *Annals of the New York Academy of Sciences,* 760:35-43, 1995.

Safran JB, Butler WT, Farach-Carson MC: Modulation of osteopontin post-translational state by 1, 25-(OH)2-vitamin D3. Dependence on Ca2+ influx. *Journal of Biological Chemistry,* 273(45):29935-29941, 1998.

Sahai A, Mei C, Schrier RW, Tannen RL: Mechanisms of chronic hypoxia-induced renal cell growth. *Kidney International,* 56(4):1277-1281, 1999.

Saitoh Y, Kuratsu J, Takeshima H, Yamamoto S, Ushio Y: Expression of osteopontin in human glioma. Its correlation with the malignancy. *Laboratory Investigations,* 72(1):55-63, 1995.

Sakagami M, Takemura T, Umemoto M, Kubo T: [Application of non-radioisotopic in situ hybridization to the inner ear—expression of osteopontin]. *Nippon Jibiinkoka Gakkai Kaiho,* 97(4):674-679, 1994.

Sakai T, Tanaka H, Shirasawa T: Two distinct epithelial responses may compensate for the ureteral obstruction in early and late phase of unilateral ureteral obstruction-treated rat: Cellular proliferation in acute phase and osteopontin expression in chronic phase. *Nephron,* 77(3):340-345, 1997.

Sakamoto A, Oda Y, Iwamoto Y, Tsuneyoshi M: A comparative study of fibrous dysplasia and osteofibrous dysplasia with regard to expressions of c-fos and c-jun products and bone matrix proteins: A clinicopathologic review and immunohistochemical study of c-fos, c-jun, type I collagen, osteonectin, osteopontin, and osteocalcin. *Human Pathology,* 30(12):1418-1426, 1999.

Sakata M, Tsuruha JI, Masuko-Hongo K, Nakamura H, Matsui T, Sudo A, Nishioka K, Kato T: Autoantibodies to osteopontin in patients with osteoarthritis and rheumatoid arthritis. *Journal of Rheumatology,* 28(7): 1492-1495, 2001.

Sakoda K, Fujiwara M, Arai S, Suzuki A, Nishikawa J, Imagawa M, Nishihara T: Isolation of a genomic DNA fragment having negative vitamin D response element. *Biochemical and Biophysical Research Communications,* 219(1):31-35, 1996.

Saksela O, Rifkin DB: Cell-associated plasminogen activation: Regulation and physiological functions. *Annual Reviews of Cellular Biology,* 4:93-126, 1988.

Salih E, Ashkar S, Gerstenfeld LC, Glimcher MJ: Identification of the in vivo phosphorylated sites of secreted osteopontin from cultured chicken osteoblasts. *Annals of the New York Academy of Sciences,* 760:357-360, 1995.

Salih E, Ashkar S, Gerstenfeld LC, Glimcher MJ: Protein kinases of cultured osteoblasts: Selectivity for the extracellular matrix proteins of bone and their catalytic competence for osteopontin. *Journal of Bone Minerals Research,* 11(10):1461-1473, 1996.

Salih E, Ashkar S, Gerstenfeld LC, Glimcher MJ: Identification of the phosphorylated sites of metabolically 32P-labeled osteopontin from cultured chicken osteoblasts. *Journal of Biological Chemistry,* 272(21):13966-13973, 1997.

Salih E, Ashkar S, Zhou HY, Gerstenfeld L, Glimcher MJ: Protein kinases of cultured chicken osteoblasts that phosphorylate extracellular bone proteins. *Connective Tissue Research,* 5(1-4):207-213, 1996.

Salih E, Huang JC, Strawich E, Gouverneur M, Glimcher MJ: Enamel specific protein kinases and state of phosphorylation of purified amelogenins. *Connective Tissue Research,* 38(1-4):225-235; discussion 241-246, 1998.

Salih E, Zhou HY, Glimcher MJ: Phosphorylation of purified bovine bone sialoprotein and osteopontin by protein kinases. *Journal of Biological Chemistry,* 271(28):16897-16905, 1996.

Salit IE: Precipitating factors for the chronic fatigue syndrome. *Journal of Psychiatric Research,* 31(1):59-65, 1997.

Sammons RL, el Haj AJ, Marquis PM: Novel culture procedure permitting the synthesis of proteins by rat calvarial cells cultured on hydroxyapatite particles to be quantified. *Biomaterials,* 15(7):536-542, 1994.

Sandhu H, Dehnen W, Roller M, Abel J, Unfried K: mRNA expression patterns in different stages of asbestos-induced carcinogenesis in rats. *Carcinogenesis,* 21(5):1023-1029, 2000.

Santoro TJ, Portanova JP, Kotzin BL: The contribution of L3T4+ T cells to lymph proliferation and autoantibody production in MRL-lpr/lpr mice. *Journal of Experimental Medicine,* 167(5):1713-1718, 1988.

Sasaguri K, Jiang H, Chen J: The effect of altered functional forces on the expression of bone-matrix proteins in developing mouse mandibular condyle. *Archives of Oral Biology,* 43(1):83-92, 1998.

Sasaki H, Harada H, Handa Y, Morino H, Suzawa M, Shimpo E, Katsumata T, Masuhiro Y, Matsuda K, Ebihara K, et al.: Transcriptional activity of a fluorinated vitamin D analog on VDR-RXR-mediated gene expression. *Biochemistry,* 34(1):370-377, 1995.

Sasaki T, Amizuka N, Irie K, Ejiri S, Ozawa H: Localization of alkaline phosphatase and osteopontin during matrix mineralization in the developing cartilage of coccygeal vertebrae. *Archives of Histology and Cytology,* 63(3):271-284, 2000.

Sasano Y, Zhu JX, Kamakura S, Kusunoki S, Mizoguchi I, Kagayama M: Expression of major bone extracellular matrix proteins during embryonic osteogenesis in rat mandibles. *Anatomy and Embryology (Berlin),* 202(1):31-37, 2000.

Sato M, Grasser W, Harm S, Fullenkamp C, Gorski JP: Bone acidic glycoprotein 75 inhibits resorption activity of isolated rat and chicken osteoclasts. *FASEB Journal,* 6(11):2966-2976, 1992.

Sato M, Iga H, Yoshioka N, Fukui K, Kawamata H, Yoshida H, Hirota S, Kitamura Y: Emergence of osteoblast-like cells in a neoplastic human salivary cancer cell line after treatment with 22-oxa-1alpha, 25-dihydroxyvitamin D3. *Cancer Letters,* 115(2):149-160, 1997.

Sato M, Morii E, Komori T, Kawahata H, Sugimoto M, Terai K, Shimizu H, Yasui T, Ogihara H, Yasui N, et al.: Transcriptional regulation of osteopontin gene in vivo by PEBP2alphaA/CBFA1 and ETS1 in the skeletal tissues. *Oncogene,* 17(12):1517-1525, 1998.

Sato M, Yasui N, Nakase T, Kawahata H, Sugimoto M, Hirota S, Kitamura Y, Nomura S, Ochi T: Expression of bone matrix proteins mRNA during distraction osteogenesis. *Journal of Bone Minerals Research,* 13(8):1221-1231, 1998.

Sato S, Kubota T, Suzuki Y: Composition and function of noncollagenous proteins in alveolar bone. *Bulletin of the Kanagawa Dentistry College,* 18(2):119-125, 1990.

Sauk JJ, Van Kampen CL, Norris K, Foster R, Somerman MJ: Expression of constitutive and inducible HSP70 and HSP47 is enhanced in cells persistently spread on OPN1 or collagen. *Biochemical and Biophysical Research Communications,* 172(1):135-142, 1990.

Sauk JJ, Van Kampen CL, Norris K, Moehring J, Foster RA, Somerman MJ: Persistent spreading of ligament cells on osteopontin/bone sialoprotein-I or collagen enhances tolerance to heat shock. *Experimental Cell Research,* 188(1):105-110, 1990.

Sawaya BP, Koszewski NJ, Qi Q, Langub MC, Monier-Faugere MC, Malluche HH: Secondary hyperparathyroidism and vitamin D receptor binding to vitamin D response elements in rats with incipient renal failure. *Journal of the American Society of Nephrology,* 8(2):271-278, 1997.

Saygin NE, Tokiyasu Y, Giannobile WV, Somerman MJ: Growth factors regulate expression of mineral associated genes in cementoblasts. *Journal of Periodontology,* 71(10):1591-1600, 2000.

Scatena M, Almeida M, Chaisson ML, Fausto N, Nicosia RF, Giachelli CM: NF-kappaB mediates alphavbeta3 integrin-induced endothelial cell survival. *Journal of Cellular Biology,* 141(4):1083-1093, 1998.

Schaumberg-Lever G, Gehring B, Kaiserling E: Ultrastructural localization of factor XIIIa. *Journal of Cutaneous Pathology,* 21(2):129-134, 1994.

Scheid C, Honeyman T, Kohjimoto Y, Cao LC, Jonassen J: Oxalate-induced changes in renal epithelial cell function: Role in stone disease. *Molecular Urology,* 4(4):371-382, 2000.

Schiller PC, D'Ippolito G, Balkan W, Roos BA, Howard GA: Gap-junctional communication is required for the maturation process of osteoblastic cells in culture. *Bone,* 28(4):362-369, 2001.

Schluederberg A, Straus SE, Peterson P, Blumenthal S, Komaroff AL, Spring SB, Landay A, Buchwald D: Chronic fatigue syndrome research: Definition and medical outcome research. *Annals of Internal Medicine,* 117(4):325-331, 1992.

Schnapp LM, Hatch N, Ramos DM, Klimanskaya IV, Sheppard D, Pytela R: The human integrin alpha 8 beta 1 functions as a receptor for tenascin, fibronectin, and vitronectin. *Journal of Biological Chemistry,* 270(39):23196-23202, 1995.

Schnee JM, Hsueh WA: Angiotensin II, adhesion, and cardiac fibrosis. *Cardiovascular Research,* 46(2):264-268, 2000.

Schrader JW, Ziltener HJ, Leslie KB: Structural homologies among the hematopoietin proteins. *Proceedings of the National Academy of Sciences of the United States of America,* 83(8):2458-2462, 1986.

Schrader M, Muller KM, Carlberg C: Specificity and flexibility of vitamin D signaling. Modulation of the activation of natural vitamin D response elements by thyroid hormone. *Journal of Biological Chemistry,* 269(8):5501-5504, 1994.

Schulz A, Loreth B, Battmann A, Knoblauch B, Stahl U, Pollex U, Bohle RM: [Bone matrix production in osteosarcoma]. *Verhalt Deutsche Gessamte Pathologie,* 82:144-153, 1998.

Schulze E, Witt M, Kasper M, Lowik CW, Funk RH: Immunohistochemical investigations on the differentiation marker protein E11 in rat calvaria, calvaria cell culture and the osteoblastic cell line ROS 17/2.8. *Histochemistry and Cellular Biology,* 111(1):61-69, 1999.

Scott JA, Weir ML, Wilson SM, Xuan JW, Chambers AF, McCormack DG: Osteopontin inhibits inducible nitric oxide synthase activity in rat vascular tissue. *American Journal of Physiology,* 275(6 Pt 2):H2258-H2265, 1998.

Seitz PK, Zhang RW, Simmons DJ, Cooper CW: Effects of C-terminal parathyroid hormone-related peptide on osteoblasts. *Mineral and Electrolyte Metabolism,* 21(1-3):180-183, 1995.

Senger DR, Asch BA, Smith BD, Perruzzi CA, Dvorak HF: A secreted phosphoprotein marker for neoplastic transformation of both epithelial and fibroblastic cells. *Nature,* 302(5910):714-715, 1983.

Senger DR, Brown LF, Perruzzi CA, Papadopoulos-Sergiou A, Van de Water L: Osteopontin at the tumor/host interface. Functional regulation by thrombin-cleavage and consequences for cell adhesion. *Annals of the New York Academy of Sciences,* 760:83-100, 1995.

Senger DR, Ledbetter SR, Claffey KP, Papadopoulos-Sergiou A, Peruzzi CA, Detmar M: Stimulation of endothelial cell migration by vascular permeability factor/vascular endothelial growth factor through cooperative mechanisms involving the alphavbeta3 integrin, osteopontin, and thrombin. *American Journal of Pathology,* 149(1):293-305, 1996.

Senger DR, Perruzzi CA: Cell migration promoted by a potent GRGDS-containing thrombin-cleavage fragment of osteopontin. *Biochimica et Biophysica Acta,* 1314(1-2):13-24, 1996.

Senger DR, Perruzzi CA, Gracey CF, Papadopoulos A, Tenen DG: Secreted phosphoproteins associated with neoplastic transformation: Close homology with plasma proteins cleaved during blood coagulation. *Cancer Research,* 48(20):5770-5774, 1988.

Senger DR, Perruzzi CA, Papadopoulos A: Elevated expression of secreted phosphoprotein I (osteopontin, 2ar) as a consequence of neoplastic transformation. *Anticancer Research,* 9(5):1291-1299, 1989.

Senger DR, Perruzzi CA, Papadopoulos A, Tenen DG: Purification of a human milk protein closely similar to tumor-secreted phosphoproteins and osteopontin. *Biochimica et Biophysica Acta,* 1996(1-2):43-48, 1989.

Senger DR, Perruzzi CA, Papadopoulos-Sergiou A, Van de Water L: Adhesive properties of osteopontin: Regulation by a naturally occurring thrombin-cleavage in close proximity to the GRGDS cell-binding domain. *Molecular Biology of the Cell,* 5(5):565-574, 1994.

Seto H, Aoki K, Kasugai S, Ohya K: Trabecular bone turnover, bone marrow cell development, and gene expression of bone matrix proteins after low calcium feeding in rats. *Bone,* 25(6):687-695, 1999.

Severson AR, Ingram RT, Fitzpatrick LA: Matrix proteins associated with bone calcification are present in human vascular smooth muscle cells grown in vitro. *In Vitro Cell Developmental Biology of Animals,* 31(11):853-857, 1995.

Shah AK, Lazatin J, Sinha RK, Lennox T, Hickok NJ, Tuan RS: Mechanism of BMP-2 stimulated adhesion of osteoblastic cells to titanium alloy. *Biology of the Cell,* 91(2):131-142, 1999.

Shalhoub V, Bettencourt B, Jackson ME, MacKay CA, Glimcher MJ, Marks SC Jr, Stein GS, Lian JB: Abnormalities of phosphoprotein gene expression in three osteopetrotic rat mutations: Elevated mRNA transcripts, protein synthesis, and accumulation in bone of mutant animals. *Journal of Cellular Physiology,* 158(1): 110-120, 1994.

Shalhoub V, Bortell R, Jackson ME, Marks SC Jr, Stein JL, Lian JB, Stein GS: Transcriptionally active nuclei isolated from intact bone reflect modified levels of gene expression in skeletal development and pathology. *Journal of Cellular Biochemistry,* 55(2):182-189, 1994.

Shalhoub V, Conlon D, Tassinari M, Quinn C, Partridge N, Stein GS, Lian JB: Glucocorticoids promote development of the osteoblast phenotype by selectively modulating expression of cell growth and differentiation associated genes. *Journal of Cellular Biochemistry,* 50(4):425-440, 1992.

Shanahan CM, Cary NR, Metcalfe JC, Weissberg PL: High expression of genes for calcification-regulating proteins in human atherosclerotic plaques. *Journal of Clinical Investigation,* 93(6):2393-2402, 1994.

Shanahan CM, Cary NR, Salisbury JR, Proudfoot D, Weissberg PL, Edmonds ME: Medial localization of mineralization-regulating proteins in association with Monckeberg's sclerosis: evidence for smooth muscle cell-mediated vascular calcification. *Circulation,* 100(21):2168-2176, 1999.

Shanahan CM, Weissberg PL, Metcalfe JC: Isolation of gene markers of differentiated and proliferating vascular smooth muscle cells. *Circulation Research,* 73(1):193-204, 1993.

Shanmugam V, Chackalaparampil I, Kundu GC, Mukherjee AB, Mukherjee BB: Altered sialylation of osteopontin prevents its receptor-mediated binding on the surface of oncogenically transformed tsB77 cells. *Biochemistry,* 36(19):5729-5738, 1997.

Shao H, Pandey A, Seldin M, O'Shea KS, Dixit VM: Characterization of B61, the ligand for the Eck receptor protein-tyrosine kinase. *Journal of Biological Chemistry,* 270:5636-5641, 1995.

Sharp JA, Sung V, Slavin J, Thompson EW, Henderson MA: Tumor cells are the source of osteopontin and bone sialoprotein expression in human breast cancer. *Laboratory Investigations,* 79(7):869-877, 1999.

Shaw JP, Kamens R: A conserved AU sequence from the 3' untranslated region of GM-CSF mRNA mediates selective mRNA degradation. *Cell,* 46:659, 1986.

Shaw JP, Utz P, Durand DB, Toole JJ, Emmel EA, Crabtree GR: Identification of a putative regulator of early T cell activation genes. *Science,* 241(4862):202-205, 1988.

Shelly JA, Laborde AL: Interleukin-1 binding, internalization, and processing in a murine osteoblastic cell line, MC3T3.E1. *European Cytokine Network,* 3(5):469-475, 1992.

Shen M, Carpentier SM, Berrebi AJ, Chen L, Martinet B, Carpentier A: Protein adsorption of calcified and noncalcified valvular bioprostheses after human implantation. *Annals of Thoracic Surgery,* 7(Suppl 5):S406-S407, 2001.

Shen M, Marie P, Farge D, Carpentier S, De Pollak C, Hott M, Chen L, Martinet B, Carpentier A: Osteopontin is associated with bioprosthetic heart valve calcification in humans. *Comptes Rendue au Academie des Sciences III,* 320(1):49-57, 1997.

Shi S, Kirk M, Kahn AJ: The role of type I collagen in the regulation of the osteoblast phenotype. *Journal of Bone Minerals Research,* 11(8):1139-1145, 1996.

Shi X, Bai S, Li L, Cao X: Hoxa-9 represses transforming growth factor-beta-induced osteopontin gene transcription. *Journal of Biological Chemistry,* 276(1):850-855, 2001.

Shi X, Yang X, Chen D, Chang Z, Cao X: Smad1 interacts with homeobox DNA-binding proteins in bone morphogenetic protein signaling. *Journal of Biological Chemistry,* 274(19):13711-13717, 1999.

Shibata Y, Fujita S, Takahashi H, Yamaguchi A, Koji T: Assessment of decalcifying protocols for detection of specific RNA by non-radioactive in situ hybridization in calcified tissues. *Histochemistry and Cell Biology,* 113(3):153-159, 2000.

Shigeyama Y, Grove TK, Strayhorn C, Somerman MJ: Expression of adhesion molecules during tooth resorption in feline teeth: A model system for aggressive osteoclastic activity. *Journal of Dentistry Research,* 75(9):1650-1657, 1996.

Shijubo N, Uede T, Kon S, Maeda M, Segawa T, Imada A, Hirasawa M, Abe S: Vascular endothelial growth factor and osteopontin in stage I lung adenocarcinoma. *American Journal of Respiration and Critical Care Medicine,* 160(4):1269-1273, 1999.

Shijubo N, Uede T, Kon S, Nagata M, Abe S: Vascular endothelial growth factor and osteopontin in tumor biology. *Critical Reviews in Oncogenesis,* 11(2):135-146, 2000.

Shin SL, Cha JH, Chun MH, Chung JW, Lee MY: Expression of osteopontin mRNA in the adult rat brain. *Neuroscience Letters,* 273(2):73-76, 1999.

Shioi A, Nishizawa Y, Jono S, Koyama H, Hosoi M, Morii H: Beta-glycerophosphate accelerates calcification in cultured bovine vascular smooth muscle cells. *Arteriosclerosis and Thrombosis Vascular Biology,* 15(11):2003-2009, 1995.

Shioide M, Noda M: Endothelin modulates osteopontin and osteocalcin messenger ribonucleic acid expression in rat osteoblastic osteosarcoma cells. *Journal of Cellular Biochemistry,* 53(2):176-180, 1993.

Shiraga H, Min W, VanDusen WJ, Clayman MD, Miner D, Terrell CH, Sherbotie JR, Foreman JW, Przysiecki C, Neilson EG, et al.: Inhibition of calcium oxalate crystal growth in vitro by uropontin: Another member of the aspartic acid-rich protein superfamily. *Proceedings of the National Academy of Sciences of the United States of America,* 89(1):426-430, 1992.

Shukunami C, Ohta Y, Sakuda M, Hiraki Y: Sequential progression of the differentiation program by bone morphogenetic protein-2 in chondrogenic cell line ATDC5. *Experimental Cell Research,* 241(1):1-11, 1998.

Shyng YC, Devlin H, Riccardi D, Sloan P: Expression of cartilage-derived retinoic acid-sensitive protein during healing of the rat tooth-extraction socket. *Archives of Oral Biology,* 44(9):751-757, 1999.

Sibalic V, Fan X, Loffing J, Wuthrich RP: Upregulated renal tubular CD44, hyaluronan, and osteopontin in kdkd mice with interstitial nephritis. *Nephrology, Dialysis, and Transplantation,* 12(7):1344-1353, 1997.

Sieling PA, Chatterjee D, Porcelli SA, Prigozy TI, Mazzaccaro RJ, Soriano T, Bloom BR, Brenner MB, Kronenberg M, Brennan PJ, et al.: CD1-restricted T-cell recognition of microbial lipoglycan antigens. *Science,* 269:227-230, 1995.

Siggelkow H, Niedhart C, Kurre W, Ihbe A, Schulz A, Atkinson MJ, Hufner M: In vitro differentiation potential of a new human osteosarcoma cell line (HOS 58). *Differentiation,* 63(2):81-91, 1998.

Siiteri JE, Ensrud KM, Moore A, Hamilton DW: Identification of osteopontin (OPN) mRNA and protein in the rat testis and epididymis, and on sperm. *Molecular and Reproductive Development,* 40(1):16-28, 1995.

Siiteri JE, Hamilton DW: Identification of osteopontin mRNA and protein in rat epididymis and of protein on epididymal sperm. *Annals of the New York Academy of Sciences,* 760:361-362, 1995.

Silbermann M, von der Mark K, Heinegard D: An immunohistochemical study of the distribution of matrical proteins in the mandibular condyle of neonatal mice. II. Non-collagenous proteins. *Journal of Anatomy,* 170:23-31, 1990.

Simon A: [Diabetic macroangiopathy in humans]. *Therapie,* 52(5):423-428, 1997.

Singh K, Balligand JL, Fischer TA, Smith TW, Kelly RA: Glucocorticoids increase osteopontin expression in cardiac myocytes and microvascular endothelial cells. Role in regulation of inducible nitric oxide synthase. *Journal of Biological Chemistry,* 270(47):28471-28478, 1995.

Singh K, Deonarine D, Shanmugam V, Senger DR, Mukherjee AB, Chang PL, Prince CW, Mukherjee BB: Calcium-binding properties of osteopontin derived from non-osteogenic sources. *Journal of Biochemistry (Tokyo),* 114(5):702-707, 1993.

Singh K, DeVouge MW, Mukherjee BB: Physiological properties and differential glycosylation of phosphorylated and nonphosphorylated forms of osteopontin secreted by normal rat kidney cells. *Journal of Biological Chemistry,* 265(30): 18696-18701, 1990.

Singh K, Mukherjee AB, De Vouge MW, Mukherjee BB: Differential processing of osteopontin transcripts in rat kidney- and osteoblast-derived cell lines. *Journal of Biological Chemistry,* 267(33):23847-23851, 1992.

Singh K, Sirokman G, Communal C, Robinson KG, Conrad CH, Brooks WW, Bing OH, Colucci WS: Myocardial osteopontin expression coincides with the development of heart failure. *Hypertension,* 33(2):663-670, 1999.

Singh RP, Patarca R, Schwartz J, Singh P, Cantor H: Definition of a specific interaction between the early T lymphocyte activation 1 (Eta-1) protein and murine macrophages in vitro and its effect upon macrophages in vivo. *Journal of Experimental Medicine,* 171(6):1931-1942, 1990.

Singh SU, Casper RF, Fritz PC, Sukhu B, Ganss B, Girard B Jr, Savouret JF, Tenenbaum HC: Inhibition of dioxin effects on bone formation in vitro by a newly described aryl hydrocarbon receptor antagonist, resveratrol. *Journal of Endocrinology,* 167(1):183-195, 2000.

Singhal H, Bautista DS, Tonkin KS, O'Malley FP, Tuck AB, Chambers AF, Harris JF: Elevated plasma osteopontin in metastatic breast cancer associated with increased tumor burden and decreased survival. *Clinical Cancer Research,* 3(4):605-611, 1997.

Slack JH, Hang L, Barkely J, Fulton RJ, D'Hoostelaere L, Robinson A, Dixon FJ: Isotypes of spontaneous and mitogen-induced autoantibodies in SLE-prone mice. *Journal of Immunology,* 132(3):1271-1275, 1984.

Smith JH, Denhardt DT: Molecular cloning of a tumor promoter-inducible mRNA found in JB6 mouse epidermal cells: Induction in stable at high, but not at low cell densities. *Journal of Cellular Biochemistry,* 34(1):13-22, 1987.

Smith LL, Cheung HK, Ling LE, Chen J, Sheppard D, Pytela R, Giachelli CM: Osteopontin N-terminal domain contains a cryptic adhesive sequence recognized by alpha9beta1 integrin. *Journal of Biological Chemistry,* 271(45):28485-28491, 1996.

Smith LL, Giachelli CM: Structural requirements for alpha 9 beta 1-mediated adhesion and migration to thrombin-cleaved osteopontin. *Experimental Cell Research,* 242(1):351-360, 1998.

Smith LL, Greenfield BW, Aruffo A, Giachelli CM: CD44 is not an adhesive receptor for osteopontin. *Journal of Cellular Biochemistry,* 73(1):20-30, 1999.

Snyder WR, Hoover J, Khoury R, Farach-Carson MC: Effect of agents used in perforation repair on osteoblastic cells. *Journal of Endodontics,* 23(3):158-161, 1997.

Sodek J, Chen J, Nagata T, Kasugai S, Todescan R Jr, Li IW, Kim RH: Regulation of osteopontin expression in osteoblasts. *Annals of the New York Academy of Sciences,* 760:223-241, 1995.

Sodek J, Ganss B, McKee MD: Osteopontin. *Critical Reviews in Oral Biology Medicine,* 11(3):279-303, 2000.

Sodek KL, Tupy JH, Sodek J, Grynpas MD: Relationships between bone protein and mineral in developing porcine long bone and calvaria. *Bone,* 26(2):189-198, 2000.

Sodhi CP, Batlle D, Sahai A: Osteopontin mediates hypoxia-induced proliferation of cultured mesangial cells: Role of PKC and p38 MAPK. *Kidney International,* 58(2):691-700, 2000.

Sodhi CP, Phadke SA, Batlle D, Sahai A: Hypoxia and high glucose cause exaggerated mesangial cell growth and collagen synthesis: Role of osteopontin. *American Journal of Physiology and Renal Physiology,* 280(4):F667-F674, 2001a.

Sodhi CP, Phadke SA, Batlle D, Sahai A: Hypoxia stimulates osteopontin expression and proliferation of cultured vascular smooth muscle cells: Potentiation by high glucose. *Diabetes,* 50(6):1482-1490, 2001b.

Somerman MJ, Berry JE, Khalkhali-Ellis Z, Osdoby P, Simpson RU: Enhanced expression of alpha v integrin subunit and osteopontin during differentiation of HL-60 cells along the monocytic pathway. *Experimental Cell Research,* 216(2):335-341, 1995.

Somerman MJ, Fisher LW, Foster RA, Sauk JJ: Human bone sialoprotein I and II enhance fibroblast attachment in vitro. *Calcified Tissue International,* 43(1):50-53, 1988.

Somerman MJ, Foster RA, Imm GM, Sauk JJ, Archer SY: Periodontal ligament cells and gingival fibroblasts respond differently to attachment factors in vitro. *Journal of Periodontology,* 60(2):73-77, 1989.

Somerman MJ, Shroff B, Agraves WS, Morrison G, Craig AM, Denhardt DT, Foster RA, Sauk JJ: Expression of attachment proteins during cementogenesis. *Jiornale di Biologia Buccale,* 18(3):207-214, 1990.

Somerman MJ, Shroff B, Foster RA, Butler WT, Sauk JJ: Mineral-associated adhesion proteins are linked to root formation. *Proceedings of the Finnish Dentistry Society,* 88(Suppl 1):451-461, 1992.

Somerman MJ, Young MF, Foster RA, Moehring JM, Imm G, Sauk JJ: Characteristics of human periodontal ligament cells in vitro. *Archives of Oral Biology,* 35(3):241-247, 1990.

Sommer B, Bickel M, Hofstetter W, Wetterwald A: Expression of matrix proteins during the development of mineralized tissues. *Bone,* 19(4):371-380, 1996.

Song F, Matsuzaki G, Mitsuyama M, Nomoto K: In vitro generation of IFN-gamma-producing Listeria-specific T cells is dependent on IFN-gamma production by non-NK cells. *Cellular Immunology,* 160(2):211-216, 1995.

Sorensen ES, Hojrup P, Petersen TE: Posttranslational modifications of bovine osteopontin: Identification of twenty-eight phosphorylation and three O-glycosylation sites. *Protein Sciences,* 4(10):2040-2049, 1995.

Sorensen ES, Justesen SJ, Johnsen AH: Identification of a macromolecular crystal growth inhibitor in human urine as osteopontin. *Urology Research,* 23(5):327-334, 1995.

Sorensen ES, Petersen TE: Purification and characterization of three proteins isolated from the proteose peptone fraction of bovine milk. *Journal of Dairy Research,* 60(2):189-197, 1993.

Sorensen ES, Petersen TE: Identification of two phosphorylation motifs in bovine osteopontin. *Biochemical and Biophysical Research Communications,* 198(1):200-205, 1994.

Sorensen ES, Petersen TE: Phosphorylation, glycosylation, and transglutaminase sites in bovine osteopontin. *Annals of the New York Academy of Sciences,* 760:363-366, 1995.

Sorensen ES, Rasmussen LK, Moller L, Jensen PH, Hojrup P, Petersen TE: Localization of transglutaminase-reactive glutamine residues in bovine osteopontin. *Biochemical Journal,* 304 (Pt 1):13-16, 1994.

Srivatsa SS, Fitzpatrick LA, Tsao PW, Reilly TM, Holmes DR Jr, Schwartz RS, Mousa SA: Selective alpha v beta 3 integrin blockade potently limits neointimal hyperplasia and lumen stenosis following deep coronary arterial stent injury: Evidence for the functional importance of integrin alpha v beta 3 and osteopontin expression during neointima formation. *Cardiovascular Research,* 36(3):408-428, 1997.

Srivatsa SS, Harrity PJ, Maercklein PB, Kleppe L, Veinot J, Edwards WD, Johnson CM, Fitzpatrick LA: Increased cellular expression of matrix proteins that regulate mineralization is associated with calcification of native human and porcine xenograft bioprosthetic heart valves. *Journal of Clinical Investigation,* 99(5):996-1009, 1997.

Staal A, Birkenhager JC, Pols HA, Buurman CJ, Vink-van Wijngaarden T, Kleinekoort WM, van den Bemd GJ, van Leeuwen JP: Transforming growth factor beta-induced dissociation between vitamin D receptor level and 1,25-dihydroxyvitamin D3 action in osteoblast-like cells. *Bone Minerals,* 26(1):27-42, 1994.

Staal A, van den Bemd GJ, Birkenhager JC, Pols HA, van Leeuwen JP: Consequences of vitamin D receptor regulation for the 1,25-dihydroxyvitamin D3-induced 24-hydroxylase activity in osteoblast-like cells: Initiation of the C24-oxidation pathway. *Bone,* 20(3):237-243, 1997.

Staal A, Van Wijnen AJ, Birkenhager JC, Pols HA, Prahl J, DeLuca H, Gaub MP, Lian JB, Stein GS, van Leeuwen JP, et al.: Distinct conformations of vitamin D receptor/retinoid X receptor-alpha heterodimers are specified by dinucleotide differences in the vitamin D-responsive elements of the osteocalcin and osteopontin genes. *Molecular Endocrinology,* 10(11):1444-1456, 1996.

Staal A, Van Wijnen AJ, Desai RK, Pols HA, Birkenhager JC, Deluca HF, Denhardt DT, Stein JL, Van Leeuwen JP, Stein GS, et al.: Antagonistic effects of transforming growth factor-beta on vitamin D3 enhancement of osteocalcin and osteopontin transcription: reduced interactions of vitamin D receptor/retinoid X receptor complexes with vitamin E response elements. *Endocrinology,* 137(5):2001-2011, 1996.

Staege H, Brauchlin A, Schoedon G, Schaffner A: Two novel genes FIND and LIND differentially expressed in deactivated and Listeria-infected human macrophages. *Immunogenetics,* 53(2):105-113, 2001.

Staeheli P, Danielson O, Haller O, Sutcliffe JG: Transcriptional activation of the mouse *Mx* gene by type I interferon. *Molecular and Cellular Biology,* 6(12):4770-4774, 1986.

Stanford CM, Welsch F, Kastner N, Thomas G, Zaharias R, Holtman K, Brand RA: Primary human bone cultures from older patients do not respond at continuum levels of in vivo strain magnitudes. *Journal of Biomechanics,* 33(1):63-71, 2000.

Stark M, Danielsson O, Griffiths WJ, Jornvall H, Johansson J: Peptide repertoire of human cerebrospinal fluid: Novel proteolytic fragments of neuroendocrine proteins. *Journal of Chromatography and Biomedical Sciences Applications,* 754(2):357-367, 2001.

St-Arnaud R, Prud'homme J, Leung-Hagesteijn C, Dedhar S: Constitutive expression of calreticulin in osteoblasts inhibits mineralization. *Journal of Cellular Biology,* 131(5):1351-1359, 1995.

Stein GS, Lian JB, Gerstenfeld LG, Shalhoub V, Aronow M, Owen T, Markose E: The onset and progression of osteoblast differentiation is functionally related to cellular proliferation. *Connective Tissue Research,* 20(1-4):3-13, 1989.

Stein GS, Lian JB, Owen TA: Relationship of cell growth to the regulation of tissue-specific gene expression during osteoblast differentiation. *FASEB Journal,* 4(13): 3111-3123, 1990.

Steinberg AD, Roths JB, Murphy ED, Steinberg RT, Raveche ES: Effects of thymectomy or androgen administration upon the autoimmune disease of MRL/Mp-lpr/lpr mice. *Journal of Immunology,* 125:871-876, 1980.

Sterling H, Saginario C, Vignery A: CD44 occupancy prevents macrophage multinucleation. *Journal of Cellular Biology,* 143(3):837-847, 1998.

Stern DN, Glimcher MJ, Saavedra RA: Localization of osteopontin during mouse development. *Annals of the New York Academy of Sciences,* 760:367-370, 1995.

Stern PH, Tatrai A, Semler DE, Lee SK, Lakatos P, Strieleman PJ, Tarjan G, Sanders JL: Endothelin receptors, second messengers, and actions in bone. *Journal of Nutrition,* 125(Suppl 7):2028S-2032S, 1995.

Stocchetto S, Marin O, Carignani G, Pinna LA: Biochemical evidence that Saccharomyces cerevisiae YGR262c gene, required for normal growth, encodes a novel Ser/Thr-specific protein kinase. *FEBS Letters,* 414(1):171-175, 1997.

Strauss PG, Closs EI, Schmidt J, Erfle V: Gene expression during osteogenic differentiation in mandibular condyles in vitro. *Journal of Cellular Biology,* 110(4): 1369-1378, 1990.

Strayhorn CL, Garrett JS, Dunn RL, Benedict JJ, Somerman MJ: Growth factors regulate expression of osteoblast-associated genes. *Journal of Periodontology,* 70(11):1345-1354, 1999.

Stubbs JT III: Generation and use of recombinant human bone sialoprotein and osteopontin for hydroxyapatite studies. *Connective Tissue Research,* 35(1-4):393-399, 1996.

Sturm SA, Strauss PG, Adolph S, Hameister H, Erfle V: Amplification and rearrangement of c-myc in radiation-induced murine osteosarcomas. *Cancer Research,* 50(13):4146-4153, 1990.

Su L, Mukherjee AB, Mukherjee BB: Expression of antisense osteopontin RNA inhibits tumor promoter-induced neoplastic transformation of mouse JB6 epidermal cells. *Oncogene,* 10(11):2163-2169, 1995.

Su ZZ, Austin VN, Zimmer SG, Fisher PB: Defining the critical gene expression changes associated with expression and suppression of the tumorigenic and metastatic phenotype in Ha-ras-transformed cloned rat embryo fibroblast cells. *Oncogene,* 8(5):1211-1219, 1993.

Suda T, Takahashi N, Abe E: Role of vitamin D in bone resorption. *Journal of Cellular Biochemistry,* 49(1):53-58, 1992.

Suehiro K, Smith JW, Plow EF: The ligand recognition specificity of beta3 integrins. *Journal of Biological Chemistry,* 271(17):10365-10371, 1996.

Sugimoto M, Hirota S, Sato M, Kawahata H, Tsukamoto I, Yasui N, Kitamura Y, Ochi T, Nomura S: Impaired expression of noncollagenous bone matrix protein mRNAs during fracture healing in ascorbic acid-deficient rats. *Journal of Bone Minerals Research,* 13(2):271-278, 1998.

Sukhu B, Rotenberg B, Binkert C, Kohno H, Zohar R, McCulloch CA, Tenenbaum HC: Tamoxifen attenuates glucocorticoid actions on bone formation in vitro. *Endocrinology,* 138(8):3269-3275, 1997.

Sun Y, Kandel R: Deep zone articular chondrocytes in vitro express genes that show specific changes with mineralization. *Journal of Bone Minerals Research,* 14(11): 1916-1925, 1999.

Sun ZL, Fang DN, Wu XY, Ritchie HH, Begue-Kirn C, Wataha JC, Hanks CT, Butler WT: Expression of dentin sialoprotein (DSP) and other molecular determinants by a new cell line from dental papillae, MDPC-23. *Connective Tissue Research,* 37(3-4):251-261, 1998.

Sun ZL, Wataha JC, Hanks CT: Effects of metal ions on osteoblast-like cell metabolism and differentiation. *Journal of Biomedical Materials Research,* 34(1):29-37, 1997.

Sung V, Gilles C, Murray A, Clarke R, Aaron AD, Azumi N, Thompson EW: The LCC15-MB human breast cancer cell line expresses osteopontin and exhibits an invasive and metastatic phenotype. *Experimental Cell Research,* 241(2):273-284, 1998.

Suva LJ, Seedor JG, Endo N, Quartuccio HA, Thompson DD, Bab I, Rodan GA: Pattern of gene expression following rat tibial marrow ablation. *Journal of Bone Minerals Research,* 8(3):379-388, 1993.

Suwanwalaikorn S, Ongphiphadhanakul B, Braverman LE, Baran DT: Differential responses of femoral and vertebral bones to long-term excessive L-thyroxine administration in adult rats. *European Journal of Endocrinology,* 134(5):655-659, 1996.

Suzuki K: [Inhibitors in calcium oxalate crystals]. *Nippon Hinyokika Gakkai Zasshi,* 90(3):411-420, 1999.

Suzuki Y, Kubota T, Koizumi T, Satoyoshi M, Teranaka T, Kawase T, Ikeda T, Yamaguchi A, Saito S, Mikuni-Takagaki Y: Extracellular processing of bone and dentin proteins in matrix mineralization. *Connective Tissue Research,* 35(1-4):223-229, 1996.

Swanink CM, Stolk-Engelaar VM, van der Meer JW, Vercoulen JH, Bleijenberg G, Fennis JM, Galama JM, Hoogkamp-Korstanje JA: *Yersinia enterocolitica* and the chronic fatigue syndrome. *Journal of Infection,* 36(3):269-272, 1998.

Swanson GJ, Nomura S, Hogan BL: Distribution of expression of 2AR (osteopontin) in the embryonic mouse inner ear revealed by in situ hybridisation. *Hearing Research,* 41(2-3):169-177, 1989.

Tagami T, Lutz WH, Kumar R, Jameson JL: The interaction of the vitamin D receptor with nuclear receptor corepressors and coactivators. *Biochemical and Biophysical Research Communications,* 253(2):358-363, 1998.

Tahara E: Molecular aspects of invasion and metastasis of stomach cancer. *Verhalt des Deutsches Gessamte Pathology,* 84:43-49, 2000.

Takahashi F, Takahashi K, Maeda K, Tominaga S, Fukuchi Y: Osteopontin is induced by nitric oxide in RAW 264.7 cells. *IUBMB Life,* 49(3):217-221, 2000.

Takahashi F, Takahashi K, Okazaki T, Maeda K, Ienaga H, Maeda M, Kon S, Uede T, Fukuchi Y: Role of osteopontin in the pathogenesis of bleomycin-induced pulmonary fibrosis. *American Journal of Respiration and Cellular Molecular Biology,* 24(3):264-271, 2001.

Takahashi K, Eto H, Tanabe KK: Involvement of CD44 in matrix metalloproteinase-2 regulation in human melanoma cells. *International Journal of Cancer,* 80(3):387-395, 1999.

Takahashi K, Takahashi F, Tanabe KK, Takahashi H, Fukuchi Y: The carboxyl-terminal fragment of osteopontin suppresses arginine-glycine-asparatic acid-dependent cell adhesion. *Biochemical Molecular Biology International,* 46(6):1081-1092, 1998.

Takano S, Tsuboi K, Tomono Y, Mitsui Y, Nose T: Tissue factor, osteopontin, alphavbeta3 integrin expression in microvasculature of gliomas associated with vascular endothelial growth factor expression. *British Journal of Cancer,* 82(12): 1967-1973, 2000.

Takano-Yamamoto T, Takemura T, Kitamura Y, Nomura S: Site-specific expression of mRNAs for osteonectin, osteocalcin, and osteopontin revealed by in situ hybridization in rat periodontal ligament during physiological tooth movement. *Journal of Histochemistry and Cytochemistry,* 42(7):885-896, 1994.

Takata T, D'Errico JA, Atkins KB, Berry JE, Strayhorn C, Taichman RS, Somerman MJ: Protein extracts of dentin affect proliferation and differentiation of osteoprogenitor cells in vitro. *Journal of Periodontology,* 69(11):1247-1255, 1998.

Takemoto M, Kitahara M, Yokote K, Asaumi S, Take A, Saito Y, Mori S: NK-104, a 3-hydroxy-3-methylglutaryl coenzyme A reductase inhibitor, reduces osteopontin expression by rat aortic smooth muscle cells. *British Journal of Pharmacology,* 133(1):83-88, 2001.

Takemoto M, Tada K, Nakatsuka K, Moriyama Y, Kazui H, Yokote K, Matsumoto T, Saito Y, Mori S: [Effects of aging and hyperlipidemia on plasma osteopontin level]. *Nippon Ronen Igakkai Zasshi,* 36(11):799-802, 1999.

Takemoto M, Yokote K, Nishimura M, Shigematsu T, Hasegawa T, Kon S, Uede T, Matsumoto T, Saito Y, Mori S: Enhanced expression of osteopontin in human diabetic artery and analysis of its functional role in accelerated atherogenesis. *Arteriosclerosis and Thrombosis Vascular Biology,* 20(3):624-628, 2000.

Takemoto M, Yokote K, Yamazaki M, Ridall AL, Butler WT, Matsumoto T, Tamura K, Saito Y, Mori S: Enhanced expression of osteopontin by high glucose in cultured rat aortic smooth muscle cells. *Biochemical and Biophysical Research Communications,* 258(3):722-726, 1999.

Takemoto M, Yokote K, Yamazaki M, Ridall AL, Butler WT, Matsumoto T, Tamura K, Saito Y, Mori S: Enhanced expression of osteopontin by high glucose. Involvement of osteopontin in diabetic macroangiopathy. *Annals of the New York Academy of Sciences,* 902:357-363, 2000.

Takemura T, Sakagami M, Nakase T, Kubo T, Kitamura Y, Nomura S: Localization of osteopontin in the otoconial organs of adult rats. *Hearing Research,* 79(1-2):99-104, 1994.

Takeshita A, Imai K, Kato S, Kitano S, Hanazawa S: 1alpha,25-dehydroxyvitamin D3 synergism toward transforming growth factor-beta1-induced AP-1 transcriptional activity in mouse osteoblastic cells via its nuclear receptor. *Journal of Biological Chemistry,* 273(24):14738-14744, 1998.

Takeshita S, Kaji K, Kudo A: Identification and characterization of the new osteoclast progenitor with macrophage phenotypes being able to differentiate into mature osteoclasts. *Journal of Bone Minerals Research,* 15(8):1477-1488, 2000.

Takeuchi E, Sugamoto K, Nakase T, Miyamoto T, Kaneko M, Tomita T, Myoui A, Ochi T, Yoshikawa H: Localization and expression of osteopontin in the rotator cuff tendons in patients with calcifying tendinitis. *Virchows Archives,* 483(6):612-617, 2001.

Tanaka F, Ozawa Y, Inage Y, Deguchi K, Itoh M, Imai Y, Kohsaka S, Takashima S: Association of osteopontin with ischemic axonal death in periventricular leukomalacia. *Acta Neuropathologica (Berlin),* 100(1):69-74, 2000.

Tanaka H, Barnes J, Liang CT: Effect of age on the expression of insulin-like growth factor-I, interleukin-6, and transforming growth factor-beta mRNAs in rat femurs following marrow ablation. *Bone,* 18(5):473-478, 1996.

Tanaka H, Liang CT: Effect of platelet-derived growth factor on DNA synthesis and gene expression in bone marrow stromal cells derived from adult and old rats. *Journal of Cellular Physiology,* 164(2):367-375, 1995.

Tanaka H, Ogasa H, Barnes J, Liang CT: Actions of bFGF on mitogenic activity and lineage expression in rat osteoprogenitor cells: Effect of age. *Molecular and Cellular Endocrinology,* 150(1-2):1-10, 1999.

Tanaka H, Quarto R, Williams S, Barnes J, Liang CT: In vivo and in vitro effects of insulin-like growth factor-I (IGF-I) on femoral mRNA expression in old rats. *Bone,* 15(6):647-653, 1994.

Tang KT, Capparelli C, Stein JL, Stein GS, Lian JB, Huber AC, Braverman LE, DeVito WJ: Acidic fibroblast growth factor inhibits osteoblast differentiation in vitro: Altered expression of collagenase, cell growth-related, and mineralization-associated genes. *Journal of Cellular Biochemistry,* 61(1):152-166, 1996.

Tani-Ishii N, Tsunoda A, Umemoto T: Osteopontin antisense deoxyoligonucleotides inhibit bone resorption by mouse osteoclasts in vitro. *Journal of Periodontal Research,* 32(6):480-486, 1997.

Taooka Y, Chen J, Yednock T, Sheppard D: The integrin alpha9beta1 mediates adhesion to activated endothelial cells and transendothelial neutrophil migration through interaction with vascular cell adhesion molecule-1. *Journal of Cellular Biology,* 145(2):413-420, 1999.

Tashiro K, Sephel GC, Weeks B, Sasaki M, Martin GR, Kleinman HK, Yamada Y: A synthetic peptide containing the IKVAV sequence from the A chain of laminin mediates cell attachment, migration and neurite outgrowth. *Journal of Biological Chemistry,* 264:16174, 1989.

Tavassoli J, Benghuzzi H, Tucci M: The effects of sustained delivery of growth promoting hormones on the proliferation of MG63 cells in culture. *Biomedical Sciences Instrumentation,* 37:269-274, 2001.

Tawada T, Fujita K, Sakakura T, Shibutani T, Nagata T, Iguchi M, Kohri K: Distribution of osteopontin and calprotectin as matrix protein in calcium-containing stone. *Urology Research,* 27(4):238-242, 1999.

Terai K, Takano-Yamamoto T, Ohba Y, Hiura K, Sugimoto M, Sato M, Kawahata H, Inaguma N, Kitamura Y, Nomura S: Role of osteopontin in bone remodeling caused by mechanical stress. *Journal of Bone Minerals Research,* 14(6):839-849, 1999.

Termine JD: Non-collagen proteins in bone. *Ciba Foundation Symposia,* 136:178-202, 1988.

Termine JD: Cellular activity, matrix proteins, and aging bone. *Experimental Gerontology,* 25(3-4):217-221, 1990.

Teti A, Farina AR, Villanova I, Tiberio A, Tacconelli A, Sciortino G, Chambers AF, Gulino A, Mackay AR: Activation of MMP-2 by human GCT23 giant cell tumour cells induced by osteopontin, bone sialoprotein and GRGDSP peptides is RGD and cell shape change dependent. *International Journal of Cancer,* 77(1): 82-93, 1998.

Teti A, Taranta A, Migliaccio S, Degiorgi A, Santandrea E, Villanova I, Faraggiana T, Chellaiah M, Hruska KA: Colony stimulating factor-1-induced osteoclast spreading depends on substrate and requires the vitronectin receptor and the c-src proto-oncogene. *Journal of Bone Minerals Research,* 13(1):50-58, 1998.

Tezuka K, Denhardt DT, Rodan GA, Harada Si: Stimulation of mouse osteopontin promoter by v-Src is mediated by a CCAAT box-binding factor. *Journal of Biological Chemistry,* 271(37):22713-22717, 1996.

Tezuka K, Sato T, Kamioka H, Nijweide PJ, Tanaka K, Matsuo T, Ohta M, Kurihara N, Hakeda Y, Kumegawa M: Identification of osteopontin in isolated rabbit osteoclasts. *Biochemical and Biophysical Research Communications,* 186(2):911-917, 1992.

Thalmann GN, Sikes RA, Devoll RE, Kiefer JA, Markwalder R, Klima I, Farach-Carson CM, Studer UE, Chung LW: Osteopontin: Possible role in prostate cancer progression. *Clinical Cancer Research,* 5(8):2271-2277, 1999.

Thalmeier K, Meissner, P, Moosmann S, Sagebiel S, Wiest I, Huss R: Mesenchymal differentiation and organ distribution of human stromal cell lines in NOD/SCID mice. *Acta Haematologica,* 105(3):159-165, 2001.

Thayer JM, Giachelli CM, Mirkes PE, Schwartz SM: Expression of osteopontin in the head process late in gastrulation in the rat. *Journal of Experimental Zoology,* 272(3):240-244, 1995.

Thayer JM, Schoenwolf GC: Early expression of osteopontin in the chick is restricted to rhombomeres 5 and 6 and to a subpopulation of neural crest cells that arise from these segments. *Anatomy Records,* 250(2):199-209, 1998.

Theofilopoulos AN, Balderas RS, Shawler DL, Lee S, Dixon FJ: The influence of thymic genotype of the SLE-like disease and T-cell proliferation of MRL/Mp-lpr/lpr mice. *Journal of Experimental Medicine,* 153:1405-1410, 1981.

Theofilopoulos AN, Dixon FJ: Murine models of systemic lupus erythematosus. *Advances in Immunology,* 37:269-390, 1985.

Thiebaud D, Guenther HL, Porret A, Burckhardt P, Fleisch H, Hofstetter W: Regulation of collagen type I and biglycan mRNA levels by hormones and growth factors in normal and immortalized osteoblastic cell lines. *Journal of Bone Minerals Research,* 9(9):1347-1354, 1994.

Thomas GP, Bourne A, Eisman JA, Gardiner EM: Species-divergent regulation of human and mouse osteocalcin genes by calciotropic hormones. *Experimental Cell Research,* 258(2):395-402, 2000.

Thomas SE, Anderson S, Gordon KL, Oyama TT, Shankland SJ, Johnson RJ: Tubulointerstitial disease in aging: Evidence for underlying peritubular capillary damage, a potential role for renal ischemia. *Journal of the American Society of Nephrology,* 9(2):231-242, 1998.

Thomas SE, Lombardi D, Giachelli C, Bohle A, Johnson RJ: Osteopontin expression, tubulointerstitial disease, and essential hypertension. *American Journal of Hypertension,* 11(8 Pt 1):954-961, 1998.

Thompson PD, Hsieh JC, Whitfield GK, Haussler CA, Jurutka PW, Galligan MA, Tillman JB, Spindler SR, Haussler MR: Vitamin D receptor displays DNA binding and transactivation as a heterodimer with the retinoid X receptor, but not with the thyroid hormone receptor. *Journal of Cellular Biochemistry,* 75(3):462-480, 1999.

Thompson PD, Jurutka PW, Haussler CA, Whitfield GK, Haussler MR: Heterodimeric DNA binding by the vitamin D receptor and retinoid X receptors is enhanced by 1,25-dihydroxyvitamin D3 and inhibited by 9-cis-retinoic acid. Evidence for allosteric receptor interactions. *Journal of Biological Chemistry,* 273(14):8483-8491, 1998.

Thorens B, Mermod JJ, Vassalli P: Phagocytosis and inflammatory stimuli induce GM-CSF mRNA in macrophages through posttranscriptional regulation. *Cell,* 48(4):671-679, 1987.

Thyberg J, Hultgardh-Nilsson A, Kallin B: Inhibitors of ADP-ribosylation suppress phenotypic modulation and proliferation of smooth muscle cells cultured from rat aorta. *Differentiation,* 59(4):243-252, 1995.

Tian JY, Sorensen ES, Butler WT, Lopez CA, Sy MS, Desai NK, Denhardt DT: Regulation of no synthesis induced by inflammatory mediators in RAW264.7 cells: Collagen prevents inhibition by osteopontin. *Cytokine,* 12(5):450-457, 2000.

Tiniakos DG, Yu H, Liapis H: Osteopontin expression in ovarian carcinomas and tumors of low malignant potential (LMP). *Human Pathology,* 29(11):1250-1254, 1998.

Tintut Y, Parhami F, Bostrom K, Jackson SM, Demer LL: cAMP stimulates osteoblast-like differentiation of calcifying vascular cells. Potential signaling pathway for vascular calcification. *Journal of Biological Chemistry,* 273(13):7547-7553, 1998.

Tokiyasu Y, Takata T, Saygin E, Somerman M: Enamel factors regulate expression of genes associated with cementoblasts. *Journal of Periodontology,* 71(12):1829-1839, 2000.

Tokunaga K, Ogose A, Endo N, Nomura S, Takahashi HE: Human osteosarcoma (OST) induces mouse reactive bone formation in xenograft system. *Bone,* 19(5):447-454, 1996.

Tolbert T, Oparil S: Cardiovascular effects of estrogen. *American Journal of Hypertension,* 14(6 Pt 2):186S-193S, 2001.

Toma CD, Ashkar S, Gray ML, Schaffer JL, Gerstenfeld LC: Signal transduction of mechanical stimuli is dependent on microfilament integrity: Identification of osteopontin as a mechanically induced gene in osteoblasts. *Journal of Bone Minerals Research,* 12(10):1626-1636, 1997.

Toma CD, Schaffer JL, Meazzini MC, Zurakowski D, Nah HD, Gerstenfeld LC: Developmental restriction of embryonic calvarial cell populations as characterized by their in vitro potential for chondrogenic differentiation. *Journal of Bone Minerals Research,* 12(12):2024-2039, 1997.

Tong HS, Sakai DD, Sims SM, Dixon SJ, Yamin M, Goldring SR, Snead ML, Minkin C: Murine osteoclasts and spleen cell polykaryons are distinguished by mRNA phenotyping. *Journal of Bone Minerals Research,* 9(4):577-584, 1994.

Towler DA, Bidder M, Latifi T, Coleman T, Semenkovich CF: Diet-induced diabetes activates an osteogenic gene regulatory program in the aortas of low density lipoprotein receptor-deficient mice. *Journal of Biological Chemistry,* 273(46):30427-30434, 1998.

Towler DA, Gordon JI, Adams SP, Glaser L: The biology and enzymology of eukaryotic protein acetylation. *Annual Reviews of Biochemistry,* 57:69-99, 1988.

Tozawa K, Yamada Y, Kawai N, Okamura T, Ueda K, Kohri K: Osteopontin expression in prostate cancer and benign prostatic hyperplasia. *Urology International,* 62(3):155-158, 1999.

Traianedes K, Findlay DM, Martin TJ, Gillespie MT: Modulation of the signal recognition particle 54-kDa subunit (SRP54) in rat preosteoblasts by the extracellular matrix. *Journal of Biological Chemistry,* 270(36):20891-20894, 1995.

Traianedes K, Martin TJ, Findlay DM: Regulation of osteopontin expression by type I collagen in preosteoblastic UMR201 cells. *Connective Tissue Research,* 34(1):63-74, 1996.

Traianedes K, Ng KW, Martin TJ, Findlay DM: Cell substratum modulates responses of preosteoblasts to retinoic acid. *Journal of Cellular Physiology,* 157(2):243-252, 1993.

Trueblood NA, Xie Z, Communal C, Sam F, Ngoy S, Liaw L, Jenkins AW, Wang J, Sawyer DB, Bing OH, et al.: Exaggerated left ventricular dilation and reduced collagen deposition after myocardial infarction in mice lacking osteopontin. *Circulation Research,* 88(10):1080-1087, 2001.

Truong LD, Sheikh-Hamad D, Chakraborty S, Suki WN: Cell apoptosis and proliferation in obstructive uropathy. *Seminars in Nephrology,* 18(6):641-651, 1998.

Tsuji K, Ito Y, Noda M: Expression of the PEBP2alphaA/AML3/CBFA1 gene is regulated by BMP4/7 heterodimer and its overexpression suppresses type I collagen and osteocalcin gene expression in osteoblastic and nonosteoblastic mesenchymal cells. *Bone,* 22(2):87-92, 1998.

Tuck AB, Arsenault DM, O'Malley FP, Hota C, Ling MC, Wilson SM, Chambers AF: Osteopontin induces increased invasiveness and plasminogen activator expression of human mammary epithelial cells. *Oncogene,* 18(29):4237-4246, 1999.

Tuck AB, Elliott BE, Hota C, Tremblay E, Chambers AF: Osteopontin-induced, integrin-dependent migration of human mammary epithelial cells involves activation of the hepatocyte growth factor receptor (Met). *Journal of Cellular Biochemistry,* 78(3):465-475, 2000.

Tuck AB, O'Malley FP, Singhal H, Harris JF, Tonkin KS, Kerkvliet N, Saad Z, Doig GS, Chambers AF: Osteopontin expression in a group of lymph node negative breast cancer patients. *International Journal of Cancer,* 79(5):502-508, 1998.

Tuck AB, O'Malley FP, Singhal H, Tonkin KS, Harris JF, Bautista D, Chambers AF: Osteopontin and p53 expression are associated with tumor progression in a case of synchronous, bilateral, invasive mammary carcinomas. *Archives of Pathology and Laboratory Medicine,* 121(6):578-584, 1997.

Tuck AB, Wilson SM, Khokha R, Chambers AF: Different patterns of gene expression in ras-resistant and ras-sensitive cells. *Journal of the National Cancer Institute,* 83(7):485-491, 1991.

Tucker MA, Chang PL, Prince CW, Gillespie GY, Mapstone TB: TPA-mediated regulation of osteopontin in human malignant glioma cells. *Anticancer Research,* 18(2A):807-812, 1998.

Tufty RH, Kretsinger RH: Troponin and parvalbumin calcium binding regions predicted in myosin light chain and T4 lysozyme. *Science,* 187(4172):167-169, 1975.

Tunio GM, Hirota S, Nomura S, Kitamura Y: Possible relation of osteopontin to development of psammoma bodies in human papillary thyroid cancer. *Archives of Pathology and Laboratory Medicine,* 122(12):1087-1090, 1998.

Turner RT, Colvard DS, Spelsberg TC: Estrogen inhibition of periosteal bone formation in rat long bones: Down-regulation of gene expression for bone matrix proteins. *Endocrinology,* 127(3):1346-1351, 1990.

Ue T, Yokozaki H, Kitadai Y, Yamamoto S, Yasui W, Ishikawa T, Tahara E: Co-expression of osteopontin and CD44v9 in gastric cancer. *International Journal of Cancer,* 79(2):127-132, 1998.

Ueda Y, Sakane T, Tsunematsu T: Hyperreactivity of activated B cells to B-cell growth factors in patients with SLE. *Journal of Immunology,* 143(12):3988-3993, 1989.

Uede T, Katagiri Y, Iizuka J, Murakami M: Osteopontin, a coordinator of host defense system: A cytokine or an extracellular adhesive protein? *Microbiology and Immunology,* 41(9):641-648, 1997.

Uemura T, Liu YK, Kuboki Y: Preliminary communication. MRNA expression of MT1-MMP, MMP-9, cathepsin K, and TRAP in highly enriched osteoclasts cultured on several matrix proteins and ivory surfaces. *Bioscience, Biotechnology, and Biochemistry,* 64(8):1771-1773, 2000.

Uemura T, Nemoto A, Deng HY: [Differentiation and function of bone cells induced by bone matrix proteins: Osteopontin in bone remodeling]. *Tanpakushitsu Kakusan Koso,* 44(2):143-148, 1999.

Ueno H, Murakami M, Okumura M, Kadosawa T, Uede T, Fujinaga T: Chitosan accelerates the production of osteopontin from polymorphonuclear leukocytes. *Biomaterials,* 22(12):1667-1673, 2001.

Ullman KS, Northrop JP, Verwij CL, Crabtree GR: Transmission of signals form the T lymphocyte antigen receptor to the genes responsible for cell proliferation and immune function: The missing link. *Annual Reviews of Immunology,* 8:421-452, 1990.

Ullrich O, Mann K, Haase W, Koch-Brandt C: Biosynthesis and secretion of an osteopontin-related 20-kDa polypeptide in the Madin-Darby canine kidney cell line. *Journal of Biological Chemistry,* 266(6):3518-3525, 1991.

Umekawa T: [Structural characteristics of osteopontin for calcium oxalate crystal]. *Nippon Hinyokika Gakkai Zasshi,* 90(3):436-444, 1999.

Umekawa T, Kohri K, Kurita T, Hirota S, Nomura S, Kitamura Y: Expression of osteopontin messenger RNA in the rat kidney on experimental model of renal stone. *Biochemistry and Molecular Biology International,* 35(1):223-230, 1995.

Umekawa T, Yamate T, Amasaki N, Kohri K, Kurita T: Osteopontin mRNA in the kidney on an experimental rat model of renal stone formation without renal failure. *Urology International,* 55(1):6-10, 1995.

Uno Y, Horii A, Umemoto M, Hasegawa T, Doi K, Uno A, Takemura T, Kubo T: Effects of hypergravity on morphology and osteopontin expression in the rat otolith organs. *Journal of Vestibular Research,* 10(6):283-289, 2000.

Urusov AG, Sadof'ev LA, Podgornaia OI: [Two proteins from the nuclear matrix bind osteopontin gene promoter]. *Tsitologiia,* 40(7):627-632, 1998.

Vanacker JM, Delmarre C, Guo X, Laudet V: Activation of the osteopontin promoter by the orphan nuclear receptor estrogen receptor related alpha. *Cellular Growth and Differentiation,* 9(12):1007-1014, 1998.

Vanacker JM, Pettersson K, Gustafsson JA, Laudet V: Transcriptional targets shared by estrogen receptor-related receptors (ERRs) and estrogen receptor (ER) alpha, but not by ERbeta. *EMBO Journal,* 18(15):4270-4279, 1999.

VandenBos T, Bronckers AL, Goldberg HA, Beertsen W: Blood circulation as source for osteopontin in acellular extrinsic fiber cementum and other mineralizing tissues. *Journal of Dentistry Research,* 78(11):1688-1695, 1999.

van der Pluijm, Vloedgraven H, Papapoulos S, Lowick C, Grzesik W, Kerr J, Robey PG: Attachment characteristics and involvement of integrins in adhesion of breast cancer cell lines to extracellular bone matrix components. *Laboratory Investigations,* 77(6):665-675, 1997.

Van Deventer SJH, Hart M, van der Poll T, Hack CE, Aarden LA: Endotoxin and tumor necrosis factor-α-induced interleukin-8 release in humans. *Journal of Infectious Diseases,* 167:461-464, 1993.

van Dijk S, D'Errico JA, Somerman MJ, Farach-Carson MC, Butler WT: Evidence that a non-RGD domain in rat osteopontin is involved in cell attachment. *Journal of Bone Minerals Research,* 8(12):1499-1506, 1993.

Van Snick J: Interleukin 6: An overview. *Annual Reviews of Immunology,* 8:253-278, 1990.

Vary CP, Li V, Raouf A, Kitching R, Kola I, Franceschi C, Venanzoni M, Seth A: Involvement of Ets transcription factors and targets in osteoblast differentiation and matrix mineralization. *Experimental Cell Research,* 257(1):213-222, 2000.

Vaskuring VV, Vaskuring J: The development of the pathophysiological concept of calciphylaxis in experiment and clinic. *Pathophysiology,* 7(4):231-244, 2001.

Veenstra TD, Benson LM, Craig TA, Tomlinson AJ, Kumar R, Naylor S: Metal mediated sterol receptor-DNA complex association and dissociation determined by electrospray ionization mass spectrometry. *Nature Biotechnology,* 16(3):262-266, 1998.

Veinot JP, Srivatsa S, Carlson P: Beta3 integrin—a promiscuous integrin involved in vascular pathology. *Canadian Journal of Cardiology,* 15(7):762-770, 1999.

Verstrepen WA, Persy VP, Verhulst A, Dauwe S, De Broe ME: Renal osteopontin protein and mRNA upregulation during acute nephrotoxicity in the rat. *Nephrology, Dialysis, and Transplantation,* 16(4):712-724, 2001.

Vojdani A, Choppa PC, Tagle C, Andrin R, Samimi B, Lapp CW: Detection of *Mycoplasma* genus and *Mycoplasma fermentans* by PCR in patients with chronic fatigue syndrome. *FEMS Immunology and Medical Microbiology,* 22(4):355-365, 1998.

Vulliet PR, Hall FL, Mitchell JP, Hardie DG: Identification of a novel proline-directed serine/threonine protein kinase in rat pheochromocytoma. *Journal of Biological Chemistry,* 264(27):16292-16298, 1989.

Wada T, McKee MD, Steitz S, Giachelli CM: Calcification of vascular smooth muscle cell cultures: Inhibition by osteopontin. *Circulation Research,* 84(2):166-178, 1999.

Waite JH, Qin X: Polyphosphoprotein from the adhesive pads of *Mytilus edulis. Biochemistry,* 40(9):2887-2893, 2001.

Wakisaka A, Tanaka H, Barnes J, Liang CT: Effect of locally infused IGF-I on femoral gene expression and bone turnover activity in old rats. *Journal of Bone Minerals Research,* 13(1):13-19, 1998.

Walker LM, Preston MR, Magnay JL, Thomas PB, El Haj AJ: Nicotinic regulation of c-fos and osteopontin expression in human-derived osteoblast-like cells and human trabecular bone organ culture. *Bone,* 28(6):603-608, 2001.

Walker LM, Publicover SJ, Preston MR, Said Ahmed MA, El Haj AJ: Calcium-channel activation and matrix protein upregulation in bone cells in response to mechanical strain. *Journal of Cellular Biochemistry,* 79(4):648-661, 2000.

Wallin R, Wajih N, Greenwood GT, Sane DC: Arterial calcification: A review of mechanisms, animal models, and the prospects for therapy. *Medical Research Reviews,* 21(4):274-301, 2001.

Wang D, Yamamoto S, Hijiya N, Benveniste EN, Gladson CL: Transcriptional regulation of the human osteopontin promoter: Functional analysis and DNA-protein interactions. *Oncogene,* 19(50):5801-5809, 2000.

Wang J, Glimcher MJ, Mah J, Zhou HY, Salih E: Expression of bone microsomal casein kinase II, bone sialoprotein, and osteopontin during the repair of calvarial defects. *Bone,* 22(6):621-628, 1998.

Wang W, Mo S, Chan L: Mycophenolic acid inhibits PDGF-induced osteopontin expression in rat mesangial cells. *Transplantation Proceedings,* 31(1-2):1176-1177, 1999.

Wang X, Louden C, Ohlstein EH, Stadel JM, Gu JL, Yue TL: Osteopontin expression in platelet-derived growth factor-stimulated vascular smooth muscle cells and carotid artery after balloon angioplasty. *Arteriosclerosis and Thrombosis Vascular Biology,* 16(11):1365-1372, 1996.

Wang X, Louden C, Yue TL, Ellison JA, Barone FC, Solleveld HA, Feuerstein GZ: Delayed expression of osteopontin after focal stroke in the rat. *Journal of Neurosciences,* 18(6):2075-2083, 1998.

Wang Y, Mochida S, Kawashima R, Inao M, Matsui A, YouLuTuZ Y, Nagoshi S, Uede T, Fujiwara K: Increased expression of osteopontin in activated Kupffer cells and hepatic macrophages during macrophage migration in *Propionibacterium acnes*-treated rat liver. *Journal of Gastroenterology,* 35(9):696-701, 2000.

Wang ZQ, Grigoriadis AE, Wagner EF: Stable murine chondrogenic cell lines derived from c-fos-induced cartilage tumors. *Journal of Bone Minerals Research,* 8(7):839-847, 1993.

Waterhouse P, Parhar RS, Guo X, Lala PK, Denhardt DT: Regulated temporal and spatial expression of the calcium-binding proteins calcyclin and OPN (osteopontin) in mouse tissues during pregnancy. *Molecular Reproduction and Development,* 32(4):315-323, 1992.

Watson KE, Bostrom K, Ravindranath R, Lam T, Norton B, Demer LL: TGF-beta 1 and 25-hydroxycholesterol stimulate osteoblast-like vascular cells to calcify. *Journal of Clinical Investigation,* 93(5):2106-2113, 1994.

Weber GF, Ashkar S: Molecular mechanisms of tumor dissemination in primary and metastatic brain cancers. *Brain Research Bulletin,* 53(4):421-424, 2000.

Weber GF, Ashkar S, Cantor H: Interaction between CD44 and osteopontin as a potential basis for metastasis formation. *Proceedings of the Association of American Physicians,* 109(1):1-9, 1997.

Weber GF, Ashkar S, Glimcher MJ, Cantor H: Receptor-ligand interaction between CD44 and osteopontin (Eta-1). *Science,* 271(5248):509-512, 1996.

Weber GF, Cantor H: The immunology of Eta-1/osteopontin. *Cytokine Growth Factor Reviews,* 7(3):241-248, 1996.

Weinreb M, Shinar D, Rodan GA: Different pattern of alkaline phosphatase, osteopontin, and osteocalcin expression in developing rat bone visualized by in situ hybridization. *Journal of Bone Minerals Research,* 5(8):831-842, 1990.

Weintraub AS, Giachelli CM, Krauss RS, Almeida M, Taubman MB: Autocrine secretion of osteopontin by vascular smooth muscle cells regulates their adhesion to collagen gels. *American Journal of Pathology,* 149(1):259-272, 1996.

Weintraub AS, Schnapp LM, Lin X, Taubman MB: Osteopontin deficiency in rat vascular smooth muscle cells is associated with an inability to adhere to collagen and increased apoptosis. *Laboratory Investigations,* 80(11):1603-1615, 2000.

Weissberg PL, Cary NR, Shanahan CM: Gene expression and vascular smooth muscle cell phenotype. *Blood Pressure Supplement,* 2:68-73, 1995.

Wennberg C, Hessle L, Lundberg P, Mauro S, Narisawa S, Lerner UH, Millan JL: Functional characterization of osteoblasts and osteoclasts from alkaline phosphatase knockout mice. *Journal of Bone Minerals Research,* 15(10):1879-1888, 2000.

Wernert N, Raes MB, Lasalle P, Dehouck MP, Gosselin B, Vandenbunder B, Stehelin D: c-ets 1 proto-oncogene is a transcription factor expressed in endothelial cells during tumor vascularization and other forms of angiogenesis in humans. *American Journal of Pathology,* 140(1):119-127, 1992.

Wesolowski G, Duong LT, Lakkakorpi PT, Nagy RM, Tezuka K, Tanaka H, Rodan GA, Rodan SB: Isolation and characterization of highly enriched, prefusion mouse osteoclastic cells. *Experimental Cell Research,* 219(2):679-686, 1995.

Wesson JA, Worcester EM, Wiessner JH, Mandel NS, Kleinman JG: Control of calcium oxalate crystal structure and cell adherence by urinary macromolecules. *Kidney International,* 53(4):952-957, 1998.

Whitfield GK, Hsieh JC, Jurutka PW, Selznick SH, Haussler CA, MacDonald PN, Haussler MR: Genomic actions of 1,25-dihydroxyvitamin D3. *Journal of Nutrition,* 125(Suppl 6):1690S-1694S, 1995.

Wiener J, Lombardi DM, Su JE, Schwartz SM: Immunohistochemical and molecular characterization of the differential response of the rat mesenteric microvasculature to angiotensin-II infusion. *Journal of Vascular Research,* 33(3):195-208, 1996.

Williams EB, Halpert I, Wickline S, Davison G, Parks WC, Rottman JN: Osteopontin expression is increased in the heritable cardiomyopathy of Syrian hamsters. *Circulation,* 92(4):705-709, 1995.

Williams GR, Bland R, Sheppard MC: Retinoids modify regulation of endogenous gene expression by vitamin D3 and thyroid hormone in three osteosarcoma cell lines. *Endocrinology,* 136(10):4304-4314, 1995.

Williams S, Barnes J, Wakisaka A, Ogasa H, Liang CT: Treatment of osteoporosis with MMP inhibitors. *Annals of the New York Academy of Sciences,* 878:191-200, 1999.

Willing M, Sowers M, Aron D, Clark MK, Burns T, Bunten C, Crutchfield M, D'Agostino D, Jannausch M: Bone mineral density and its change in white women: Estrogen and vitamin D receptor genotypes and their interaction. *Journal of Bone Minerals Research,* 13(4):695-705, 1998.

Winn SR, Randolph G, Uludag H, Wong SC, Hair GA, Hollinger JO: Establishing an immortalized human osteoprecursor cell line: OPC1. *Journal of Bone Minerals Research,* 14(10):1721-1733, 1999.

Winnard RG, Gerstenfeld LC, Toma CD, Franceschi RT: Fibronectin gene expression, synthesis and accumulation during in vitro differentiation of chicken osteoblasts. *Journal of Bone Minerals Research,* 10(12):1969-1977, 1995.

Wisner-Lynch LA, Shalhoub V, Marks SC Jr: Administration of colony stimulating factor-1 to toothless osteopetrotic rats normalizes osteoblast, but not osteoclast, gene expression. *Bone,* 16(6):611-618, 1995.

Woitge HW, Kream BE: Calvariae from fetal mice with a disrupted Igf1 gene have reduced rates of collagen synthesis but maintain responsiveness to glucocorticoids. *Journal of Bone Minerals Research,* 15(10):1956-1964, 2000.

Woitge HW, Seibel MJ: Biochemical markers to survey bone turnover. *Rheumatic Diseases Clinics of North America,* 27(1):49-80, 2001.

Wong A, Hwang SM, McDevitt P, McNulty D, Stadel JM, Johanson K: Studies on alpha v beta 3/ligand interactions using a [3H]SKandF-107260 binding assay. *Molecular Pharmacology,* 50(3):529-537, 1996.

Wong IH, Chan AT, Johnson PJ: Quantitative analysis of circulating tumor cells in peripheral blood of osteosarcoma patients using osteoblast-specific messenger RNA markers: A pilot study. *Clinical Cancer Research,* 6(6):2183-2188, 2000.

Woodard JC, Donovan GA, Fisher LW: Pathogenesis of vitamin (A and D)-induced premature growth-plate closure in calves. *Bone,* 21(2):171-182, 1997.

Woods A, Couchman JR: Focal adhesions and cell matrix interactions. *Collagen Related Research,* 8(2):155-182, 1988.

Worcester EM: Urinary calcium oxalate crystal growth inhibitors. *Journal of the American Society of Nephrology,* 5(5 Suppl 1):S46-S53, 1994.

Worcester EM, Beshensky AM: Osteopontin inhibits nucleation of calcium oxalate crystals. *Annals of the New York Academy of Sciences,* 760:375-377, 1995.

Worcester EM, Blumenthal SS, Beshensky AM, Lewand DL: The calcium oxalate crystal growth inhibitor protein produced by mouse kidney cortical cells in culture is osteopontin. *Journal of Bone Minerals Research,* 7(9):1029-1036, 1992.

Worcester EM, Kleinman JG, Beshensky AM: Osteopontin production by cultured kidney cells. *Annals of the New York Academy of Sciences,* 760:266-278, 1995.

Wozniak M, Fausto A, Carron CP, Meyer DM, Hruska KA: Mechanically strained cells of the osteoblast lineage organize their extracellular matrix through unique sites of alphavbeta3-integrin expression. *Journal of Bone Minerals Research,* 15(9):1731-1745, 2000.

Wrana JL, Kubota T, Zhang Q, Overall CM, Aubin JE, Butler WT, Sodek J: Regulation of transformation-sensitive secreted phosphoprotein (SPPI/osteopontin) expression by transforming growth factor-beta. Comparisons with expression of SPARC (secreted acidic cysteine-rich protein). *Biochemical Journal,* 273(Pt 3):523-531, 1991.

Wrana JL, Zhang Q, Sodek J: Full length cDNA sequence of porcine secreted phosphoprotein-I (SPP-I, osteopontin). *Nucleic Acids Research,* 17(23):10119, 1989.

Wu CB, Pan YM, Simizu Y: Microsomal casein kinase II in endoplasmic reticulum- and Golgi apparatus-rich fractions of ROS 17/2.8 osteoblast-like cells: An enzyme that modifies osteopontin. *Calcified Tissue International,* 57(4):285-292, 1995.

Wu CB, Shimizu Y, Ng A, Pan YM: Characterization and partial purification of microsomal casein kinase II from osteoblast-like cells: An enzyme that phosphorylates osteopontin and phosphophoryn. *Connective Tissue Research,* 34(1): 23-32, 1996.

Wu D, Ikezawa K, Parker T, Saito M, Narayanan AS: Characterization of a collagenous cementum-derived attachment protein. *Journal of Bone Minerals Research,* 11(5):686-692, 1996.

Wu LN, Ishikawa Y, Sauer GR, Genge BR, Mwale F, Mishima H, Wuthier RE: Morphological and biochemical characterization of mineralizing primary cultures of avian growth plate chondrocytes: Evidence for cellular processing of Ca2+ and Pi prior to matrix mineralization. *Journal of Cellular Biochemistry,* 57(2):218-237, 1995.

Wu S, Ren S, Chen H, Chun RF, Gacad MA, Adams JS: Intracellular vitamin D binding proteins: Novel facilitators of vitamin D-directed transactivation. *Molecular Endocrinology,* 14(9):1387-1397, 2000.

Wu Y, Denhardt DT, Rittling SR: Osteopontin is required for full expression of the transformed phenotype by the ras oncogene. *British Journal of Cancer,* 83(2):156-163, 2000.

Wuthrich RP: The complex role of osteopontin in renal disease. *Nephrology, Dialysis, and Transplantation,* 13(10):2448-2450, 1998.

Wuthrich RP, Fan X, Ritthaler T, Sibalic V, Yu DJ, Loffing J, Kaissling B: Enhanced osteopontin expression and macrophage infiltration in MRL-Fas(lpr) mice with lupus nephritis. *Autoimmunity,* 28(3):139-150, 1998.

Xie Y, Nishi S, Iguchi S, Imai N, Sakatsume M, Saito A, Ikegame M, Iino N, Shimada H, Ueno M, et al.: Expression of osteopontin in gentamicin-induced acute tubular necrosis and its recovery process. *Kidney International,* 59(3):959-974, 2001.

Xie Z, Pimental DR, Lohan S, Vasertriger A, Pligavko C, Colucci WS, Singh K. Regulation of angiotensin II-stimulated osteopontin expression in cardiac microvascular endothelial cells: Role of p42/44 mitogen-activated protein kinase and reactive oxygen species. *Journal of Cellular Physiology,* 188(1):132-138, 2001.

Xuan JW, Hota C, Chambers AF: Recombinant GST-human osteopontin fusion protein is functional in RGD-dependent cell adhesion. *Journal of Cellular Biochemistry,* 54(2):247-255, 1994.

Xuan JW, Hota C, Shigeyama Y, D'Errico JA, Somerman MJ, Chambers AF: Site-directed mutagenesis of the arginine-glycine-aspartic acid sequence in osteopontin destroys cell adhesion and migration functions. *Journal of Cellular Biochemistry,* 57(4):680-690, 1995.

Yabe T, Nemoto A, Uemura T: Recognition of osteopontin by rat bone marrow derived osteoblastic primary cells. *Bioscience, Biotechnology and Biochemistry,* 61(4):754-756, 1997.

Yagisawa T, Chandhoke PS, Fan J, Lucia S: Renal osteopontin expression in experimental urolithiasis. *Journal of Endourology,* 12(2):171-176, 1998.

Yamada S: [Expression of c-myc and N-myc in mouse embryos during craniofacial development]. *Kokubyo Gakkai Zasshi,* 57(1):83-105, 1990.

Yamada T, Abe M, Higashi T, Yamamoto H, Kihara-Negishi F, Sakurai T, Shirai T, Oikawa T: Lineage switch induced by overexpression of Ets family transcription factor PU.1 in murine erythroleukemia cells. *Blood,* 97(8):2300-2307, 2001.

Yamagishi S, Fujimori H, Yonekura H, Tanaka N, Yamamoto H: Advanced glycation endproducts accelerate calcification in microvascular pericytes. *Biochemical and Biophysical Research Communications,* 258(2):353-357, 1999.

Yamagiwa H, Endo N, Tokunaga K, Hayami T, Hatano H, Takahashi HE: In vivo bone-forming capacity of human bone marrow-derived stromal cells is stimulated by recombinant human bone morphogenetic protein-2. *Journal of Bone Mineral Metabolism,* 19(1):20-28, 2001.

Yamagiwa H, Tokunaga K, Hayami T, Hatano H, Uchida M, Endo N, Takahashi HE: Expression of metalloproteinase-13 (Collagenase-3) is induced during fracture healing in mice. *Bone,* 25(2):197-203, 1999.

Yamamoto M, Aoyagi M, Azuma H, Yamamoto K: Changes in osteopontin mRNA expression during phenotypic transition of rabbit arterial smooth muscle cells. *Histochemistry and Cell Biology,* 107(4):279-287, 1997.

Yamamoto S, Hijiya N, Setoguchi M, Matsuura K, Ishida T, Higuchi Y, Akizuki S: Structure of the osteopontin gene and its promoter. *Annals of the New York Academy of Sciences,* 760:44-58, 1995.

Yamamoto S, Nasu K, Ishida T, Setoguchi M, Higuchi Y, Hijiya N, Akizuki S: Effect of recombinant osteopontin on adhesion and migration of P388D1 cells. *Annals of the New York Academy of Sciences,* 760:378-380, 1995.

Yamashita DS, Dodds RA: Cathepsin K and the design of inhibitors of cathepsin K. *Current Pharmaceutical Design,* 6(1):1-24, 2000.

Yamate T, Kohri K, Umekawa T, Amasaki N, Amasaki N, Isikawa Y, Iguchi M, Kurita T: The effect of osteopontin on the adhesion of calcium oxalate crystals to Madin-Darby canine kidney cells. *European Urology,* 30(3):388-393, 1996.

Yamate T, Kohri K, Umekawa T, Iguchi M, Kurita T: Osteopontin antisense oligonucleotide inhibits adhesion of calcium oxalate crystals in Madin-Darby canine kidney cell. *Journal of Urology,* 160(4):1506-1512, 1998.

Yamate T, Kohri K, Umekawa T, Konya E, Ishikawa Y, Iguchi M, Kurita T: Interaction between osteopontin on Madin-Darby canine kidney cell membrane and calcium oxalate crystal. *Urology International,* 62(2):81-86, 1999.

Yamate T, Mocharla H, Taguchi Y, Igietseme JU, Manolagas SC, Abe E: Osteopontin expression by osteoclast and osteoblast progenitors in the murine bone marrow: Demonstration of its requirement for osteoclastogenesis and its increase after ovariectomy. *Endocrinology,* 138(7):3047-3055, 1997.

Yamate T, Tsuji H, Amasaki N, Iguchi M, Kurita T, Kohri K: Analysis of osteopontin DNA in patients with urolithiasis. *Urology Research,* 28(3):159-166, 2000.

Yamate T, Umekawa T, Iguchi M, Kurita T, Kohri K: Detection of osteopontin as matrix protein in calcium-containing urinary stones. *Hinyokika Kiyo,* 43(9):623-627, 1997.

Yamauchi M: [Effects of intermittent compressive force on transforming growth factor beta and osteopontin synthesis in cultured bone cells]. *Kanagawa Shigaku,* 24(4):716-729, 1990.

Yamazaki M, Nakajima F, Ogasawara A, Moriya H, Majeska RJ, Einhorn TA: Spatial and temporal distribution of CD44 and osteopontin in fracture callus. *Journal of Bone and Joint Surgery of Britain,* 81(3):508-515, 1999.

Yanaka N, Akatsuka H, Kawai E, Omori K: 1,25-Dihydroxyvitamin D3 upregulates natriuretic peptide receptor-C expression in mouse osteoblasts. *American Journal of Physiology,* 275(6 Pt 1):E965-E973, 1998.

Yang R, Gotoh Y, Moore MA, Rafidi K, Gerstenfeld LC: Characterization of an avian bone sialoprotein (BSP) cDNA: Comparisons to mammalian BSP and identification of conserved structural domains. *Journal of Bone Minerals Research,* 10(4):632-640, 1995.

Yang W, Hyllner SJ, Christakos S: Interrelationship between signal transduction pathways and 1,25(OH)(2)D(3) in UMR106 osteoblastic cells. *American Journal of Physiology, Endocrinology and Metabolism,* 281(1):E162-E170, 2001.

Yang X, Ji X, Shi X, Cao X: Smad1 domains interacting with Hoxc-8 induce osteoblast differentiation. *Journal of Biological Chemistry,* 275(2):1065-1072, 2000.

Yao KL, Todescan R Jr, Sodek J: Temporal changes in matrix protein synthesis and mRNA expression during mineralized tissue formation by adult rat bone marrow cells in culture. *Journal of Bone Minerals Research,* 9(2):231-240, 1994.

Yasui T, Fujita K, Hayashi Y, Ueda K, Kon S, Maeda M, Uede T, Kohri K: Quantification of osteopontin in the urine of healthy and stone-forming men. *Urology Research,* 27(4):225-230, 1999.

Yasui T, Fujita K, Sasaki S, Iguchi M, Hirota S, Nomura S, Azuma Y, Ohta T, Kohri K: Alendronate inhibits osteopontin expression enhanced by parathyroid hormone-related peptide (PTHrP) in the rat kidney. *Urology Research,* 26(5):355-360, 1998.

Yasui T, Fujita K, Sasaki S, Sato M, Sugimoto M, Hirota S, Kitamura Y, Nomura S, Kohri K: Expression of bone matrix proteins in urolithiasis model rats. *Urology Research,* 27(4):255-261, 1999.

Yasui T, Fujita K, Sato M, Sugimoto M, Iguchi M, Nomura S, Kohri K: The effect of takusha, a kampo medicine, on renal stone formation and osteopontin expression in a rat urolithiasis model. *Urology Research,* 27(3):194-199, 1999.

Yasui T, Sato M, Fujita K, Ito Y, Nomura S, Kohri K: Effects of allopurinol on renal stone formation and osteopontin expression in a rat urolithiasis model. *Nephron,* 87(2):170-176, 2001.

Yasui T, Sato M, Fujita K, Tozawa K, Nomura S, Kohri K: Effects of citrate on renal stone formation and osteopontin expression in a rat urolithiasis model. *Urology Research,* 29(1):50-56, 2001.

Yeh JK, Evans JF, Chen MM, Aloia JF: Effect of hypophysectomy on the proliferation and differentiation of rat bone marrow stromal cells. *American Journal of Physiology,* 276(1 Pt 1):E34-E42, 1999.

Yen PM, Liu Y, Sugawara A, Chin WW: Vitamin D receptors repress basal transcription and exert dominant negative activity on triiodothyronine-mediated transcriptional activity. *Journal of Biological Chemistry,* 271(18):10910-10916, 1996.

Yokosaki Y, Matsuura N, Sasaki T, Murakami I, Schneider H, Higashiyama S, Saitoh Y, Yamakido M, Taooka Y, Sheppard D: The integrin alpha(9)beta(1) binds to a novel recognition sequence (SVVYGLR) in the thrombin-cleaved amino-terminal fragment of osteopontin. *Journal of Biological Chemistry,* 274(51):36328-36334, 1999.

Yokasaki Y, Sheppard D: Mapping of the cryptic integrin-binding site in osteopontin suggests a new mechanism by which thrombin can regulate inflammation and tissue repair. *Trends in Cardiovascular Medicine,* 10(4):155-159, 2000.

Yokogawa K, Miya K, Sekido T, Higashi Y, Nomura M, Fujisawa R, Morito K, Masamune Y, Waki Y, Kasugai S, et al.: Selective delivery of estradiol to bone by aspartic acid oligopeptide and its effects on ovariectomized mice. *Endocrinology,* 142(3):1228-1233, 2001.

Yokota M, Nagata T, Ishida H, Wakano Y: Clonal dental pulp cells (RDP4-1, RPC-C2A) synthesize and secrete osteopontin (SPP1, 2ar). *Biochemical and Biophysical Research Communications,* 189(2):892-898, 1992.

Yoon K, Buenaga R, Rodan GA: Tissue specificity and developmental expression of rat osteopontin. *Biochemical and Biophysical Research Communications,* 148(3):1129-1136, 1987.

Yoshida E, Noshiro M, Kawamoto T, Tsutsumi S, Kuruta Y, Kato Y: Direct inhibition of Indian hedgehog expression by parathyroid hormone (PTH)/PTH-related peptide and up-regulation by retinoic acid in growth plate chondrocyte cultures. *Experimental Cell Research,* 265(1):64-72, 2001.

Yoshitake H, Rittling SR, Denhardt DT, Noda M: Osteopontin-deficient mice are resistant to ovariectomy-induced bone resorption. *Proceedings of the National Academy of Sciences of the United States of America,* 96(14):8156-8160, 1999.

Yoshizawa T, Handa Y, Uematsu Y, Takeda S, Sekine K, Yoshihara Y, Kawakami T, Arioka K, Sato H, Uchiyama Y, et al.: Mice lacking the vitamin D receptor exhibit impaired bone formation, uterine hypoplasia and growth retardation after weaning. *Nature Genetics,* 16(4):391-396, 1997.

You J, Reilly GC, Zhen X, Yellowley CE, Chen Q, Donahue HJ, Jacobs CR: Osteopontin gene regulation by oscillatory fluid flow via intracellular calcium mobilization and activation of mitogen-activated protein kinase in MC3T3-E1 osteoblasts. *Journal of Biological Chemistry,* 276(16):13365-13371, 2001.

You J, Yellowley CE, Donahue HJ, Zhang Y, Chen Q, Jacobs CR: Substrate deformation levels associated with routine physical activity are less stimulatory to bone cells relative to loading-induced oscillatory fluid flow. *Journal of Biomechanical Engineering,* 122(4):387-393, 2000.

Young BA, Burdmann EA, Johnson RJ, Alpers CE, Giachelli CM, Eng E, Andoh T, Bennett WM, Couser WG: Cellular proliferation and macrophage influx precede interstitial fibrosis in cyclosporine nephrotoxicity. *Kidney International,* 48(2):439-448, 1995.

Young MF, Kerr JM, Ibaraki K, Heegaard AM, Robey PG: Structure, expression, and regulation of the major noncollagenous matrix proteins of bone. *Clinical Orthopedics,* 281:275-294, 1992.

Young MF, Kerr JM, Termine JD, Wewer UM, Wang MG, McBride OW, Fisher LW: cDNA cloning, mRNA distribution and heterogeneity, chromosomal location, and RFLP analysis of human osteopontin (OPN). *Genomics,* 7(4):491-502, 1990.

Yu XQ, Fan JM, Nikolic-Paterson DJ, Yang N, Mu W, Pichler R, Johnson RJ, Atkins RC, Lan HY: IL-1 up-regulates osteopontin expression in experimental crescentic glomerulonephritis in the rat. *American Journal of Pathology,* 154(3): 833-841, 1999.

Yu XQ, Nikolic-Paterson DJ, Mu W, Giachelli CM, Atkins RC, Johnson RJ, Lan HY: A functional role for osteopontin in experimental crescentic glomerulonephritis in the rat. *Proceedings of the Association of American Physicians,* 110(1):50-64, 1998.

Yu XQ, Wu LL, Huang XR, Yang N, Gilbert RE, Cooper ME, Johnson RJ, Lai KN, Lan HY: Osteopontin expression in progressive renal injury in remnant kidney: Role of angiotensin II. *Kidney International,* 58(4):1469-1480, 2000.

Yue TL, McKenna PJ, Ohlstein EH, Farach-Carson MC, Butler WT, Johanson K, McDevitt P, Feuerstein GZ, Stadel JM: Osteopontin-stimulated vascular smooth muscle cell migration is mediated by beta 3 integrin. *Experimental Cell Research,* 214(2):459-464, 1994.

Zayzafoon M, Stell C, Irwin R, McCabe LR: Extracellular glucose influences osteoblast differentiation and c-Jun expression. *Journal of Cellular Biochemistry,* 79(2):301-310, 2000.

Zhang DE, Hetherington CJ, Gonzalez DA, Chen HM, Tenen DG: Regulation of CD14 expression during monocytic differentiation induced with 1 alpha,25-dihydroxyvitamin D3. *Journal of Immunology,* 153(7):3276-3284, 1994.

Zhang L, Zhang M, Zhou Q, Chen J, Zeng F: Solution properties of antitumor sulfated derivative of alpha-(1→3)-D-glucan from *Ganoderma lucidum. Bioscience, Biotechnology and Biochemistry,* 64(10):2172-2178, 2000.

Zhang Q, Domenicucci C, Goldberg HA, Wrana JL, Sodek J: Characterization of fetal porcine bone sialoproteins, secreted phosphoprotein I (SPPI, osteopontin), bone sialoprotein, and a 23-kDa glycoprotein. Demonstration that the 23-kDa glycoprotein is derived from the carboxyl terminus of SPPI. *Journal of Biological Chemistry,* 265(13):7583-7589, 1990.

Zhang Q, Fan M, Bian Z, Chen Z, Zhu Q: Immunohistochemistry of bone sialoprotein and osteopontin during reparative dentinogenesis in vivo. *Chinese Journal of Dental Research,* 3(2):38-43, 2000.

Zhang Q, Wrana JL, Sodek J: Characterization of the promoter region of the porcine opn (osteopontin, secreted phosphoprotein 1) gene. Identification of positive and negative regulatory elements and a "silent" second promoter. *European Journal of Biochemistry,* 207(2):649-659, 1992.

Zhang R, Supowit SC, Klein GL, Lu Z, Christensen MD, Lozano R, Simmons DJ: Rat tail suspension reduces messenger RNA level for growth factors and osteopontin and decreases the osteoblastic differentiation of bone marrow stromal cells. *Journal of Bone Minerals Research,* 10(3):415-423, 1995a.

Zhang RW, Supowit SC, Xu X, Li H, Christensen MD, Lozano R, Simmons DJ: Expression of selected osteogenic markers in the fibroblast-like cells of rat marrow stroma. *Calcified Tissue International,* 56(4):283-291, 1995b.

Zheng DQ, Woodard AS, Tallini G, Languino LR: Substrate specificity of alpha(v)beta(3) integrin-mediated cell migration and phosphatidylinositol 3-kinase/AKT pathway activation. *Journal of Biological Chemistry,* 275(32):24565-24574, 2000.

Zhou H, Choong P, McCarthy R, Chou ST, Martin TJ, Ng KW: In situ hybridization to show sequential expression of osteoblast gene markers during bone formation in vivo. *Journal of Bone Minerals Research,* 9(9):1489-1499, 1994.

Zhou H, Hammonds RG Jr, Findlay DM, Fuller PJ, Martin TJ, Ng KW: Retinoic acid modulation of mRNA levels in malignant, nontransformed, and immortalized osteoblasts. *Journal of Bone Minerals Research,* 6(7):767-777, 1991.

Zhou H, Hammonds RG Jr, Findlay DM, Martin TJ, Ng KW: Differential effects of transforming growth factor-beta 1 and bone morphogenetic protein 4 on gene expression and differentiated function of preosteoblasts. *Journal of Cellular Physiology,* 155(1):112-119, 1993.

Zhu JX, Sasano Y, Takahashi I, Mizoguchi I, Kagayama M: Temporal and spatial gene expression of major bone extracellular matrix molecules during embryonic mandibular osteogenesis in rats. *Histochemistry Journal,* 33(1):25-35, 2001.

Zhu X, Luo C, Ferrier JM, Sodek J: Evidence of ectokinase-mediated phosphorylation of osteopontin and bone sialoprotein by osteoblasts during bone formation in vitro. *Biochemistry Journal,* 323(Pt 3):637-643, 1997.

Zimolo Z, Wesolowski G, Tanaka H, Hyman JL, Hoyer JR, Rodan GA: Soluble alpha v beta 3-integrin ligands raise [Ca2+]i in rat osteoclasts and mouse-derived osteoclast-like cells. *American Journal of Physiology,* 266(2 Pt 1):C376-C381, 1994.

Zipfel PF: Hemolytic uremic syndrome: How do factor H mutants mediate endothelial damage? *Trends in Immunology,* 22(7):345-348, 2001.

Zohar R, Cheifetz S, McCulloch CA, Sodek J: Analysis of intracellular osteopontin as a marker of osteoblastic cell differentiation and mesenchymal cell migration. *European Journal of Oral Sciences,* 106(Suppl 1):401-407, 1998.

Zohar R, Lee W, Arora P, Cheifetz S, McCulloch C, Sodek J: Single cell analysis of intracellular osteopontin in osteogenic cultures of fetal rat calvarial cells. *Journal of Cellular Physiology,* 170(1):88-100, 1997.

Zohar R, McCulloch CA, Sampath K, Sodek J: Flow cytometric analysis of recombinant human osteogenic protein-1 (BMP-7) responsive subpopulations from fetal rat calvaria based on intracellular osteopontin content. *Matrix Biology,* 16(6):295-306, 1998.

Zohar R, Sodek J, McCulloch CA: Characterization of stromal progenitor cells enriched by flow cytometry. *Blood,* 90(9):3471-3481, 1997.

Zohar R, Suzuki N, Suzuki K, Arora P, Glogauer M, McCulloch CA, Sodek J: Intracellular osteopontin is an integral component of the CD44-ERM complex involved in cell migration. *Journal of Cellular Physiology,* 184(1):118-130, 2000.

Zreiqat H, Evans P, Howlett CR: Effect of surface chemical modification of bioceramic on phenotype of human bone-derived cells. *Journal of Biomedical Materials Research,* 44(4):389-396, 1999.

Zreiqat H, Howlett CR: Titanium substrata composition influences osteoblastic phenotype: In vitro study. *Journal of Biomedical Materials Research,* 47(3):360-366, 1999.

Zreiqat H, Markovic B, Walsh WR, Howlett CR: A novel technique for quantitative detection of mRNA expression in human bone derived cells cultured on biomaterials. *Journal of Biomedical Materials Research,* 33(4):217-223, 1996.

Zreiqat H, McFarland C, Howlett CR: The effect of polymeric chemistry on the expression of bone-related mRNAs and proteins by human bone-derived cells in vitro. *Journal of Biomaterial Science, Polymer Edition,* 10(2):199-216, 1999.

Index

Page numbers followed by the letter "t" indicate tables.